Contents

List of Tables xiii

Preface xv

Introduction: The Art and Science of Yoga Sequencing 1

Part One: Foundations and Principles 5

Chapter One: Philosophy and Principles of Sequencing 7

Traditional Approaches to Yoga Sequencing 10

Parinamavada and Vinyasa Krama 15

Principle One: Moving from Simple to Complex 19

Principle Two: Moving from Dynamic to Static Exploration, or
Moving into Stillness 21

Principle Three: Cultivating Energetic Balance 22

Principle Four: Integrating the Effects of Actions 25

Principle Five: Cultivating Sustainable Self-Transformation 26

Chapter Two: The Arc Structure of Yoga Classes 29

Initiating the Yogic Process 32

Sidebar: Creating a Theme-Oriented Class 36

Warming and Awakening the Body 39

The Pathway to the Peak 43

Exploring the Peak 49

Integrating the Practice 50

Sidebar: Deepening the Integration of Asana 52

Chapter Three: Sequencing Within and Across Asana Families 55

The General Properties of Asanas 56

Standing Asanas 57

Core Awakening 61

Arm Support Asanas 63

Sidebar: Healthy Wrist Sequence 64

Sidebar: Healthy Shoulder Sequence 65

Back Bends 69

Twists 75

Forward Bends 77

Hip Openers 81

Inversions 84

Savasana 88

The Next Step in Sequencing 92

Chapter Four: Sequencing Asana Instructions 93

Teaching What You Know 94

Step One: Demonstrating Asanas 95

Step Two: Transitioning into Asanas 97

Step Three: Refining Asanas 102

Step Four: Transitioning out of Asanas 109

Step Five: Absorbing and Integrating the Effects of Asanas 111

Sequencing Cues Within Asana Families 112

Sidebar: Down Dog as the Foundational Arm Support Asana 115

Part Two: Designing Beginning, Intermediate, and Advanced Classes 123

Chapter Five: Surya Namaskara—Sun Salutations 125

General Properties of Surya Namaskara 127

Classical Surya Namaskara 128

Classical Surya Namaskara (Sequence 1) 130

Surya Namaskara A 131

Surya Namaskara A (Sequence 2) 135

Surya Namaskara B 136

Surya Namaskara B (Sequence 3) 139

Sidebar: Dancing Warrior 140

Dancing Warrior (Sequence 4) 141

Yoga
Sequencing

Yoga
Sequencing

DESIGNING TRANSFORMATIVE YOGA CLASSES

MARK STEPHENS

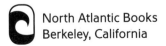
North Atlantic Books
Berkeley, California

Published by
North Atlantic Books
Berkeley, California

Cover photos by DiAnna Van Eycke
Cover photo collage by Paula Morrison
Cover and book design by Suzanne Albertson

Printed in the United States of America

Yoga Sequencing: Designing Transformative Yoga Classes is sponsored and published by the Society for the Study of Native Arts and Sciences (dba North Atlantic Books), an educational nonprofit based in Berkeley, California, that collaborates with partners to develop cross-cultural perspectives, nurture holistic views of art, science, the humanities, and healing, and seed personal and global transformation by publishing work on the relationship of body, spirit, and nature.

North Atlantic Books' publications are available through most bookstores. For further information, visit our website at www.northatlanticbooks.com or call 800-733-3000.

Library of Congress Cataloging-in-Publication Data

Stephens, Mark, 1958–
    Yoga sequencing: designing transformative yoga classes / Mark Stephens.
        p. cm.
    Includes bibliographical references and index.
    Summary: "Written for a broad yoga market that includes teachers, teacher trainers, studio owners, and students, *Yoga Sequencing* presents the essential principles of sequencing along with sixty-seven sequences of poses designed for a range of yoga student experience and offers a comprehensive resource for designing and refining yoga classes."—Provided by publisher.
    ISBN 978-1-58394-497-4
    1. Yoga. 2. Yoga—Study and teaching. I. Title.
    RA781.7.S7277 2012
    613.7'046—dc23   2011048182

9 10 11 12 SHERIDAN 20 19 18
Printed on recycled paper

North Atlantic Books is committed to the protection of our environment.
We partner with FSC-certified printers using soy-based inks
and print on recycled paper whenever possible.

To teachers and students on the path of sustainable, transformational, and joyful yoga.

Chapter Six: Introductory and Beginning-Level Classes 143

Creating and Teaching Beginning-Level Sequences 147

Beginning Class Sequences 149

Basic Introduction to Yoga Class (Sequence 5) 149

Introduction to Yoga Workshop for More Physically Fit
Students (Sequence 6) 151

Beginning Level—Focus on Back Bends (Sequence 7) 153

Beginning Level—Focus on Hip Opening (Sequence 8) 156

Beginning Level—Focus on Twisting (Sequence 9) 157

Beginning Level—Focus on Standing Balance (Sequence 10) 159

Beginning Level—Focus on Arm Support (Sequence 11) 161

Beginning Level—Focus on Forward Bends (Sequence 12) 163

Beginning Level—Focus on Inversion (Sequence 13) 165

Chapter Seven: Intermediate-Level Classes 167

Creating and Teaching Intermediate-Level Sequences 170

Intermediate Class Sequences 173

Intermediate Level—Focus on Back Bends I (Sequence 14) 173

Intermediate Level—Focus on Back Bends II (Sequence 15) 176

Intermediate Level—Focus on Hip Opening (Sequence 16) 179

Intermediate Level—Focus on Twisting (Sequence 17) 181

Intermediate Level—Focus on Standing Balance
(Sequence 18) 184

Intermediate Level—Focus on Arm Support I (Sequence 19) 187

Intermediate Level—Focus on Arm Support II (Sequence 20) 189

Intermediate Level—Focus on Forward Bends (Sequence 21) 192

Intermediate Level—Focus on Inversions (Sequence 22) 194

Chapter Eight: Advanced-Level Classes 197

Creating and Teaching Advanced-Level Sequences 200

Advanced Level Sequences 203

Advanced Level—Focus on Back Bends I (Sequence 23) 203

Advanced Level—Focus on Back Bends II (Sequence 24) 206

Advanced Level—Focus on Hip Opening (Sequence 25) 208

Advanced Level—Focus on Twisting (Sequence 26) 211

Advanced Level—Focus on Standing Balance (Sequence 27) 214
Advanced Level—Focus on Arm Support I (Sequence 28) 217
Advanced Level—Focus on Arm Support II (Sequence 29) 220
Advanced Level—Focus on Forward Bends (Sequence 30) 222
Advanced Level—Focus on Inversions (Sequence 31) 225

Part Three: Sequencing Across the Life Cycle 229

Chapter Nine: Yoga Sequencing for Kids 231

Yoga for Elementary School–Age Children (Sequence 32) 235
Yoga for Middle School–Age Children (Sequence 33) 237
Yoga for High School–Age Youth (Sequence 34) 239

Chapter Ten: Sequencing for Special Conditions of Women 243

Practicing Yoga During Menstruation 246
Yoga for Easing Menstrual Discomfort (Sequence 35) 246
Practicing Yoga During and After Pregnancy 248
Yoga Sequences by Stage of Pregnancy 251
Yoga in the First Trimester of Pregnancy—New to Yoga
(Sequence 36) 252
Yoga in the First Trimester of Pregnancy—Healthy and
Experienced Yogini (Sequence 37) 253
Yoga in the Second Trimester of Pregnancy—New to Yoga
(Sequence 38) 257
Yoga in the Second Trimester of Pregnancy—Healthy and
Experienced Yogini (Sequence 39) 259
Yoga in the Third Trimester of Pregnancy—New to Yoga
(Sequence 40) 262
Yoga in the Third Trimester of Pregnancy—Healthy and
Experienced Yogini (Sequence 41) 263
Yoga in the Third Trimester of Pregnancy—During Labor
(Sequence 42) 265
Yoga for Postpartum Reintegration (Sequence 43) 266
Yoga Sequences for Menopause 267
Yoga for Symptoms of Hot Flashes (Sequence 44) 269

Yoga for Bone Health—Preventing Osteoporosis
(Sequence 45) 270
Yoga for Reducing Mood Swings (Sequence 46) 272

Chapter Eleven: Yoga Sequencing for Seniors 275

Creating and Teaching Yoga Sequences for Seniors 277
Yoga Sequences for Seniors 278
Yoga for Seniors with Arthritis (Sequence 47) 278
Yoga for Seniors with Osteoporosis (Sequence 48) 280
Yoga for Seniors with Difficulty Balancing (Sequence 49) 282
Yoga for Seniors with Heart Disease (Sequence 50) 283

Part Four: Sequencing for More Radiant Health and Well-Being 285

Chapter Twelve: Cultivating Emotional and Mental Health 287

Simple Relaxation Class for Beginning–Intermediate Students
(Sequence 51) 289
Relax Deeply Class for Intermediate–Advanced Students
(Sequence 52) 290
Mildly Stimulating Class for Beginning–Intermediate Students
(Sequence 53) 291
Mildly Stimulating Class for Intermediate–Advanced Students
(Sequence 54) 292

Chapter Thirteen: Chakra Sequences 295

Muladhara Chakra 297
Muladhara Chakra Class (Sequence 55) 297
Svadhisthana Chakra 299
Svadhisthana Chakra Class (Sequence 56) 300
Manipura Chakra 303
Manipura Chakra Class (Sequence 57) 304
Anahata Chakra 306
Anahata Chakra Class (Sequence 58) 307
Vishuddha Chakra 309
Vishuddha Chakra Class (Sequence 59) 309

Ajna Chakra   311

   Ajna Chakra Class (Sequence 60)   312

Sahasrara Chakra   313

   Sahasrara: An Integrated Chakra Class (Sequence 61)   314

Chapter Fourteen: Ayurvedic Yoga Sequencing   317

Yoga Sequences for Dosha Balancing   319

   Vata Balancing Class (Sequence 62)   319

   Pitta Balancing Class (Sequence 63)   322

   Kapha Balancing Class (Sequence 64)   324

Part Five: Bringing It All Together 327

Chapter Fifteen: Further Tips on Yoga Sequencing   329

   Soulful Vinyasa Yoga—An Integrated Level 1–2 Class (Sequence 65)   335

   Soulful Vinyasa Yoga—An Integrated Level 2–3 Class (Sequence 66)   339

   Soulful Vinyasa Yoga—An Integrated Level 3+ Class (Sequence 67)   344

Appendix A: Glossary   347

Appendix B: The Constituent Elements of Asanas   359

Appendix C: Yoga Class Sequencing Worksheet   457

Appendix D: Popular Hatha Yoga Sequences   461

Appendix E: Additional Resources   469

Notes   471

References   479

Index   489

About the Author   507

Tables

In Chapters

 2.1. Basic Template for a Complete Arc Class 32

 3.1. Asana Families 56

 3.2. Basic Arc Template Applied to Different-Level Yoga Classes 89

 4.1. Cueing Oppositional Actions 105

 4.2. Roots and Extension 107

 4.3. Deeper Refining Cues 108

 5.1. Twelve Asanas in the Surya Namaskara Family 126

 5.2. Sequencing Cues for Breath and Movement in Classical Surya Namaskara 129

 6.1. When and to Whom to Teach Pranayama 146

In Appendix D

 D.1. Anusara Sequence—Basic Template 461

 D.2. Ashtanga Vinyasa Sequence (Primary Series) 462

 D.3. Bikram Sequence—Beginning Class 463

 D.4. Iyengar Sequence—Basic Class 464

 D.5. Kripalu Sequence—Sun Flow 464

 D.6. Power Yoga Sequence 465

 D.7. Prana Flow Sequence for Natarajasana 466

 D.8. Sivananda Sequence 467

 D.9. White Lotus Sequence 467

Preface

Yoga is alive and well as a globalized practice for cultivating overall health and well-being. With tens of millions of people now doing yoga all over the world, the yoga teaching profession has finally begun to establish clearer and stronger standards of competence for teachers. As yoga teacher training programs proliferate, there is a growing need for training resources that support these standards. My previous book, *Teaching Yoga: Essential Foundations and Techniques* (2010), offers a comprehensive text for yoga teachers, covering the main subject areas in which teachers should have at least basic knowledge and skills. While many other books in the vast marketplace of yoga literature go into further depth on a variety of topics, including yoga philosophy, anatomy, and specific asana techniques, in-depth guidance on planning and sequencing classes is largely nonexistent.

Countless yoga teachers and teacher trainers have expressed the need for comprehensive guidance on designing yoga classes, inspiring me the write this book. While it is easy to find published sequences for a variety of yoga styles or for exploring some specific asanas, the essential missing ingredient for crafting yoga classes is a thorough resource covering the principles and methods for designing sequences for a variety of levels, conditions, and settings. This book is an attempt to offer that resource to the yoga community.

After completing yoga teacher training in 1995, I started teaching public classes at Malibu Yoga and soon thereafter at the original Yoga Works in Santa Monica, California. A couple of years into teaching, I founded the Yoga Inside Foundation along with several friends to establish ongoing yoga programs in alternative settings across North America. Soon we were teaching in prisons, juvenile institutions, drug rehabilitation centers, mental health treatment facilities, and schools. Our collective experience revealed that the yoga sequencing concepts we learned in teacher training and refined in regular public classes were very limited and often left us ill-prepared for working with the more diverse student needs and interests we encountered through Yoga Inside. This led to deeper reflection on how to obtain or develop that preparation, which in turn led to deeper study of the elements of *asana, pranayama*, and meditation. The insights gained through this experience soon informed not only our service work in alternative settings but how to approach yoga sequencing in all settings, including regular public yoga classes offered in yoga studios and fitness centers as well as at yoga institutes and conferences. Many more years of practice, deep study, observation, and experimentation led to further refinement of the principles and techniques for planning and sequencing yoga classes. This book is the culmination of that process.

My personal yoga practice became consistent just over twenty years ago after I met Erich Schiffmann, who taught me the method of being "guided from within" that he learned from Joel Kramer. Over the years I dove deeply into Ashtanga Vinyasa, took innumerable workshops with brilliantly insightful Iyengar teachers, and opened to the effusive spirit of Vinyasa Flow and the transformative potential of tantra; I also came to appreciate the refined insights of those working in the field of yoga therapy and those who draw from deep knowledge of functional anatomy, biomechanics, and kinesiology in making yoga accessible and sustainable for all who choose to do it. Amid it all, the intuitive yoga sensibilities of Erich Schiffmann and Joel Kramer are still resonating with me, even as I design and teach yoga to classrooms of yoga students.

The apparent contradiction between planned classes and intuitive practice unravels when we appreciate that students benefit from learning principles and techniques of practice in a way that makes it easier and more natural for them to discover and honor the best teacher they will ever have, the one dancing inside their bodymind to the rhythms of the breath and the beats of the heart. What I offer here is in the spirit of teaching in a way that empowers students to ultimately become their own teacher, intelligently guided from within.

Everything in this book has benefited from the lively exchanges over the years among participants in my "Art and Science of Yoga Sequencing" workshops that are required in my yoga teacher certification program. Hundreds of teachers-in-training along with experienced teachers have explored, discussed, debated, and shared about yoga sequencing with one another in these intensives; I have done my best to listen and learn from each and every one of them. Their contributions are embedded in every word printed on these pages, for which I take sole responsibility while honoring the gift of their wide-ranging insights.

Teaching yoga is one of the most joyful and rewarding parts of my life. Much of the joy arises from the sense of connection with students from myriad backgrounds who come to yoga for a wide variety of reasons. My students are my teachers, each giving me unique insights into the practice. I am particularly appreciative of my students and fellow teachers in the Santa Cruz yoga community who have shared with and have been supportive of me during my retreats into writing. Anne Tharpe, Alison Mitchell, Sean Lang, and all the teachers at Santa Cruz Yoga ensured that our yoga studio thrived when my attention was focused on this work.

Writing a book can easily tempt one away from the discipline and healthy benefits of daily yoga practice. It is all about balance. I am indebted to Ganga White, Sally Kempton, Joel Kramer, Diana Alstad, Erich Schiffmann, James Wvinner, James G. Bailey, and Shiva Rea not only for their supportive friendship but for offering living models of how staying in the practice for decades allows one to stay in balance even amid the turbulence of life. Each encouraged me in their unique way to stay with this project and also offered invaluable suggestions.

My research assistants—yoga teachers Tony Agostinelli, Anne Tharpe, and Cindy Cheung—were instrumental in helping me gather and organize many of the resources provided here. Karen Bassi, Anne Tharpe, and Melinda Stephens-Bukey read and critiqued the manuscript, offering a variety of helpful suggestions. DiAnna Van Eycke and I shot all the photographs shown in the sequences. James Wvinner provided the photographs that appear elsewhere in the book.

Bailey Johnson, Brenna Mackin, Erika Abrahamian, Emily Perry, Greta Mitchell, Jeanette Lehouillier, Jennifer Stanley, Malia Rawlings, Marcia Charland, Mary Maleta, Naomi Hegenbart, Ray Charland, Rowan Rawlings, Seana Messina, and Tony Agostinelli graciously, patiently, and playfully modeled for the images shown in the sequences.

Working with North Atlantic Books is always a delight. My project editor, Jessica Sevey, expertly guided me though the entire process of translating a manuscript into a book, helping to ensure greater coherence and clarity throughout. My copy editor, Christopher Church, masterfully edited the entire manuscript, making it clearer, simpler, and easier to read. Suzanne Albertson's beautiful design speaks for itself.

I am deeply grateful for the loving support of my family and close friends, especially DiAnna Van Eycke, Jennifer Stanley, Mike Rotkin, Michael Stephens, Melinda Stephens-Bukey, John Bukey, Reatha White, Ralph Quinn, James Wvinner, and Siddha.

A Note on Language

Yoga originated in India, where much of its development was expressed through the ancient Sanskrit language. The meaning of many yoga concepts is still best stated in Sanskrit, and wherever there is translation there is concern about accuracy. This might not be an issue for teachers whose approach eschews all reference to yoga's ancient roots. Many other teachers (as well as books, periodicals, and electronic media) do draw from the ancient teachings and also employ the Sanskrit terms for concepts and asanas (which means "to take one seat"). Learning the Sanskrit terms does not imply belief in any particular philosophy; rather, it gives greater access to participation in the global conversation and practice of yoga.

The most commonly accepted and used terms for asanas and other aspects of yoga are drawn from the global influence of yoga teachers B. K. S. Iyengar, Pattabhi Jois, and T. K. V. Desikachar. *Yoga Journal* and *Yoga International* magazines, along with scores of books, have further popularized this terminology (and the related spelling forms). Throughout this book we use these terms and forms, providing the English translation with each first instance of the Sanskrit term. With asana names, we give the Sanskrit and English names at the first instance of the asana in the narrative section of each chapter and only the Sanskrit name thereafter. All yoga-related terms, whether in English or Sanskrit, are in the glossary, and all asanas are additionally listed in Appendix B with their Sanskrit and English names.

Introduction

The Art and Science of Yoga Sequencing

Doing yoga and teaching yoga are inextricably intertwined. The experiences we have on our yoga mats help us to refine our personal practice and provide insights into how we might best share yoga with others. The farther we go in our practice, the more we discover the vast universe of elements that are at play in yoga's incredible potential for enhancing our lives. In the interrelation of these elements we come to specific practices—sequences of actions—that have different effects depending on how it all flows together. This brings us to several questions: What are the elements of a complete practice? How are they best structured to make the practice most accessible, sustainable, and transforming? What are the best ways to begin a yoga practice session? What should each session include? What are the best ways to sequence different asanas, breathing practices, and meditations? What is the relationship between this asana and that asana? How does this asana affect that asana? What are the effects of asanas ordered in a particular way compared to the same asanas ordered differently? What are the relationships within and between families of asanas—standing asanas, core asanas, arm balances, back bends, twists, forward bends, hip openers, and inversions? What about pranayama (conscious breathing) and meditation practices? What affects them, and how in turn do they affect what follows? On what basis—other than habit, intuition, or whim—should one determine the overall structure and sequence of a complete class? What about moving from one class to the next across the span of a week, a month, a year, or a lifetime? What are the best ways to design classes for a lifetime of yoga?

Superficially simple, these questions about sequencing decisions are as complex as the beautifully diverse mosaic of human beings doing yoga. Age, genetics, lifestyle, physical and mental condition, environmental setting, personal intention, and spiritual philosophy all come into play in doing yoga. Moreover, some of these variables can change from day to day, inviting or even requiring us to modify what we're doing—or at least how we do what we're doing. Taking a holistic perspective on yoga, it's vitally important to give experiential and thoughtful consideration to all of these myriad elements, which, when properly blended together, lead to healthy, wholesome, and sustainable yoga practices in which students more and more come to a place of balance along their yoga path and in their larger lives.

The primary roles of a yoga teacher are showing students a yogic pathway and offering them guidance along that path. Doing this with inspiration, knowledge, skill, patience, compassion, and creativity defines a good teacher. The many elements of teaching—creating a safe space for self-exploration, crafting class sequences that take students on physical and energetic journeys, cueing students in their process of refinement, offering practical guidance in meditation, offering examples for extending the practice off the mat— collectively lead to the same thing: yoga as a process for awakening to the truth of one's being, to an abiding sense of equanimity amid the shifting tides of daily experience and the seasons of one's life.[1]

If yoga were a practice of attainment in which we were all aiming for a certain goal, the role of the teacher would be much simpler. We would tell students what to do and how to do it. Sequences would be prescribed even as we would draw from our knowledge of yoga philosophy, energetics, anatomy, and psychology to craft classes and instructions that correctly orient students in moving toward the goal. In the physical practice, instruction would focus on the perfection poses; in pranayama we would teach the perfection of breath and energetic balance; in meditation we would teach students to still the mind. But yoga is not a practice of attainment; it is an unending *process of self-discovery and self-transformation*. In this process, teachers are facilitators and guides who offer insightful encouragement to each student along his or her unique path as it evolves, breath by breath.

The art and science of teaching yoga is creatively expressed in how you craft asana, pranayama, and meditation sequences that honor the needs and intentions of the students in your classes. Your creativity is given form by yoga philosophy, the style of yoga you are teaching, the biomechanics and energetic requirements and effects of asanas, and by your personal sense of purpose in meaningfully sharing yoga. Here we look to use our full palette of knowledge and skills to create classes that resonate with the needs and expressed intentions of students, offering them a clearer pathway to more radiant well-being.

This book offers yoga students and teachers a set of resources for creating a rich array of yoga sequences. To make the most of these resources, you will ideally be in or have already completed a yoga teacher training program that teaches the fundamentals of yoga practice. While books, DVDs, and the seemingly infinite resources available online are all useful in learning more about the art and science of teaching yoga, learning to teach yoga is best done through direct interaction with others in a setting wholly dedicated to acquiring, developing, and refining the skills and knowledge that will make you the best possible teacher that you can be. The purpose of this book is to help support that process.

Part One covers the foundations and principles of sequencing. Just as there are many yoga paths dating back to the very origins of yoga in India some five thousand years ago, so too is there a vast sea of philosophical, spiritual, and intellectual orientations to the specific elements of yoga practice. This diverse world of yoga is briefly reviewed in my earlier work (Stephens 2010) and will not be explored in any further depth here. Here we will explore specifically the kernels of wisdom and insight bearing directly on sequencing, including materials found in the ancient archives of Indian thought and experience as well as contemporary sources that shed further light on yoga practice. Through each successive chapter, we will funnel our exploration from broad principles of sequencing to increasingly specific methods and techniques for crafting classes that are designed for different students, spaces, conditions, and intentions, culminating in how best to sequence the verbal cues given to students in approaching and refining movements and energetic actions in asanas.

In Part Two, we turn our attention to designing classes for different levels of yoga students. We start by looking at Surya Namaskaras, the Sun Salutations that are often the initiating part of other yoga sequences along with more complex "dancing warrior" sequences. Then, using the ubiquitous distinction of beginning, intermediate, and advanced to distinguish practice levels, each of the next chapters first defines the level and then discusses the elements and qualities of practice appropriate to it. We then consider which asanas are most appropriately taught at that level and how to place them in relation to each other in each of several thematically oriented classes (such as hip-opening, heart-opening, balancing, calming, and stimulating). Here we will also address the pranayama and meditation techniques appropriate to each level and how they are best sequenced in relation to the asanas.

Part Three focuses on designing classes for students across the span of the life cycle, starting with Chapter Nine on yoga sequences for children, with sequencing guidelines given for elementary school, middle school, and high school–age kids. In Chapter Ten we turn our attention to the special condition of women in yoga, looking closely at yoga sequencing for menstruation, pregnancy (with separate sequences given for new and experienced yoga students in each trimester of pregnancy and postpartum), and moving into menopause. Chapter Eleven addresses yoga for seniors, exploring how best to adapt yoga sequences that help with circulation, arthritis, osteoporosis, physical balance, and heart disease.

Part Four explores creating more specialized classes that help take the practice to a deeper energetic level, starting in Chapter Twelve with sequencing for emotional and mental conditions that lead to stress, anxiety, and depression. Chapter Thirteen focuses on designing yoga sequences around the chakras, including using the chakras as symbolic tropes for getting at emotional and psychological issues as well as considering their more traditional concepts. In Chapter Fourteen we look at how the insights of ayurveda can be applied to creating energetically balancing sequences of asanas and pranayamas for each of the three doshic constitutions.

In bringing it all together, Part Five—Chapter Fifteen—offers further thoughts on creating yoga classes along with a few of my favorite Soulful Vinyasa class sequences.

Appendix A provides a glossary of yoga-related terms. Appendix B provides thumbnail pictures of the asanas to ease their identification as part of an extensive resource giving the constituent elements of 125 asanas. Appendix C is a class planning worksheet to assist in planning yoga class sequences. Appendix D gives representative sequences from several popular styles of Hatha yoga. Appendix E provides information on the Teaching Yoga Resource Center at www.markstephensyoga.com.

Part One

Foundations and Principles

Chapter One

Philosophy and Principles
of Sequencing

A grand adventure is about to begin.
—WINNIE THE POOH

There are as many approaches to planning and sequencing yoga classes as there are styles, traditions, and brands of yoga. Add the creative expression of yoga teachers fashioning their own classes and we find a dizzying array of class designs across the vast landscape of hatha, or physical, yoga.[1] As the yoga movement continues to expand, we can anticipate the further evolution of yoga practices, some consciously harnessed to ancient teachings and others decidedly not. This is part of the sublime beauty of yoga: it is alive and evolving each and every time someone steps onto a mat, explains a technique, or guides students through a class.

While a few yoga styles insist that they offer the true, original, best, most effective, or otherwise most ideal approach, there is no absolutely correct or incorrect sequence (although, as we shall see, some are dangerously risky or otherwise go against the grain of even the most basic sequencing principles). Rather, different sequences make more or less sense in terms of how yoga works for different people in various life situations and conditions, what is being emphasized in a particular style or tradition of yoga, or with respect to the intention of an individual student or teacher. Thus, yoga teachers have tremendous freedom is designing and teaching different sequences, freedom that also carries responsibility for ensuring that the sequences are sensible. Crafting sequences that give structure, coherence, meaning, and transformative potential to yoga classes, you have an opportunity to draw from and apply everything you have learned about yoga, from anatomy to philosophy, asana to pranayama, self-acceptance to self-realization.

Most classes are not planned; commonly (and usually problematically) they reflect random creativity. Random creativity can be a wonderful source of discovery. If it is just you coming to your yoga mat and following your senses, then such spontaneous sequencing might give you the perfect practice. Many yoga students choose a home practice that is informed less by what some style or system of yoga prescribes than an intuitive sense of being guided from within. This is a wonderful way to approach your personal practice. But if you are designing a sequence for others to do, the random approach is likely to lead students into unnecessary confusion, difficulty, and even injury. Even in one's personal practice, random or purely intuitively informed sequences can lead to greater difficulty in cultivating the stability and ease that we want throughout the practice. Moving from one particular pose to another might make sense in terms of efficiency or relatively seamless and fluid transition, but it can create unnecessary and potentially risky obstacles over the longer term, can lead to energetic imbalances, or can cause physical strain or injury.

In some yoga styles and traditions, most notably Ashtanga Vinyasa and Bikram, the order of poses is already set. One benefit of this approach is that the asanas, and in some styles even the specific actions for transitioning between them, are like a perfect mirror onto the practitioner because the only thing that changes from one practice to the next is the practitioner, thus making the experience of doing the sequence somewhat more a reflection of the person doing it than the sequence itself. Do you feel different doing the practice from one day to the next? According to the set sequence approach, that difference is primarily you, not the sequence, thus giving the practitioner an opportunity for deeper insight into the process of personal awakening, evolution, and self-transformation that is yoga.

In doing set sequences, you know where you are headed. Some find this leads to greater anticipation of what's ahead and detracts from the experience of being fully present in the current moment in connecting breath, body, and mind. Others find that knowing what is coming next leads to deeper absorption in what is happening right now. These tendencies, which tend to arise in any style of practice, are typically greater in set sequence practices.

The more significant issue that arises in doing set sequences is the potential strain caused by doing repetitive actions. For instance, in the primary (beginning) series of Ashtanga Vinyasa yoga, the sequence calls for flowing through Chaturanga Dandasana (Four-Limbed Staff Pose) over fifty times. Even if one is properly aligned and engaging effective energetic actions, this can be a very challenging sequence that, done repetitively, can strain the shoulder and wrist joints as well as the lower back, knees, hips, elbows, and neck. If a student approaches the set sequence with clear intention to practice with *sthira* and *sukham*—the steadiness and ease that the ancient yogic sage Patanjali posits as the essential interrelated qualities of asana practice—repetitive stress might be reduced or even eliminated. Nonetheless, the repetitive nature of practically any set sequence, especially one devoid of counterposes that systematically address the tension that naturally accumulates along the way, can itself cause physical strain, mental fatigue, and energetic imbalance.

In between random creativity and set sequences we find a plethora of classes loosely based on a template found in a book, teacher training manual, or online site or adapted from observation of other teachers' classes. While these templates can be an effective way to get started in crafting unique and well-informed classes, the tendency is to apply the template or observed sequence in cookie-cutter fashion, teaching it to students or in settings for which it was never intended. Another tendency is to change the sequence in ways that disrupt the integrity with which it addresses the biomechanics of movement or flexibility, the energetics of the sequence, or some other integral aspect that made the original sequence make sense. While creativity is beautiful, it is ideally expressed in keeping with the basic sequencing principles that make physical yoga beneficial and sustainable.

Traditional Approaches to Yoga Sequencing

Looking far back into the history of yoga, we find a variety of specific prescriptions for how to sequence one's yoga practice. Considering yoga in the broadest sense as a practice of awakening and integration, the prescriptions range from what do to across the span of many lifetimes to how to order a specific session. Focusing on yoga across the span of one's life in this world, we

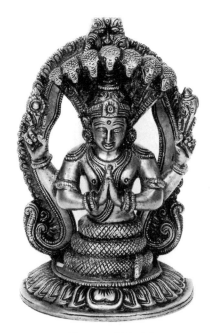

The sage Patanjali

find in Patanjali's Yoga Sutras four levels of yogic evolution in practices that are designed to control the mind (*chitta vritti nirodaha,* "to calm the fluctuations of the mind") and open one to bliss.[2] Predating the development of Hatha yoga (yoga that involves doing multiple asanas and pranayamas), Patanjali offers a step-by-step process for these practices, with variations offered that make the practices more accessible to different temperaments and conditions.

To make the path to bliss more accessible, Patanjali offers an eight-stage process: (1) *yama,* (2) *niyama,* (3) *asana,* (4) *pranayama,* (5) *pratyahara,* (6) *dharana,* (7) *dhyana,* and (8) *samadhi.*[3] In this model, one begins with yama to establish a moral foundation for the deeper practices to follow, then proceeds to niyama, self-purification and self-study practices, before attempting asana. It is said that to begin asana before yama and niyama will result in further mental disturbance and negate the benefits of asana practice. At the time—Patanjali wrote around 200 CE—asana was the practice of sitting (literally, "to take one seat"), and all that Patanjali added to this definition were the essential asana qualities of sthira (steadiness) and sukham (ease).[4] Still, mastery of asana was considered the essential preparation for doing pranayama, with severe consequences (injury or even death) if one violates the prescribed order. Thus, each stage is preparation for the next, with pranayama opening the subtle energetic pathways for more balanced energy that make pratyahara, "relieving the senses of external distraction," possible, which leads to focused concentration in dharana and then a sense of oneness in dhyana. One then dissolves into samadhi, a state of bliss.

Several hundred years later, we find the first evidence of physical yoga, a practice involving several asanas and other practices that came to be called Hatha yoga. In the earliest literature on Hatha yoga, specifically Swami Swatmarama's fourteenth-century CE Hatha Yoga Pradipika (Muktibodhananda 1993, 566–74) and the Siva Samhita (Mallinson 2004, 28), we are given four different evolutionary stages of yoga that are said to apply to learning all yogic practices (in the Siva Samhita, these stages are given specifically for pranayama practice). Together they are known as *bhava*, suggesting a spontaneous evolution in which the quality of body-breath-mind experience is more and more deeply refined. These four stages give us the traditional delineation of beginning, intermediate, advanced, and beyond advanced yoga.

1. Arambha Avastha—Beginning Stage: Here one is first becoming familiar with one's body, exploring yoga asanas at the level of gross anatomy as one learns the basic forms and actions within the asanas. B. K. S. Iyengar (2009, 168) refers to this stage as "scratching the surface." The objective is to get a feeling for the wholeness of each asana, cultivating steadiness and ease while exploring how to expand and refine the breath.

2. Ghata Avastha—Vessel Stage: Here one begins to explore more deeply how qualities of mind are affected by changes in the body. The practice moves into more subtle awareness of breath, sound, and overall sensation, refining the vessel that contains the bodymind. Moving more internally, one begins to apply breath retention practices, gradually doing more complex pranayamas with an abiding commitment to refining the flow of breath as a means of developing more refined awareness.

3. Parichaya Avastha—Increase Stage: Having refined the temple of the body through beginning and intermediate asanas and the instrument of the breath through pranayamas, one now enters the stage of becoming intimately acquainted with the mind. Staying in the asana and pranayama practices, one can now explore the embodiment of consciousness, bringing refined awareness into every cell of one's being, and with it gain a sense of overall integration of bodymind.

4. Nispattia Avastha—Consummation Stage: With body-breath-mind refined into a seamless quality of pure being, everything one does and experiences in life is a moving meditation, with the very

distinction between the body and consciousness disappearing as one comes to be in a state of bliss.

In the beginning stage (Arambha Avastha) of Hatha yoga as taught in these early texts, the student of yoga begins with *shatkarma* practices that help establish an initial harmony in the bodymind[5] that makes Patanjali's path, which starts with yama, niyama, and asana, more accessible. From there, one moves along the same path as given in the Yoga Sutras, with asana preceding pranayama and both preceding the four stages of meditation practice. Many traditional and contemporary teachings prescribe just this sequence.

The ancient teachings offer still other approaches to moving from where one is to an awareness of enlightened being. An overarching concept in ancient writings on yoga is that the energy of each embodied being is contained in a set of five interrelated sheaths or *koshas*. First mentioned in the Taittiriya Upanishad (Gambhirananda 1989), the kosha model helps to map the inner journey of yoga as a sequence of increasingly subtle yet integrated awareness and being. There are five koshas: *annamaya, pranamaya, manomaya, vijnanamaya,* and *anandamaya.* Starting on the periphery of the physical body and moving toward the core of your being as an embodied soul, the koshas are not a literal anatomical model of the body but rather, as Shiva Rea (1997, 43) puts it, "a metaphor that helps describe what it feels like to do yoga from the inside—the process of aligning what in contemporary language we often call the 'mind, body, and spirit' or 'mind-body connection.'"

Using the kosha typology to conceptualize and explore the nature of being, yoga helps bring the body, breath, mind, wisdom, and spirit (bliss) into harmony. Existing as an energetic whole, all aspects of all five sheaths are simultaneously present, interwoven like a tapestry. Hatha yoga offers a sequential method for becoming consciously aware of this interwoven fabric of existence, connecting the

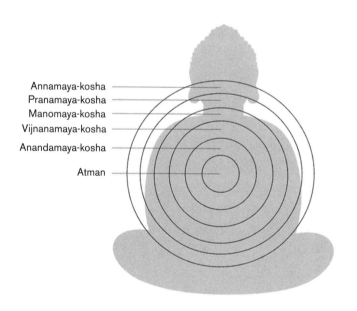

Annamaya-kosha
Pranamaya-kosha
Manomaya-kosha
Vijnanamaya-kosha
Anandamaya-kosha
Atman

A two-dimensional model of the koshas

physical and subtle bodies while bringing awareness more and more to a place of blissful being. In this model, the annamaya kosha is the sheath of the physical self, named for its quality of being nourished by food (*anna* means "food"; *maya* means "full of"). Yoga starts to happen as we begin to explore and experience the physical body in its manifold connections with the energetic, intellectual, wisdom, and blissful bodies. Looking through the lens of traditional Hatha yoga, this is the beginning stage, Arambha Avastha, in a lifelong yoga sequence.

The pranamaya kosha, or "energy sheath," connects the physical body with the other koshas, vitalizing and holding together the body and mind. Composed of *prana,* the vital life force, it pervades the whole organism, physically manifesting in the constant flow and movement of breath. Part of the subtle body, prana cannot be seen or physically touched as it moves through thousands of *nadis,* or energy channels, sustaining the entire physical and energetic system. The pranamaya kosha is associated on a physiological level with the respiratory and circulatory systems but is neither reducible to, nor coterminous with, them. In doing pranayama, we are expanding and directing this energy to cultivate a more fluid and harmonious interaction among the koshas, integrating body, mind, and spirit. Working with the breath in the physical body in exploration of asanas—playing with the asanas, holding them, refining them, letting them go—expands our awareness beyond the physical body. With prana as the source and guide, we begin to discover its more subtle expressions, called *prana-vayus,* each with a unique movement and effect. This can be seen as the vessel stage (Ghata Avastha) in Hatha yoga.

Going more deeply into a kosha sequence, we come to the manomaya kosha, from *manos,* or "mind," and the five sensory faculties, conveying the powers of thought and judgment. Here one is coming into the stage of increase (Parichaya Avastha). Associated with the brain and nervous system, manomaya kosha distinguishes humans from other living organisms. Endowed with the ability to differentiate, it is the cause of distinctions such as "I" and "mine," from which it creates freedom or bondage. Breath mediates the interaction between this sheath and the physical body, which we sense when mental strain compromises breath and wellness, or when the breath leads to a sense of oneness between body and mind and a sense of inner peace. Going deeper, we experience the vijnanamaya kosha, meaning "composed of *vijnana*" (wisdom), referring to the reflective aspect of consciousness that discriminates, determines, or wills. The reflective aspect of consciousness, vijnanamaya is present to our consciousness when we begin to experience deeper insight into the world and ourselves. Sometimes referred to as the "wisdom sheath," vijnanamaya is still identified with the body, subject to change, sentient, and thinking. As the physical and subtle bodies are felt as one, there is a deepening insight into the unity of self and nature, ego and the divine. When this experience is shrouded over by memories—manos—the identity is still with the ego, the vijnanamaya kosha, not the supreme Self. But when "the witness of the experience dissolves into the experience of the moment," as Shiva Rea puts it, anandamaya is shining through.

From *ananda,* meaning "bliss," in the Upanishads, the anandamaya kosha is known as *karana sharira,* or the "causal body." It is the consciousness that is always there, that always has been and always will be there, even when the mind, senses, and body are sleeping. It manifests itself by catching a reflection of the divine, which is absolute bliss, felt in moments of calm inner peace and tranquility. In the traditional Hatha yoga model of stages, this is the consummation stage (Nispattia Avastha).

It is important to note that these traditional approaches to yoga sequencing are given for practices one undertakes as part of walking a wider path of spiritual awakening and transformation that is said to ultimately lead to transcending the cycles of birth-life-death-rebirth. While many students come to yoga with this interest or intention, many more come to yoga with less profound or grandiose intentions: to reduce stress, to develop more balance in life, to increase strength and flexibility, and to cultivate a happier outlook on life and a greater sense of overall well-being. Fundamentalist yogis typically dismiss such intentions as arising from *maya,* "illusion," specifically the illusion that the everyday world of diversity and individuality is not real, indeed, that *you* are not real.

Here we take this world and our experience in it as altogether real, even if often clouded by illusions arising from a diseased bodymind or the cultural clutter than filters much of our personal experience and thoughts about life. Starting from the idea that we do live in a real world and in real bodies, we can then look to fashion yoga sequences that meet a wide array of needs, interests, and intentions that make practical sense in this life.

Parinamavada and Vinyasa Krama

A complete and effective yoga sequence is one that allows students to progress steadily, safely, and simply from one place to another in their personal practice. Every student comes to yoga somewhat uniquely and also changes from day to day and practice to practice. Here we are blending two essential philosophical concepts at the heart of planning yoga classes: (1) *parinamavada,* the understanding that constant change is an inherent part of the cause and effect nature of life; and (2) *vinyasa krama,* from *vinyasa,* which means "to place in a special way," and *krama,* which means "proceeding step by step according to a regular order," referring to the informed and sequential arrangement and pacing of asanas, pranayamas, and other yoga techniques to accommodate different intentions and abilities (Krishnamacharya 1934, 160). Let's explore this further.

If we accept the constancy of change, we are still left with the question of how to consciously participate in the changes that are happening. This question applies in every phase of a yoga practice, from setting intention at the beginning, to refining how you do what you are doing, to settling into Savasana (Corpse Pose) and moving back out into the larger world. The concept of change is of particular significance in sequencing because it encourages us to appreciate where we are and how we feel in the present moment and then to chart a course of action based on cultivating intended changes that are realistic given our immediate circumstances. In crafting and teaching sequences to others, it calls on us to more fully assess, anticipate, and honor the realities of students in our classes, thereby offering them a pathway that makes yoga work for them. The idea is to begin from where you are, and for a student to begin his or her practice based on his or her present physical, emotional, and mental condition.

The power of this insight is in its simplicity: acknowledge where you are and progress from there, as opposed to jumping ahead at the expense of stability and ease. For a teacher, this means letting go of preconceptions about students and classes in favor of observing where they are and offering guidance based on that observed reality. It also means crafting and teaching sequences that make sense in terms of the students actually in a class rather than teaching a preconceived sequence that could be too easy, too hard, too complex, or otherwise inappropriate for that particular class on that particular day. For students doing a yoga practice, this means exploring consciously, one breath at a time, and moving with stability and ease along the path toward a deeper, more self-transforming practice.

The concept of vinyasa krama is from the teachings of Tiramulai Krishnamacharya, whose famous students T. K. V. Desikachar, Indra Devi, B. K. S. Iyengar, and Pattabhi Jois became among the most influential yoga teachers in the world in the mid to late twentieth century. Although these teachers have expressed the quality of vinyasa krama in somewhat different ways, all emphasize the importance of offering a step-by-step practice based on the needs of the individual student or class. Vinyasa krama thus asks us to approach yoga with a systematic method, integrating breath, mind, and body while moving sequentially into a deeper practice. It also asks us to take an expanded view of "vinyasa," which unfortunately is commonly reduced to "Chaturanga, Up Dog, Down Dog" in the popular yoga lexicon.

Vinyasas are variations and movements in which we consciously connect the breath, mind, and body in relation to one another. By "connect" we refer to yoga itself, from its root word *yuj*, "to yoke." Thus we are gradually moving into more elaborate and complex forms of practice while continuously yoking the mind and body through the medium of the breath.[6]

The breath becomes this medium when we utilize the essential yogic breathing technique of *ujjayi pranayama:* slow, smooth, lightly audible, conscious breathing through the nose. Ujjayi pranayama offers a prism or barometer through which to maintain awareness of how one is doing in one's yoga practice. If the breath is strained, it is a sure sign to slow down or even retreat from the intensity or form of action in which one is engaging. Using the breath in this way allows one to proceed with a clearer awareness of steadiness and ease, the twin fundamental qualities of asana described in the Yoga Sutras of Patanjali.

By exploring the practice breath by conscious breath, each and every movement becomes a vinyasa sequence unto itself. Even the simplest of movements are vinyasas. For example, we do a vinyasa when moving from standing in Tadasana (Mountain Pose) to sweeping the arms out and up overhead into the Urdhva Hastasana (Upward Hands Pose). Indeed, there is a vinyasa in simply taking in a single breath and being conscious of the movement of the breath-body-mind amid this flow. From the smallest microsequences such as this to the macrosequence of one's life, we develop the yoga practice breath by breath, step by step, sequence by sequence, class by class, each breath and movement drawing from what came just before just as it prepares us for what may come next. This is the essence of vinyasa krama.

The concepts of parinamavada and vinyasa krama apply equally to planned group classes and individual instruction (as well as in one's personal practice, in which one is listening inside for intuitive guidance). The teacher's role in this process is threefold: (1) to intelligently plan the route based on the realities of the terrain and the students in class; (2) to observe and communicate with students in order to ascertain when they have integrated the experience with stability and ease; and (3) to provide informed guidance and inspiration along the path.

In this book we are primarily focused on the first of these roles—designing and teaching classes that are accessible, meaningful, and sustainable. In applying the concepts of parinamavada and vinyasa krama, we are led to create sequences that are informed, effective, efficient, beautiful, and integrated.[7] Let's briefly explore each of these terms as they relate to planning and sequencing yoga practices:

Informed: By *informed* we mean that one draws from accurate information and knowledge about the elements of the practice one is doing or teaching.

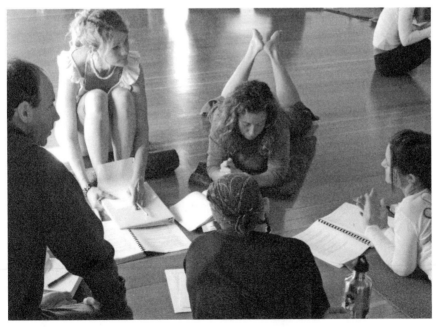

Designing good classes requires study, practice, and refinement.

Yoga is informed by many sources of knowledge and wisdom, including introspection, spiritual philosophy, subtle energetics, functional anatomy, and the sciences of biomechanics and kinesiology, to name just a few. Given the vastness of each of these sources of insight and the complex diversity of human beings, there is really no limit to how much one can learn and apply in the art and science of sequencing. While this can seem overwhelming, by taking the large perspective of yoga as a lifelong practice, one can approach the various methods and techniques one open-minded breath at a time, thereby making possible some new insight in every moment of the practice.

Effective: By *effective* we mean that the sequence is successful in bringing about the intended result of the practice—whatever that intention may be— while being safe, balanced, and transformational. Different sequences can have dramatically different effects, which will also vary for different students or even for the same students in various settings or conditions. If someone is emotionally depressed and goes to a yoga class with the intention of elevating their mood, a class designed for reducing anxiety through deep, sustained forward bends can have just the opposite effect. Similarly, a student experiencing insomnia and able to practice only in the evenings after work is likely to exacerbate his or her sleep problems if the class has lots of back bends or stimulating breathing practices such as *kapalabhati* (skull-cleansing) pranayama.

Efficient: An efficient sequence moves toward the intended result in the simplest way, allowing a feeling of graceful transition into a gradually more sublime experience of yoga. This is not to say that the practice should be void of difficulty or complexity. To the contrary, it is often precisely in the experience of working through challenging situations or experiences that we move most deeply into yoga as a practice of self-transformation. But just as perseverance contributes to the yogic path, so too we benefit from surrendering in a way that allows us to more fully accept our limitations and move beyond them through patient exploration. This interrelated set of qualities—perseverance practice and letting go—allows us to more consciously chart the simplest solutions to removing the physical, emotional, and mental obstacles that we encounter in the evolution of our practice and ourselves. By crafting sequences that are informed by an understanding of how to most simply navigate the obstacles one is likely to encounter along the way, we can move from where we are to a deeper unwinding of unnecessary tension and thereby open to the deepest possible yoga practice.

Beautiful: Taking this graceful approach becomes a source of beauty as the practice comes to reflect one's inherent nature as a beautiful being. Nothing is forced. Each breath, movement, and posture is done consciously, in keeping with one's overall intention and an abiding openness to the clearer insights that emerge from doing yoga more consciously. The practice then progresses away from external sensibilities—how a pose appears or compares to others—and toward internal integrity and the integral awareness of refining the expression of one's being through conscious action. The effect is an elegant and inwardly satisfying practice that simply feels right.

Integrated: Lastly, a complete practice is an integrated practice that takes account of the whole experience. While many students come to yoga primarily for a physical workout, to reduce stress, clear the mind, or open to a more expansive sense of being, as a yoga teacher it is important to offer class sequences that offer all of these qualities, even if more focused in certain of these areas. We know that the body, mind, heart, and sense of spirit are interrelated. Given this, it is incumbent upon yoga teachers to create the space in our classes for the integration of these elements, including through how we fashion sequences and guide students through them. As students rise from Savasana or otherwise conclude their mat practice, they should feel at least a bit more whole—integrated—than when they stepped onto their mat.

Taken together, these sensibilities allow us to identify and define the core principles of sequencing that are ideally embodied in every class sequence: Moving from Simple to Complex, Moving from Dynamic to Static Exploration (or Moving into Stillness), Cultivating of Energetic Balance, Integrating Effort and Ease, and Cultivating Sustainable Self-Transformation.

Principle One: Moving from Simple to Complex

Yoga practice allows us to consciously cultivate the path of our personal change and transformation. Yet if we leap far ahead of what we are presently able to do with a sense of steadiness and ease, we tend to cut ourselves off from the conscious process that makes yoga a transformative practice. Thus, moving step by conscious step from where we are to wherever it is we might be going is an essential part of vinyasa krama. The basic principle is to move progressively from simple to complex actions that lead to the deepest and easiest possible exploration along the entire path of a practice. This gives us the basic sequencing principle of *moving from simple to complex along the path of least resistance.*

Each asana and transitional movement requires certain muscular actions, contracting or releasing in a way that supports stability, ease, and balance within the asana. Rather than creating a random sequence of asanas, it is important to place asanas in relationship to each other in a way that makes each one more accessible. Like a child learning to crawl before walking and to walk before running, yoga students benefit from first learning basic asanas before attempting complex ones, playing the edge with each breath along the way. Similarly, within a single class, students benefit from moving from simple to complex poses, each pose and breath cultivating a deeper awareness of how the body can open and stabilize in certain forms.

Every yoga asana contains elements of other poses. When we break down an asana into its constituent elements, we can identify the elements that are relatively easier or more accessible to students based on their prior preparation, condition, and intention. In identifying the most basic elements of asanas, we discover the simplest ones in which the body feels a relatively deeper sense of natural familiarity, steadiness, and ease. These simpler asanas suggest the starting points for exploring movement into more complex asanas. Moving gradually from simple to complex, the body most easily and thereby safely opens to its deepest possible expression of whatever is being explored. We can then apply the principle of moving from simple to complex to poses within a common family of asanas or to the movement across families in designing a complete class sequence in which the most complex asanas are more accessible, enabling students to go farther in their exploration.

This evolutionary learning process ideally involves anticipatory experiences along the path, giving students the opportunity to successively explore—with clear guidance from their teacher—the various alignment forms, energetic actions, and other qualities of engagement and release they will be asked to apply in more complex actions to come. By introducing the constituent elements of the peak asana in simpler form, you will help students to grasp intellectually and to embody consciously the more complex combination of elements found in the related but more complex asana.

For example, when introducing Adho Mukha Svanasana (Downward-Facing Dog Pose) in a beginning yoga class, start on all fours with the arms extended forward in the Puppy Dog variation; here you can guide students into the hand, arm, shoulder girdle, and spine elements of the full asana without the added challenge of opening through the legs and pelvis. Cat and Dog tilts can then be explored as a way to experience pelvic neutrality in relationship to the lumbar spine, while Uttanasana (Standing Forward Bend Pose) can be tapped for teaching about *pada bandha,* internal rotation of the thighs, and activation of the quadriceps. Now students will find it easier to integrate these elements when exploring the full expression of Adho Mukha Svanasana.

The ability to craft sequences that reflect this principle requires at least basic knowledge of functional anatomy and the biomechanics of movement. It is with this knowledge that you can identify the interrelations of asanas, more easily breaking each one down into its constituent elements and then seeing how it relates to others within and across the families of asanas. We will address this topic further when discussing "pathway sequences," and we will also identify many of these essential relationships in Chapter Three. You can also refer to Appendix B, which gives preparatory asanas for 125 asanas.

Principle Two: Moving from Dynamic to Static Exploration, or Moving into Stillness

We are anything but static beings. Rather, we are inherently dynamic beings. Yoga practice should allow, not suppress, this natural quality of our being. Even when as still as can be, our heart is beating, the circulatory system is functioning, nerve impulses are traveling through the body, and the breath is flowing in and out. This is part of the problem of thinking of asanas as "poses." Poses are something that models do for cameras, the results usually airbrushed to create an idealized form meant to convey some contrived meaning to the viewer. Asanas, by contrast, are about the internal experience of yoga practitioners opening to a stronger and more flexible body, more balanced energy, more open heart, and clearer awareness. Rather than thinking of long-held asanas as static, it is important to encourage very small refining movements that bring stronger stability and lighter ease to the breath and bodymind. Opening to our natural dynamism is a surer path to deeper inner peace and clarity than the determined effort to be perfectly still.

In dynamic exploration, we move in and out of asanas with the rhythmic flow of the breath, giving practical expression to the abstract concepts of parinamavada and vinyasa krama. Dynamic movement allows the body to open more slowly, gently, and deeply so that the ultimate positioning becomes more assimilated into the body. This method of practice more fully awakens the sense of connection of breath to movement, strength, and release within and between the asanas, making the breath more integral to the overall practice. This both prepares the body for safer and deeper exploration of held asanas and deepens the ultimate effects of asanas as students become more attuned to what is happening inside.

Surya Namaskaras (Sun Salutations) are the classic example of dynamic movement. In Ashtanga Vinyasa–style yoga, dynamic movement spices up the entire practice as students perform the flowing vinyasa between most of the held asanas, as follows: Tolasana (Scales Pose) to Lolasana (Dangling Earring Pose) to Chaturanga Dandasana to Urdhva Mukha Svanasana (Upward-Facing Dog Pose) to Adho Mukha Svanasana to Dandasana (Staff Pose), or to other asanas depending on where it is in the sequence or series. Yet even in classes that draw primarily from the Iyengar method, including John Friend's Anusara, Paulie Zink and Paul Grilley's Yin yoga, and Iyengar classes themselves, allowing a feeling of breathing the entire body allows students to use natural movement along the path to stillness.

Moving into stillness is a concept that applies to the entire yoga practice.[8] When we look later in this chapter and then throughout the book at various phases of practice sessions, we will want to bear in mind that there is an opportunity to move into stillness from the moment we step onto our mat, through the most intense parts of practice, to Savasana and beyond.

Principle Three: Cultivating Energetic Balance

We are always and forever subject to the forces of the universe. In Samkhya, one of six classical schools of Indian philosophy, the universe is divided into *purusha*, or consciousness, and *prakriti*, or nature/matter. Prakriti consists of three qualities known as *gunas*, which describe the natural tendencies of the mind and emotions that express the deeper qualities of the mind and wisdom. The unique expression of the gunas within each person gives that person his or her energetic composition and sense of self. This model is a useful tool in analyzing and understanding the patterns of our thoughts and emotions, with direct application in our practice and teaching of yoga. (One can tap into this source of philosophical insight without embracing the whole of Samkhya philosophy or its dualistic ontology.) The three gunas are *rajas, tamas,* and *sattva:*

- Driven by desire, rajas revolves around the feeling of needing or losing something, even to the point of becoming obsessed by it. If we do not act, we fear losing what we feel we need. If successful in attaining whatever is driving our desire, then the mind will return to a balanced sense of calm (or potentially flip into fear of loss). Rajas involves a sense of intense dynamism, stimulating you to act in the world with excitement and passion, the mind always imbued with anxiety or expectation about how things might turn out. When in balance, rajasic energy is what allows us to get out of bed in the morning and to move through the day feeling fully energized. Yet if excessive, it is also what can keep us from falling asleep at night or finding contentment in our daily lives.

- Tamas reflects a confused mind that leads to indecision, lethargy, and inaction. This is the feeling of not knowing what you are feeling or what you want or need. Caught in this tendency, your behavior can become self-destructive or harmful to others. Yet tamas also allows us to calm down, relax, and restore our energy through rest and sleep.

- Sattva describes a calm and clear state of mind, a sense of being complete and fulfilled. Filled with this sense of levity, clarity, and tranquility, one is kinder and more thoughtful toward oneself and others. Yoga philosophy describes this as our natural state of mind, albeit one that is often seemingly lost amid the shifting currents of our lives. With sattvic energy, we can act in the world with ease because our mental balance is not dependent on something external. This allows us to move about in our lives in greater harmony with our self and others.

Taken together, the three gunas are always present to some degree in everyone's life, forming each person's attitude, nature, and potential. Rather than judging these tendencies as good or bad, we can look upon them for insight into how we feel within ourselves and how we interact with others in our lives. In our normal life we tend to be attracted to things and people in the world. There is nothing wrong with this. More important is the *quality*

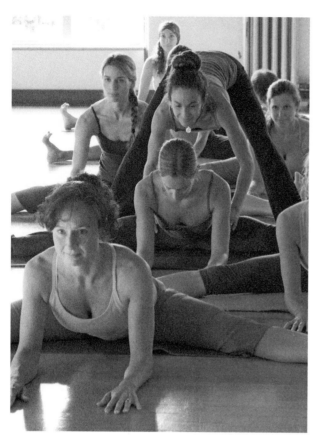

A well-balanced class allows students to be in a sattvic state throughout their practice.

of that attraction. Whatever we tend to be attracted to preoccupies our mind. If our intention is to move into a place of clarity, being aware of where our attention and energy are focused, even in the simplest of life's everyday activities, gives insight into what stands in the way of that clarity.

The essential unity of the gunas is described in the Samkhya-Karika using the analogy of an oil lamp. The heavy basin containing the oil rests stably on the ground, seemingly inert in its tamasic nature. The oil, with properties of movement or flow, symbolizes the rajasic tendency. The wick, made of clean white cotton, symbolizes sattva. The interplay of these elements produces the flame. A healthy balance in life involves all three, with one or the other dominant at the appropriate time. Without tamas, we would never sleep. Without rajas, we would never move. Without sattva, we would never calmly shine forth in the world.

Hatha yoga is a practice of moving into energetic balance amid the constancy of change in our lives. Put simply, the "ha" part of *hatha* is more energizing, the "tha" part more relaxing. Generally speaking, yoga classes should cultivate a sustainable balance of energy, a sattvic effect in which students feel fully awakened yet calm and clear. Sometimes you may want to offer a more stimulating or calming class. As we will explore later, the asanas and pranayama practices you offer in a class—as well as their order—will make a class more or less energizing or calming. On balance, it is ideal to design and teach every class in a way that enables students to most simply and deeply cultivate an overall sense of energetic balance, sending them back out into the world with a sense of being more grounded, awake, and clear.

Principle Four: Integrating the Effects of Actions

Each asana works and stretches the body in ways that create new needs and possibilities for further exploration and change. For instance, after practicing Urdhva Dhanurasana (Upward-Facing Bow Pose, sometimes called Wheel Pose), we place considerable pressure down into the hands and the fully extended (or hyperextended) wrist joints, stretch and work deeply into the shoulders, fully arch the spine, ground through the feet, work to internally rotate the thighs, and stretch deeply through the hip flexors and abdominal core. Depending on each unique student, these actions can be a source of new tension in the body, inviting the exploration of other actions that will neutralize this tension in order to integrate the prior actions and come into a new, more deeply integrated balance.

This neutralizing practice is achieved through *pratikriyasana* (*prati* meaning "against" and *kriya* meaning "action"). The objective of pratikriyasana is to integrate prior actions in a way that prepares students to move forward into the next asana, sequence, class, or later activity free of tension and as balanced and blissful as possible.

This principle is often applied with its literal meaning of "opposite action," "counterpose," or "counteraction." This can be problematic, especially when applied asana by asana. For example, in this narrow conception of pratikriyasana, one would counterpose deep back bends with deep forward bends, possibly straining the muscles and ligaments along the spine. The opposite of Sirsasana I (Headstand) would be Tadasana or Urdhva Hastasana, likely causing some students to become dizzy and possibly fall, and in any case not giving the simplest path to the release of accrued tension and thus the integration of the asana. What we want to do instead is to neutralize, integrate, refine, and deepen along a path in which successively sequenced asanas are similar, not opposite, while being attentive to releasing accumulated tension.

There are many ways to sequence asanas for effective pratikriyasana. Generally, first offer students the simplest form of a neutralizing asana, and then offer variations or successively more complex asanas to reduce accumulated tension and restore overall stability and ease. Rather than approaching pratikriyasana asana by asana, it is better to take a broader view of entire practices, considering where, in the small sequences that make up an entire class, neutralizing and opposing asanas can help students to integrate their practice. See Appendix B for neutralizing asanas.

Principle Five: Cultivating Sustainable Self-Transformation

A sustainable practice of yoga as a tool for cultivating overall health, well-being, and self-transformation requires being as conscious as possible of the balance of effort and ease while moving gradually into deeper release, openness, and clarity. It also involves a holistic approach to doing yoga in which the various elements of practice—asana, pranayama, meditation—are included in each class or session. Yet in spite of the fact that these principles are largely common knowledge among experienced yoga teachers—along with the yogic values contained in the yamas and niyamas—they are often absent from many classes. The consequence is anything but sustainable yoga as students (and often teachers) get injured, burn out, or give up the practice.

Every veteran yoga teacher I know—whether in the Vinyasa Flow, Iyengar, Power, Ashtanga, Anusara, or other traditions—has experienced an injury while practicing yoga, often setting their practice back by weeks, months, even years. Almost all of these injuries occurred in one of three ways:

1. Not practicing with *aparigraha*—instead grasping for something that is out of reach;

2. Dwelling in *avidya*—i.e., ignorance, not knowing what one is doing; or

3. Getting adjusted by a teacher with his or her own aparigraha or avidya challenges.

Let's explore this further. At the neurological center of the body, the spine carries messages back and forth to every cell and nerve. Tightness and compression in and around the spine compromises this natural internal communication system. Indeed, integrating the bodymind—the central raison d'être of yoga—significantly depends on the openness of your neurological pathways. Constrict those pathways—or ignore the messages flowing through them—and strain or injury is almost certain.

Let's consider the wrists. Why are they one of the joints most at risk of injury? While relative weakness, misalignment, and repetitive stress are often rightly cited as factors in wrist injuries, there is typically an underlying "listening" problem. When the muscles in the upper back are tight or compressed, neural communication through the shoulder girdle and into the arms is compromised. This inhibits awareness of what is happening in the wrists and hands. With neurological flow to the wrists compromised, the ability of the nerves to tell the muscles what to do is thrown off, contributing to the likelihood of injuries such as strains and sprains in and around the wrist joint.

Vinyasa is an approach to both asana and pranayama practice that is predicated on the gradual, conscious, intelligent, and compassionate opening of the body. Using functional anatomy and Kinesiology along with insights drawn from the received wisdom of tradition, yoga classes are ideally sequenced in a way that opens the body deeply and safely. Conscious yogic breathing—ujjayi pranayama—is employed to warm the body internally by warming the breath and to create a soft mantra-like sound that helps the student cultivate steadiness while moving energy through the body. Immediate neurological feedback also comes through the rhythm of the breath which is disturbed if any actions in the body are creating strain.

The key to cultivating a sustainable yoga practice begins with conscious intention to practice with intelligence and inner compassion. Within that intention, breath and simple movement can then gradually warm and open the spine before involving more intense use of other parts of the body. This is the ancient wisdom of vinyasa krama, or the wisdom of gradual progression, beginning with Surya Namaskara—bowing to the inner sun, to the truth of the heart, and letting all else unfold from there like a flower to the morning rays.

At the other end of the practice, winding down from the peak of the practice through a series of integrative pratikriyasanas, one eventually comes to Savasana, by far the most important of all the asanas in the full integration of the practice. The mental, physical, energetic, and physiological state one is in just before and after Savasana is ideal for doing pranayama and meditation. Here and now the body is less a source of distraction when tuning into and cultivating the subtle processes involved in going beyond ujjayi to deeper pranayama practices. The processes and effects of asana and deeper pranayama in turn contribute to being both calm and in an utterly sattvic state most conducive to meditation. At the close of meditation, consider setting a renewed intention for the next vinyasa, stepping off your mat and into the world. Taking the path of the practice to this completion opens us to yoga as a sustainable practice of self-transformation.

When you next step onto your mat, consider beginning with your palms together at your heart in a prayer position, *anjali mudra*. Then bring your fingertips to your forehead and set clear intention in your practice, vowing to practice consciously as a true sadhu, a yoga practitioner guided by the principles of *ahimsa* (nonhurting) and *satya* (truth). With your palms and that intention sealed at your heart, find the breath and let the warming flow begin.

Chapter Two

The Arc Structure
of Yoga Classes

You cannot stay on the summit forever; you have to
come down again. So why bother in the first place?
Just this: What is above knows what is below, but
what is below does not know what is above. One
climbs, one sees. One descends, one sees no longer,
but one has seen. There is an art of conducting oneself
in the lower regions by the memory of what one saw
higher up. When one can no longer see, one can at
least still know.

—RENÉ DAUMAL

Yoga's potential for improving or transforming our lives arises from doing it
consistently over the long span of our lives. Each and every time we step onto
our mat we have a renewed opportunity to learn more and more about the
subtleties and technical requirements of the asanas, breathing techniques, and
other elements of a full practice, including the use of *bandhas, dristana* practice,
energetic actions, playing the edge, and how to balance effort and ease. With
dedication, perseverance, patience, and a healthy dose of nonattachment, we
can make our yoga practice a lifelong Chautauqua, a learning journey in which
we discover more and more about ourselves along the path.

Like learning a new language, the languages of yoga take time and patience
to sink in as we gradually learn, breath by breath, how the various elements
unite to create an integral experience. While there are intellectual aspects of
this learning, the deeper learning happens in the practice itself as we come

to discover how we are who we are through the infinitely varied prisms of experience offered by all of the different asana, breathing, and meditation practices. In the beginning, students can have the experience of being dissociated from their bodies, as if the body and mind are separate. Staying in the practice, the physical body, sense organs, qualities of neuromuscular sensitivity, emotions, mental acuity, and consciousness itself all come slowly and gradually into greater harmony as we gain fluency with yoga. Whether a student is entirely new to yoga or a seasoned practitioner, there is no end to what one can learn, how much one can grow, or how deeply one can cultivate self-transformation.

Along with time and patience, this lifelong yogic learning process and the deepening practice that comes through it are enhanced when approached step-by-step. Even when one has a clear understanding of what is involved in doing certain types of practice, the practice itself is always a sequential one with a certain order of actions. And the order—the vinyasa krama—matters for how the practice is experienced and integrated.

In part because there are potentially infinite ways to structure a yoga class, we need guidelines for what to do, when, and in what relation to everything else. Each different sequence will have different effects on different students (as will the same sequence practiced with differing levels of intensity, pace, and duration). The challenge to the teacher is to craft sequences that give students an appropriate practice for where they are in their lives, respecting where they are in the experience of parinamavada.

In crafting sequences, yoga teachers are like mountain guides: we are taking students on a trek. We are inviting them to join in an adventure in which the experience is ultimately one of self-reflection and conscious personal evolution amid the constancy of change within and all around them. To make the most of the adventure requires proper mental and physical preparation, charting a path that makes sense in terms of the trekkers and the terrain, sufficient time to enjoy exploring the peaks of the experience, and a safe path back to where one began, thus allowing the experience to be fully and meaningfully embodied.

This metaphor points us toward the wisdom of the arc structure of yoga classes. There are five stages in the vinyasa krama arc:

1. Initiating the Yogic Process
2. Warming the Body
3. Pathway to the Peak
4. Peak Exploration
5. Integration

Here we look more closely at the essential qualities of each part of the arc and offer a variety of ways to approach and develop the practice at each of the five stages.

Yoga Class Arc Structure

The arc structure of yoga classes can take a variety of forms that generate different degrees of intensity and allow different qualities of exploration.

Table 2.1. Basic Template for a Complete Arc Class

1. Seated meditation, ujjayi pranayama	7. Arm balances (can be omitted)
2. Initial warming	8. Back bends (contraction, then leveraged)
3. Surya Namaskara (Classical, A, and B)	9. Twists
4. Standing asanas: externally rotated hips	10. Forward bends and hip openers
5. Standing asanas: internally rotated hips	11. Inversions
6. Abdominals (can be omitted)	12. Savasana

Initiating the Yogic Process

Most people are first drawn to yoga to reduce stress, develop flexibility, heal a physical or emotional injury, explore new social relationships, or pursue physical fitness. But once in the practice, connecting body-breath-mind, something starts to happen. Students begin to experience a clearer self-awareness, a sense of being more fully alive; they feel better, more in balance, more conscious, clearer. The yearning that we have as human beings for a happy, wakeful, meaningful life and a sense of connection with something greater than our individual selves starts to become a powerful motivation for practicing yoga over the course of our lives.

When used as a tool for self-transformation and awakening to clearer awareness, yoga starts the moment a student first pays attention to what he or she is doing in the practice. If a student is unsteady, falling, in pain, or distracted by discomfort, the tendency will be to go back into his or her analytical or agitated mind. Sthira and sukham—steadiness and ease—give the asanas their transformative potential. Being steady does not mean being perfectly still in a pose that you hold for a very long time. Asanas, by contrast, are alive, in each moment a unique expression of the human being doing them.[1] Opening one's self to a feeling of inner peace amid the relative intensity of the asana practice—being calm and soft while strong and stable—takes the practice to a deeper level. The breath itself starts to become a mantra in the movement meditation that is asana practice. In this way the practice is one of meditative awareness in which one is more fully and consciously attuned to what is happening in the moment.[2] This experiential process—not the religious worship of a deity or insistence on precise form in held poses—is what makes asana practice itself a transformational or spiritual practice. And it is precisely here, in creating a space that encourages the cultivation of clearer awareness, that the yoga teacher becomes an awareness facilitator.

In guiding yoga classes that encourage self-reflective awareness, each asana, each moment within and between the asanas, every breath, every sensation, and every thought and feeling become windows into the nature of the mind, consciousness, and spirit. The practice becomes a process offering insight into the "stickiness and delusions of the mind," which, Stephen Levine (1979, 69) writes, "are seen more clearly when viewed from the heart." This is where doing yoga asanas becomes a practice of self-transformation and healing, and a profound sense of conscious awakening and connection begins to emerge. It is here that we most fully initiate the internal process that is yoga.

There are many ways to encourage this more-conscious approach to yoga practice. Recognizing that some students are uncomfortable chanting "aum" while others are deeply into a bhakti (devotional) yoga practice, you need to use your judgment in deciding how to create a safe space for everyone while remaining true to your own sensibilities. How you approach this will surely change as you evolve in your teaching.

The first step in initiating the yogic process—the first step in sequencing—begins with how you greet your class. Try to greet each student as he or she enters the room. Make eye contact and be present with that one student, even if only for a brief time. When ready to start, greet the entire class by saying "Welcome" or "Namaste." Simple and perhaps obvious as this may be to many teachers, offering a welcoming gesture facilitates student trust and invites students to tune in inside and let go a little more easily.

Starting your classes with at least a few minutes of sitting still helps students to fully "arrive" and tune in to what they are feeling in their body, breath, mind, and spirit. Invite everyone in the class to come into a comfortable cross-legged or another sitting position.

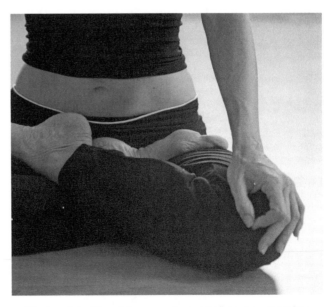

The hand position of *jnana mudra* symbolizes movement into more integrated being and wholeness.

Encourage and demonstrate the use of a bolster to elevate the sitting bones as high as it takes to bring the pelvis into a neutral position. Ask students to begin tuning in inside, to feel the simple, natural flow of their breath. Ask them to feel their sitting bones, encouraging them to more firmly nestle their sitting bones down as if into the earth, giving a greater feeling of being grounded. Then ask them to bring their attention back to their breath, feeling the natural movements in their body from the movement of their breath. Encourage them to relax their face, their eyes, between their temples. From a place of ease and stability, ask them to begin very gradually to breathe more deeply, feeling the natural effects of the breath in their body, expanding and growing taller and more spacious with each inhale, relaxing and quieting more deeply inside with each exhale. Encourage them to pay attention to the spaces between their breaths, without holding the breath in or out, and to allow the quality of sensation they feel in the pauses to come with them as the breath flows along. With the calm, steady cultivation of the breath, ask your students to listen to the breath as it flows through their throat, a sound like wind breezing through the trees or like the ocean at the seashore. Encourage them to stay attuned to the sound, sensation, and balanced flow of the breath throughout their practice.

From the soft and receptive inner space created from sitting, breathing, watching, and feeling, invite your students to draw their palms together at their hearts in anjali mudra (reverence seal, or prayer position of the palms at the heart). Encouraging your students to stay connected with the breath, ask them to bring their fingertips to their forehead, symbolically connecting their head with their heart. From this place of inner connection, ask them to take a moment to reflect inside, to remind themselves why they are there and to give themselves a clearer sense of intention, inner purpose, in their practice. Considering your own intention and the class setting, you may want to:

- Offer a few minutes of sitting in silence or with guided meditation.
- Read a poem or other writing that sets the mood or suggests a theme.
- Lead a chant, which might differ from class to class or season to season.
- Awaken with pranayama—ujjayi is a must; *nadi shodhana* and kapalabhati are good options for the beginning of intermediate to advanced classes.

Here you can also create the space for students (and yourself) to dedicate their practice to someone or something that is important to them. Allowing this to be personal and private, rather than suggesting that the dedication be to some particular concept of the spiritual, students will feel freer and more comfortable in this part of the practice. At natural intervals later in the class, such as pausing after an intense sequence of asanas, ask the students once again to bring their palms together at their heart, fingertips to their forehead, and to come back into their intention.

Most students in yoga studio classes enjoy the shared chanting of the sound of "aum." *Aum* is a mystical or sacred syllable mentioned in the Vedas, Upanishads, and Bhagavad Gita, variously described as "the essential sound of the universe," "the voice of God," and "the originating sound of creation." In some expressions of Hinduism, the letter *a* represents creation (issuing from Brahma's essence), *u* the preservation of balance in the world (as the god Vishnu balances Brahma overhead on a lotus flower), and *m* the completion of the cycle of existence (when Vishnu falls asleep and all existing things dissolve into their essence).[3] It signifies the beginning of the yoga practice, setting the tone and bringing awareness more inside. The three sounds can also be used to symbolize opening to the creative possibilities of practice, moving into a deeper source of balance in one's life and letting go of the mental obstacles standing in the way of this practice. In simpler form, you may make the sound as "om." You might find some students expressing resistance to this through their body language; let it be and continue with your class, or take the time to explain the meaning of aum and the reason for chanting it.

Bringing the qualities discussed here together initiates the process of unification that is Hatha yoga: relieving the senses of their external distractions by focusing the mind on the breath, body, and energetic awakening. Always create space for this initiation of the practice, setting the tone, intention, theme, and other overarching aspects of the class. The most fundamental part of this process is breath awareness, which extends as the unifying thread—sutra— throughout the entire class. By guiding students into a more focused inner awareness connecting body, breath, and mind, you help them to establish the fundamental foundation of their practice.

How students sit—usually in a cross-legged position or Virasana (Hero Pose)—or lie during this opening of the class should be determined by the larger class plan and your assessment of student ability. Sitting in a cross-legged position is most stable and accessible for most students. In intermediate to advanced classes, Virasana is an excellent starting asana. In restorative, prenatal and postnatal, children's, and therapeutic classes, lying on the back offers a more calming introduction to the practice. Observe and try to get a feeling for the mood, energy level, and mental focus of the class. Let this observation and intuitive assessment inform how long to sit and what to include in this initial sitting part of the practice. This is an excellent time to go into further depth with pranayama techniques that move the class more immediately toward a sattvic state of being. Stimulating pranayamas like kapalabhati will help raise the energy level of a tamasic group of students; nadi shodhana will help calm a more rajasic group. Also consider a longer meditation practice at the beginning of class; if students seem to be focused in the initial sitting, consider staying with it for several more minutes, whether as silent or guided practice.

Many yoga teachers like to start class more actively, with students standing in Tadasana (Mountain Pose) or otherwise positioned to dive right into the physical practice. Many also teach yoga primarily as a form of exercise, often in gym settings with greater time constraints. It is still possible—indeed advisable unless not part of one's sense of yoga at all—to nonetheless offer at least a brief moment in which students can quietly check-in inside, tune into the breath and a sense of how they are feeling, and set a personal intention in their practice. This does not have to involve things like drawing the palms into a prayer position or chanting anything at all. Still, all students will benefit in their practice by having the initial space to tune in and get more focused on doing yoga.

As part of this initial awakening and focusing process, consider sharing whatever theme or point of focus that you have in mind for the class.

Creating a Theme-Oriented Class

Creating fresh and meaningful yoga classes is one of the most fulfilling aspects of teaching yoga. Whether you teach a set sequence style like Ashtanga Vinyasa or Bikram or fashion your own sequences, every class is an opportunity for you and your students to contribute to the creative evolution of yoga. Yet this creative process—coming up with new, accessible, interesting and sustainable classes—can be challenging. That's where class themes come in, offering a wide array of possibilities for making yoga classes more interesting and memorable.

Themes allow us to more clearly and expansively make connections between various elements of the practice, from alignment principles to refinement of the breath to opening to clearer awareness, and can help to awaken students to greater clarity about what brought them to their mat in the first place.

In creating a themed class, start with something that resonates with your own yogic sensibilities and your embodied knowledge and skills as a teacher. Then ask yourself again why you practice yoga. Write a simple list of what's most important to you in the practice—and in your teaching. By freely opening your mind and heart to these personal yoga values, you will discover the most fertile soil in which to grow your class themes.

In designing a themed class, be attentive to applying basic sequencing principles that help ensure a safe, sustainable, and transformational practice.

Five ideas for class themes:

Action in the Body: Some asana cues can be confusing. For example, externally rotating the arms in Tadasana can seem opposite to the same action in Urdhva Hastasana (Upward Hands Pose). This confusion can be a source of strain when attempting to extend the arms overhead in poses like Utthita Parsvakonasana (Extended Side Angle Pose). Making external rotation of the arms the class theme will reduce this confusion and free students to move forward in refining other aspects of their practice. *Other examples:* external versus internal rotation of the thighs; the relationship between roots and extension; pelvic neutrality in relation to the lumbar spine as the starting point for all other movements of the spine.

Nature and the Cosmos: Let's say you value being connected to the rhythms of nature and you want to create space in your classes for students to explore this connection. Here you can play with shifts in light and energy associated with the seasons, moon phases, even the time of day. For example, in moving from the autumnal equinox toward the winter solstice, you can play with adapting the asana and pranayama practices to better preserve energy or use the idea of diminishing light as an image for exploring the sense of light and dark that pulsates through the rhythms of our lives.

Archetypes and Mythology: The verbal root *asana* includes the idea of ritual, a set of actions with symbolic significance that we can use to highlight certain

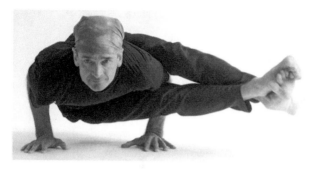
Astavakrasana tells us we can unwind the inner knots that bind us to a limited sense of possibility in our lives.

areas of personal, emotional, or spiritual experience. One source of symbolism is the vast realm of mythological figures found across the world's diverse cultural landscapes, each offering profound wisdom about the conditions and circumstances of life and consciousness. Whether you're bowing to the sun in Surya Namaskara with a sense of deepening connection to the inner sun residing in the spiritual heart center or transcending misunderstanding and complexity through the story of Astavakra and the arm balance Astavakrasana (Eight-Angle Pose), there are unlimited possibilities.

Asana Families: Emphasizing one asana family throughout a class—say, back bends—allows your students to go more deeply into that aspect of their practice. Here you can also better focus on how elements of the various asana families are interrelated. For example, rather than treating back bends as an isolated family, you can explore how these asanas gain their fullest expression when the body is naturally warmed through Surya Namaskara (Sun Salutations) and standing poses, hip flexors are opened through lunges, the spinal muscles are made more supple through twists, and the shoulder girdle is more open through specific shoulder stretches.

Chakras: Whether you relate to chakras as subtle energy centers, the emanation of divine consciousness, or useful symbols for reflecting more clearly on the bodymind, chakra-themed classes will give your students a memorable experience to take off their mats and into the world. My seven-day retreats often focus on one chakra each day, with the asana, pranayama, and meditation practices keyed to balancing each one: grounding, creating, manifesting, loving, sharing, awakening to clearer awareness, being in bliss. Part of the fun is in planning sequences that correlate with the chakras and their meaning while offering balanced practices every day.

There are as many class theme possibilities as there are creative yoga teachers. Keep exploring in the fields of spiritual philosophy, postural considerations, polarities of experience and action, subtle energetics, holidays, and even current events to offer classes that your students find help them make clearer connections on their own yoga path.

Warming and Awakening the Body

Gradually warming the body increases flexibility, reduces the risk of injury, and generates *tapas*, inner fire, to burn away toxicity and emotional gripping. In the conventional science of flexibility, warm-up is divided into two broad categories: passive, which uses an outside force such as a heated room or hot bath; and active, which is self-initiated (Alter 1996, 149–50). Studies show that passive warming, as found in Bikram-style yoga and other "hot" yoga styles, is significantly more effective than active warming in increasing hip flexion; for example, releasing into Balasana (Child's Pose) or a Uttanasana (Standing Forward Bend Pose). However, increased temperature reduces the tensile strength of connective tissue, potentially leading to muscle-fiber tears (Troels 1973, 1–126), due in part to the less conscious awareness of what is happening in the body in the case of passive sources of warming. While passive warming is helpful in preparing the body for intense activity, active warming has several added benefits in yoga: increased heart rate, which prepares the cardiovascular system for more intense activity; increased blood flow through active muscles; increased metabolic rate; increased speed of nerve impulses, which facilitates more subtle awareness of body movements; and increased reciprocal innervation, in which opposing muscles work more efficiently.

There are two types of active warming, general and targeted, both of which are given emphasis in yogic and Western exercise literature. General active warming consists of activities that bring overall warmth to the body. These warming activities should be done at the beginning of the practice, either immediately following or incorporated into the earlier initiation of the yogic process discussed above. Once the body is generally warmed, it is important to maintain this warmth along the path to the peak asana so that the spine and the body in general remain flexible and the mind focused in the practice. While in many classes it is important to provide resting places while retaining warmth, cooling asanas generally should be done after the peak asana as part of the integrative pathway to Savasana (Corpse Pose).

Here are several ways to initially warm the body in preparation for deeper exploration in the asana practice:

Ujjayi Pranayama: The basic yogic breathing technique, ujjayi pranayama involves breathing just through the nose with a very slight narrowing of the throat at the epiglottis (where you feel sensation when coughing or gargling).

This increases the vibration of the larynx, creating a soft sound like wind breezing through the trees or the sound of the sea at the seashore. Ujjayi pranayama warms the breath as it flows through the turbinates in the nose, thus warming the lungs, which warms the blood, which warms the body and helps to more easily awaken the body to natural opening in the asanas. All students can safely practice ujjayi pranayama (with caution to pregnant students not to overheat their body).

Kapalabhati Pranayama: This is a far more intense warming activity that stimulates the cardiovascular system and generates warmth throughout the body. Kapalabhati (from *kapala,* "skull," and *bhati,* "luster") pranayama energizes the entire body by tremendously oxygenating the blood supply and creating a feeling of exhilaration.[4] In natural breathing, the inhalation is active, i.e., activated by muscles, while the exhalation is passive, resulting from contraction of the elastic lungs. This is reversed in kapalabhati pranayama: the exhalations are made active and inhalations passive. After completion of an ujjayi exhalation, the breath is drawn in halfway and then rapidly and repeatedly blasted out through the nose, with a slight pause when empty of breath. The sound is in the nostrils, not the throat. Doing this for one to three minutes (and in one to three rounds) after a few minutes of ujjayi pranayama is excellent for warming the body in preparation for doing more extensive and energetic movement.

Cat and Dog Tilts: Level 1 and level 1–2 classes can effectively warm up with undulating movement through the pelvis, spine, and shoulder girdles into alternating forms called Cat and Dog Tilts. Starting on all fours with the knees aligned under the hips and the wrists shoulder distance apart about an inch forward of the shoulders, cue students to move with the breath: inhaling, rotate the pelvis forward (anterior rotation) while drawing the chest forward, then exhaling, reverse this positioning to arch the spine and draw the forehead and pubis toward each other. Continue for several rounds, gradually awakening awareness along the spine and initiating a clearer coordination of the flow of the breath with movement in the body.

Ashtanga Pranam: This dynamic movement is drawn from the Classical Surya Namaskara. Starting in Phalakasana (Plank Pose), with an exhalation, slowly release the chest and chin to the floor (eight-point prostration, "ashtanga pranam"). With the inhalation, extend the legs back—feet and pelvis rooting down, inner thighs spiraling up, tailbone pressing toward the heels—while pressing down firmly through the hands and fingers, lifting the shoulders just level with the elbows while creating a feeling of pulling the heart center forward through the window of the arms (keep the neck in neutral extension to reduce straining it). This is Salabhasana B (Locust Pose B), a wonderful pose for awakening the spinal erector muscles, hip extensors, arms, shoulders, and legs. With the exhalation, press back up onto all fours, repeating several times before resting in Balasana or transitioning to either a Puppy Dog Pose or full Adho Mukha Svanasana (Downward-Facing Dog Pose).

Surya Namaskara: The classic physical warm-up in Hatha yoga is through Surya Namaskara, the Sun Salutations. While warming the entire body, Surya Namaskara also offers targeted warming and awakening as it involves every asana family except twists: forward bends, back bends, standing poses, arm support, and inversion. The number, form, and duration of Surya Namaskaras should be varied depending on the level and overall plan of the class. Three Surya Namaskara sequences (Classical, A, B) are explained in detail in Chapter Four.

Adho Mukha Svanasana (Downward-Facing Dog Pose): Down Dog is a great initial warming asana in intermediate and advanced classes. It gently opens the shoulders, chest, upper back, hips, and the backs of the legs as well as the hands and feet. Introduce this asana with dynamic movements, including moving forward into Phalakasana and back to Adho Mukha Svanasana several times, bicycling the legs and extending one leg back and up. In flow-style classes, exploring Down Dog as an early warming exercise also allows detailed explanation of this asana prior to holding it more briefly as part of Surya Namaskara.

Plank–Chaturanga–Up Dog–Down Dog: Start in Phalakasana, holding for up to a minute to explain its basic alignment principles and energetic actions. Cue feeding the

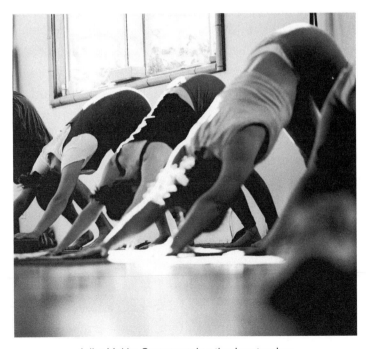

Adho Mukha Svanasana is a timeless teacher.

legs (pressing back through the heels and slightly internally rotating the thighs) while pressing down through the hands and depressing the shoulder blades against the back ribs. Here students will automatically find their abdominal muscles awakening, which, along with active legs, will keep their body in a plank form rather than sagging through the pelvis. Cue the slow transition to Chaturanga Dandasana (Four-Limbed Staff Pose) on an exhalation, stopping when the shoulders are level with the elbows, shoulder blades still rotated down against the back ribs, spacious heart, and active belly and legs. Cue the gradual transition into Urdhva Mukha Svanasana (Upward-Facing Dog Pose) with the inhalation, feet now pointed back and the legs active as in Locust B, described above, but fully off the floor, shoulders aligned over the wrists, upper spine pressing forward into the heart center, the gaze forward, up, or back. Exhale to Adho Mukha Svanasana, using the abdominal core to help lift the hips up and back. Repeat several times.

Salamba Sirsasana I (Supported Headstand): Students in popular Vinyasa-style classes are often taken aback by the idea of starting a practice in Headstand, as in most flow-style classes it is typically placed toward the end of class as part of the finishing practice. However, this is a classic warm-up pose in intermediate and advanced classes in the Iyengar method. Start in Tadasana to initially awaken the legs and stimulate length and awakening up through the body, then raise the arms overhead into Urdhva Hastasana (Upward Hand Pose)—stretch through the shoulders and arms; next, fold into Uttanasana, and hold for two to three minutes, preparing the body physiologically for the far more intense and sustained holding of Headstand. Hold Headstand for two to ten minutes before resting in Balasana or Uttanasana.

Sustained Standing Asana Sequences: Standing asanas provide an excellent way to continue generally warming the body, especially when interwoven with vinyasas of Plank–Chaturanga–Up Dog–Down Dog or transitions through arm balances. Standing asanas are powerfully grounding, bringing more awareness and warmth into the feet, legs, and pelvis while opening the hips and stimulating awareness and warm energy up through the core of the body. Here a variety of variations can give targeted warming to complex poses that will come later in the class, including positioning of the spine, shoulders, and arms in preparation for arm balances and back bends. These relationships and variations are explored further in Chapter Three, on sequencing within and between asana families.

Core Activation: Paripurna Navasana (Full Boat Pose), Tolasana (Scales Pose), Lolasana (Dangling Earring Pose), and core abdominal awakening movements such as Yogic Bicycles and Jathara Parivartanasana (Revolving Twist Pose) are excellent ways to warm the entire body. Although concentrated in the abdominal core, these dynamic core movements involve energetic actions through the legs, torso, and shoulder girdle. Offer simpler approaches to these and other core awakening and warming movements in easier-going classes. Play with including movement from all fours with one arm extended overhead and the opposite leg extended straight back from the hip, slowly abducting the opposite arm or leg away and back toward the midline several times before switching sides.

Depending on the class, setting, theme, season, and your intention with the class, there are many other ways to stimulate this initial general warming of the body: dance-like movements, qigong practices, and handstand are a few further examples. As we transition into looking at the pathway to the peak of the practice, bear in mind that this initial warming is part of the pathway and that it should be included in the specific pathway that you design based on the basic sequencing principles along with what follows here. In most classes the initial warming leads to further warming through standing asana sequences.

The Pathway to the Peak

Designing a sequence of actions leading to the peak of a practice is all about making the practice simpler, more accessible, deeper, and more sustainable. The experience along the pathway to the peak will make all the difference in the experience of the peak itself. The peak should not be confused or conflated with the point of maximum internal heat generated through prior actions and poses; it is not so much about peak heat as peak openness. While peak heat is part of how we might define the peak in certain types of practices—particularly Vinyasa Flow or Power yoga classes involving a vigorous set of asanas and transitions—the peak more specifically is *the point in the practice where prior actions and asanas have brought the bodymind to the point of being most prepared for the most challenging part of the practice.*

In crafting the sequence of asanas that comprise the pathway to the peak, you are charting a specific order of actions and positions that collectively anticipate or prefigure the actions and positions involved in the peak asana. In

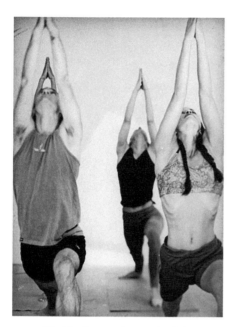

Virabhadrasana I, a moderately complex asymmetrical standing asana. What are its elements?

order to do this, start by breaking down the peak asana into its constituent elements. Constituent elements in any asana are primarily (1) the body's orientation to gravity, (2) joint positions, and (3) supportive muscular actions. For example, in Adho Mukha Vrksasana (Downward-Facing Tree Pose, more commonly called Handstand) the body is fully inverted, the arms are in full flexion and supporting the weight of the body, the spine is in neutral extension, the pelvis is neutral, the legs are fully extended, and muscles throughout the body are engaged in isometric cocontraction to stabilize the joints in maintaining the largely anatomical positioning of the body while support is on the hands in inversion. Each of these elements can be further broken down to identify more precisely what is being asked of the body in a stable Adho Mukha Vrksasana. To help you get started, in Appendix B we have provided the basic constituent elements for each of 125 asanas.

From your analysis of the constituent elements of the peak asana, the next step is to identify simpler asanas that include some of those same elements. Staying attentive to gradually warming the body, you will now order the simple to increasingly more complex asanas to gradually move toward the form and actions of the peak pose. In doing so you are crafting the pathway sequence, a series of preparatory (and integrative) asanas that are asanas in and of themselves yet the building blocks of the peak asana as well.

Along the pathway to the peak, students should get to sequentially explore and experience what it takes to move into certain forms supported by specific actions. These positions and actions should be easier and more accessible than the peak asana, thus making it easier to grasp in the bodymind what is being cued in the preparatory asanas and then applying this when exploring the peak asana. If the peak is Adho Mukha Vrksasana, ideally students will have already heard most of the relevant instructions for the hands, arms, and shoulders when in Tadasana, Urdhva Hastasana, and Adho Mukha Svanasana earlier along the path. Once at the peak, those instructions will likely be echoing about in your students' bodyminds, making your cues for Adho Mukha Vrksasana more intelligible and easier to embody in action.

There are potentially infinite pathways to any given peak asana. Different paths will give different experiences. Rather than always going along the same path to a particular peak pose, play around with varying the preparatory asanas as well as their specific order. Do this first in your own practice to feel the varying effects of alternative pathways while remaining attentive to the basic principle of moving from simple to complex and following your analysis of constituent elements of the peak. This will enhance your creativity and allow you to spice up your classes with fresh and interesting approaches to the peak asanas.

In getting at the constituent elements, start by addressing each of these questions:

- **What needs to be open?** Start by focusing on the joints that will be opening to a relatively full range of motion. Which muscles will be most stretched—asked to let go—around each of those joints? Ask the same of other joints mainly involved in the asana, even if not asked to so fully open. Which simpler asanas involve this or similar opening?

    Example: With the asymmetrical Hanumanasana (Divine Monkey Pose, colloquially called "splits"), we are asking for deep release through the hamstrings, hip flexors and extensors, hip adductors, and hip internal and external rotators. Simpler asanas that contribute to this opening include Uttanasana for the hamstrings, Utthita Trikonasana (Extended Triangle Pose) for the hamstrings and internal rotators, Prasarita Padottanasana (Spread-Leg Forward Fold Pose) for the hamstrings and hip adductors, Anjaneyasana (Low Lunge Pose) and Eka Pada Raj Kapotasana Prep (One-Leg King Pigeon Pose Prep) for the hip flexors and extensors as well as the internal rotators, and Garudasana (Eagle Pose) for the external rotators.

- **What needs to be cooperative in allowing that specific opening?** Opening in one part of the body usually involves prior opening elsewhere. For example, our ability to raise the arms fully overhead is much easier once the rhomboid muscles between the shoulder blades are warm and supple. Which simpler asanas involve this or similar cooperation?

Example: For Hanumanasana, give more targeted warming to the legs and hips through a wide variety of standing asanas, focusing especially on internally rotated standing asanas. Help open the calf muscles (specifically the gastrocnemius and soleus muscles) through Ashta Chandrasana (Crescent Pose), Virabhadrasana (Warrior) I and II, and Pada Hastasana (Hand to Foot Pose). Give more targeted emphasis to working internal rotation of the back leg.

- **What needs to be stable?** Recall the basic qualities of asana: sthira and sukham, steadiness and ease. Both of these qualities are necessary for stability; and with stability, steadiness and ease will more naturally arise. For any given peak asana, there are certain areas of the body that must be stable. What are they? Which simpler asanas involve this or similar challenges to stability?

  Example: Hanumanasana requires the pelvis and legs to be stably grounded as the foundation of the asana.

- **What are the sources of that stability?** To identify the sources of stability, start with the foundation of the asana. What is on the floor? How can it be more firmly grounded without compromising ease? Next, what are the weak links in the asana? These are areas in which the muscles have more difficulty supporting joints in the position asked for in the asana. How can these areas be stabilized (see the question on energetic actions, below)? Which simpler asanas involve this or similar stabilizing actions?

  Example: Due to tight muscles and limited range of motion, most students are not able to ground the legs and pelvis to the floor in exploring Hanumanasana. This indicates the value of a prop placed under the sitting bone area of the front leg—as tall as necessary to allow firm grounding of the sitting bone while extending the back leg straight back from its hip while moving that hip forward.

- **What are the basic postural forms and alignment principles of the peak asana?** Proper alignment of one joint in relationship to another joint is an important aspect of a safe and sustainable practice. Amid the complexity of peak asanas, maintaining proper alignment can be quite challenging. In thoroughly breaking down the alignment elements of the peak asana, identify which simpler asanas involve some of the same basic postural forms and alignments.

Example: With Hanumanasana, give primary consideration to aligning the back leg (to protect the knee and help with internal rotation of that femur) while rotating that side of the pelvis forward in order to create a more symmetrical foundation in the pelvis. Virabhadrasana I and Eka Pada Raj Kapotasana Prep are simpler asanas requiring these same alignment forms and energetic actions.

- **What are the energetic actions of the peak asana?** Maintaining steadiness and ease requires doing something amid the relative stillness of a held asana or in the transition from one asana to the next. What are those actions in the peak asana? While primarily isometric muscular engagement, include other actions such as the relative challenge of maintaining ujjayi pranayama and directing the breath into areas of tension. Then ask which other asanas have the same or similar energetic actions.

  Example: The front leg is strongly engaged with isometric contraction of the quadriceps femoris, which allows the hamstrings to more easily release. The back leg is actively internally rotating to maintain its extension and to prevent twisting forces in the knee joint; this energetic action also contributes to rotation of the pelvis to a more neutral and symmetrical position. Again, Virabhadrasana I and Eka Pada Raj Kapotasana Prep are simpler asanas requiring these similar positioning and energetic actions.

- **What tension is likely to arise in doing the asanas on the pathway to the peak?** Recall that every asana can create new areas of tension. Identify these areas of tension for each asana on the pathway to the peak.

  Example: This will depend on which specific preparatory asanas are included in the pathway sequence.

- **What asanas can address the new areas of tension along the pathway to the peak without compromising the warming and opening generated in the pathway sequence?** Identify asanas or asana variations that stretch, relax, or stabilize areas of added tension or energetic imbalance in the pathway sequence, thus bringing an integrative quality to the flow of asanas.

Knowing the constituent elements of the peak asanas, you can design a creative yet sensible pathway to the peak. This should be done in keeping with the gradual warming of the body and while moving from simple to complex asanas.

Most pathway sequences include some form of Surya Namaskara and standing poses, both of which offer a variety of opportunities for targeted warming and exploration of the elements of the peak asana. The Surya Namaskaras include every family of asana except twists, offering a number of options for guiding students into clearer awareness of the alignment principles and energetic actions found in a vast array of complex asanas. If you choose to pause amid the Surya Namaskaras to offer guided exploration of certain poses or actions related to the peak asana, it is important to counsel students to take it easy as they are still in the general warming phase of class and perhaps not ready to hold some of the asanas for more than a few breaths.

Standing poses are another perfect place for exploring targeted warming and awakening actions related to the peak asana. They continue to provide general warming while also giving more targeted emphasis to particular parts of the body. Here you can give repeated guidance that helps students better understand the actions of internal versus external rotation of the hips, movement into pelvic neutrality in relation to the lumbar spine, the quality of resilient buoyancy,[5] and the essential principle of roots-and-extension that applies in every asana. You can also blend in creative variations to better target certain areas and actions, especially with varied arm, shoulder, and torso positioning.

Your ability as a teacher to accurately analyze all the asanas in a complete class sequence requires studying the functional anatomy, biomechanics, and subtle energetics of the asanas. The complexity of the human body, particularly in a class setting with a diverse student body, makes this a lifelong process of learning and professional development. Yet from the beginning you will express your own creativity in the particular ways you structure and guide each class. As you work on developing this base of knowledge and skills, you can use the principles, guidelines, examples, methods, and templates found in this book as resources, including the sequencing matrix in Appendix B, to design pathway sequences that are informed, efficient, effective, beautiful, and integrated.

Exploring the Peak

The peak asana or asanas are simultaneously the easiest and most challenging part of the class. They are the easiest if the pathway to the peak offers a clear and simple view of the peak from the variety of perspectives offered in the preparatory asanas. If approached in this way, there are few surprises and much joy in the feeling of exhilaration in exploring what might otherwise be unimaginable or unattainable. Peak asanas are the most challenging because they require the greatest strength, openness, or balance.

Many yoga classes place back bends at the peak. This is perfectly sensible given that back bends are among the most complex asanas, but they are certainly not the only option. The peak asana can be from any asana family and chosen based on the type of class, students, theme, and other considerations. Indeed, the peak can be practically any asana; what are apparently very simple asanas to an experienced and healthy student might be very difficult for someone with significant physical limitations, and thus the seemingly simple asana deserves to be broken down into its even simpler elements is designing a class around it as a peak asana.

Once at the final approach to the peak, it is important to create space for students to completely relax, balance the breath, and tune in to their personal intention in the practice. This space might be only a few breaths long, encouraging students to relax and recenter their awareness, or a longer pause in Balasana or another resting position that ideally maintains the warmth and openness cultivated up to that point in class. It is important to appreciate that all the warmth in the world cannot completely overcome nervous tension. Try to maintain warmth, but more importantly guide students into letting go before exploring the peak.

This is a good time to remind students that yoga is not a practice of attaining idealized physical postures, but a process of self-exploration,

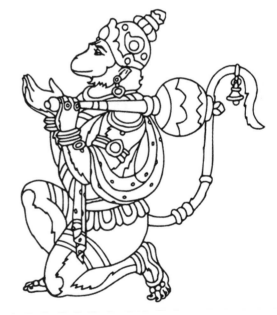

Hanumanasana, named for the monkey god Hanuman, is a complex asana best placed at the peak of practice in intermediate and advanced classes.

self-acceptance, and self-transformation. Reinforce the concept of playing the edge, encouraging students to abide by the core principle of *sthira sukham asanam*—steadiness, ease, and presence of mind. Since there are invariably students with different abilities and interests in all classes, offer appropriate modifications and variations. As you develop your skill and comfort as a teacher, you will increasingly be at ease in offering multiple options to the class while remaining responsive to what is happening with each student in the class.

In exploring the peak asana give plenty of time for students to try the asana at least a few times. If it is an asymmetrical asana (with the left and right sides of the body in somewhat different positions), guide students to alternate sides between each set of explorations. Appreciate that student familiarity and ability with the asana will likely vary considerably across the spectrum of the class, so give ample time and support to students based on their experience and needs. Some students will want to explore the asana longer than others, so be prepared with initial counterasanas in which some students can rest while others are still exploring.

Integrating the Practice

As discussed earlier, pratikriyasana applies to individual asanas, sets of asanas, and to complete class sequences. With experience, students will learn to sustain a balance of effort and ease from the beginning of each practice until completely letting go in Savasana. Still, in an arc-structured class it is important to offer more deeply integrating and restorative asanas following the peak of the practice en route to Savasana. There are four stages in this postpeak integrative process: (1) peak pratikriyasana; (2) deep and relatively more static relaxing asanas; (3) pranayama and meditation; and (4) Savasana.

Peak Pratikriyasana: Offer a sequence of asanas to neutralize any tension arising from the practice of peak asanas. Continuing with the example of Hanumanasana, the hamstrings, internal rotators, and groins are intensely stretched. The task now is to identify asanas that allow those areas to soften without being stretched. Setu Bandha Sarvangasana (Bridge Pose) is excellent in helping restore the tendinous attachment of the hamstrings at the ischial tuberosities (sitting bones). The internal rotators and groins will soften when adducting the legs in simple twists such as Ardha Matsyendrasana (Half Lord of the Fishes Pose) or Supta Parivartanasana (Reclined Revolved Pose). Depending on where you are going from the peak asana, consider blending in peak counterasanas that more naturally take the class in that direction.

Deeper Release and Integration: After neutralizing tension, teach a series of asanas that calm the body and allow students to move into deeper release and energetic balance. Seated forward folds and hip openers are excellent for calming down. Be just as aware in sequencing these asanas as you are in designing the pathway to the peak; the integrative pathway should also move from simple to complex and should still allow dynamic exploration while moving into stillness. Eventually, transition into calming inversions such as Salamba Sarvangasana (Supported Shoulder Stand), Halasana (Plow Pose), or Viparita Karani (Active Reversal Pose).

Pranayama and Meditation:[6] Here we are approaching pranayama and meditation in the context of classes that are primarily focused on asana practice. This should not be confused with doing complete pranayama or deep meditation practices, which together require at least thirty minutes and preferably an hour or longer. As related earlier, a balanced asana practice is perfect preparation for pranayama and meditation. If you are teaching a retreat or have time to teach a two-hour class, consider going further with pranayama and meditation at this stage of the practice (or after coming out of Savasana). Two pranayamas that are appropriate for most students in most public yoga classes at the close of asana practice are kapalabhati (skull cleansing) and nadi shodhana (alternate nostril breathing). For detailed guidance in teaching these techniques, see Stephens (2010). With meditation, note that a few minutes of calm sitting at the close of class is a wonderful way to segue into the next vinyasa, taking students off their mats. It is not, to be sure, sufficient to go very deeply into meditation. For deeper meditation, wait until after Savasana and explore when there is ample time (at least thirty minutes) to get deeply into it.

Savasana: Conclude all classes with at least five minutes in Savasana, the ultimate restorative asana. Remind students that Savasana allows them fully to assimilate the effects of the practice while offering a feeling of completeness, openness, and wholeness.

Deepening the Integration of Asana

Each practice is potentially a movement into deeper self-transformation. This movement occurs within each breath, each asana, and each sequence and extends across all the practices a person does in a lifetime. Cultivating a gradual, simple, expanding awakening in this process of self-transformation revolves around continuously coming back to a sense of *samasthihi*—equanimity in body, breath, mind, and spirit. This gives the asana practice a quality of *yoga chikitsa*—literally "yoga therapy"—in which the body is restructured and a person's entire energetic being is refined.[7] This is an essential element of every class, one that requires you as a teacher to create the space, sequence the asanas, and guide the class in a way that helps endow students with a practical awareness of this transformation and integration in their bodies, minds, and spirits.

Here are several ways to promote this integration of asana practice in classes and thereby maximize the benefits of each practice, building on what we have already covered in this section:

- *Create space for rest.* Toward the beginning of every class, remind students that it is important for them to feel a sense of steadiness and ease throughout the class while practicing near the edge of their ability. Give them explicit permission—even encouragement—to rest as they feel the need, creating a space in which they can rebalance their breath and energy before resuming their practice. Demonstrate Balasana, reminding them that this asana is a dear friend they can visit at will. At the conclusion of any particularly intense sequence of asanas, always offer an opportunity for rest.

- *Create space for renewed self-assessment.* Give brief or long pauses in the flow of the class in which you invite students to come back to their initial intention in the practice, to check in with how they are feeling and to stay with their intention and sense of samasthihi as you resume the asanas.

- *Apply pratikriyasana* to neutralize tension from asanas and establish balance in the body.

- *Offer energetically balanced sequences.* When planning a class, give careful consideration to the energetic arc and waves of the asana sequences to achieve the intended energetic balance for that class.

- *Savasana.* A few minutes—five or more—in Savasana is absolutely essential for the full integration and completion of a practice. Lying down with effortless breath, surrendering to gravity, and allowing the body, breath, and mind to completely settle is the most important way to integrate the practice.

- *Create space for meditation.* While the entire practice is ideally a meditative experience, students can deepen this experience when you create the space in class for moving into a deeper sense of stillness. This can be done at the beginning of class, during the flow of asanas, or at the conclusion of the asana practice (before or after Savasana).

- *Moving off the mat.* Rising from one's mat, the next vinyasa starts with being conscious and present in the next transition—back out into the world. Encourage students to pay attention to how they are moving, breathing, thinking, and feeling. Consider concluding class with a moment of reflection with the palms and fingertips together at the heart and forehead to symbolize and feel a sense of connecting the head and the heart in setting intention in moving out into the rest of the day.

Chapter Three

Sequencing Within and Across Asana Families

You must understand the whole of life, not just one little part of it. That is why you must read, that is why you must look at the skies, that is why you must sing and dance, and write poems and suffer and understand, for all that is life.

—J. KRISHNAMURTI

Sequencing begins with breaking down asanas into their constituent elements and then placing selected asanas into an order that is informed by how the actions involved in these elements are related in moving with steadiness and ease through the arc structure of an entire class. When informed by the principles presented in Chapter Two, this approach leads to the design of classes that are safe, transformational, and sustainable, allowing students to gradually move more or less seamlessly from beginning to moderate to more challenging practices. You can apply this approach to the design of any yoga class, regardless of style, level, or setting by following this three-step process:

1. Consider the general properties of different asanas and what this suggests about their sequencing.

2. Identify the constituent elements of individual asanas and what this suggests about their interrelationships and sequencing. (See Appendix B.)

3. Choose peak asanas and class themes, then design complete arc class sequences for them based on the insights discovered in steps 1 and 2. (See examples in Chapters 5–15.)

The General Properties of Asanas

For sequencing purposes, yoga asanas can be categorized into asana families that are defined as sharing basic postural and functional anatomical qualities. Within each family we can then look more closely at the general properties of the asanas in it and later at the more specific properties of individual asanas and their interrelations. We categorize asanas into the following families:

Table 3.1. Asana Families

Asana Family	Basic Distinguishing Elements
Standing	All asanas in which the weight of the body is placed primarily on one or both feet.
Core awakening	All asanas that are primarily focused on the activation of muscles in the abdominal core.
Arm support	All asanas in which the weight of the body is placed primarily on one or both hands or forearms.
Back bends	All asanas in which the spine is extended beyond anatomical position.
Twists	All non-standing positions in which the primary position is rotation of the spine.
Forward bends	All non-standing positions in which the primary action is anterior rotation of the pelvis and stretching the back of the body.
Hip openers	All non-standing positions in which there is stretching of muscles attached to the pelvis.
Inversions	All asanas in which the body is inverted.

To these families we add two further categories: Surya Namaskara (Sun Salutations), which are an assemblage of asanas from several families but widely shared as a distinct part of asana practice, and Savasana (Corpse Pose), which stands alone (or rather lies) as a wholly distinct asana.

This schema can appear to be somewhat arbitrary or problematic since most asanas have elements that meet the criteria for being in more than one category. For instance, Adho Mukha Svanasana (Downward-Facing Dog Pose) is clearly a forward bend (stretching the back of the body), hip opener (asking for ninety degrees of hip flexion), an arm support pose (the positioning of the hands, arms, shoulders, and torso akin to a handstand), and a standing pose (as the weight is increasingly placed in the feet while the legs are active in creating a foundation for lengthening the spine). Some asanas could be categorized in two or three of the twist, forward bend, or hip opener families. There are also a multitude of asana variations that further push the already somewhat blurry boundaries of these familial categories. Still, the distinctions made here are widely recognized across the mainstream of the global yoga community and provide a useful starting point for more clearly identifying what is involved in the interrelationships among asanas. Where an asana can be placed in more than one family, we have placed it in one and explained the rationale for doing so.

Standing Asanas

Standing asanas are the powerfully grounding physical foundation for the overall asana practice. Standing on their feet, students begin to experience how a stable foundation creates support up through their legs, pelvis, spine, arms, and head. They also discover that a stable foundation is resilient, beginning with the activation of pada bandha in the feet.[1] Blending sthira and sukham in the standing asanas, students begin to find samasthihi (equal standing), which invokes an attitude and awareness of equanimity as they feel the connection of body, breath, mind, and spirit. In deepening this sense of equanimity, students develop an embodied awareness of how the lightness of being depends on being grounded, allowing them to move about in their yoga practice and daily life with greater ease and joy.

Standing asanas are divided into two categories: (1) externally rotated femurs and (2) neutrally or internally rotated femurs. Externally rotated standing asanas generally stretch the inner groin and thighs while strengthening the external rotators and abductors. Internally rotated standing asanas generally strengthen the adductors and internal rotators while stretching the external rotators and abductors. (Neutral rotation is close to internal rotation in its actions and effects, but the rotational effort is very slight.) Standing balance asanas strengthen the entire standing leg and the pelvic girdle while creating an opportunity to explore the instinctual fear of falling while moving into steadier balance. Taken together, these asanas teach us about the integration of practice as we discover how the feet are connected to the legs, pelvis, spine, heart center, head, and arms—and ultimately to the breath and spirit.

Following initial warming and awakening movements (such as Cat and Dog Tilts, Surya Namaskara, or kapalabhati pranayama), standing asanas are the safest asana family for warming and opening the entire body in preparation for more complex asanas. Standing asanas are energetically stimulating, helping to focus the mind and awaken the body in the early part of the practice.

In Sequencing Standing Asanas …

- Standing asanas can be good preparation for all other asanas, with specific standing asanas and variations giving targeted preparation for particular asanas in other families.

- Tadasana (Mountain Pose) is the foundational asana for all standing asanas. Teach it first, emphasizing pada bandha, the natural physical relationship between rooting down through the feet and awakening and lengthening up through the body (the principle of roots and extension), the balance of effort and ease, and an opening to equanimity (samasthihi, meaning "equal standing").

- Use Tadasana, Adho Mukha Svanasana, or the preparatory stance of Prasarita Padottanasana (Spread-Leg Forward Fold Pose) as a starting stance for all other standing asanas.

- Separately sequence externally rotated standing asanas (e.g., Utthita Trikonasana [Extended Triangle Pose], Virabhadrasana II [Warrior II Pose], and Parsvakonasana [Extended Side Angle Pose]) and internally rotated standing asanas (e.g., Parsvottanasana [Intense Extended Side Stretch Pose], Parivrtta Trikonasana [Revolved Triangle Pose], Virabhadrasana I, and Virabhadrasana III).

- Place externally rotated-hip standing asanas before internally and neutrally rotated-hip standing asanas in keeping with the principle of moving from simple to complex. Doing externally rotated-hip standing asanas makes it is easier to establish proper alignment in the more difficult internally rotated-hip standing asanas. The significant exceptions are Tadasana, which should be taught first to cover the basic foundational actions involved in yogic standing, and the standing asanas that are included in a dynamic warming sequence (such as Anjaneyasana [Low Lunge Pose]) in classical Surya Namaskara.

- In creatively sequenced beginning and intermediate-level classes (i.e., not set sequence classes such as Ashtanga Vinyasa), refrain from moving back and forth between internally and externally rotated-hip standing asanas. This will allow students to stay present in the intelligence of actions required in one versus the other rotation while helping them to open their hips more gracefully and safely.

- When transitioning from Virabhadrasana I to Virabhadrasana II, carefully guide students to keep the knee of their front leg aligned directly above or behind the heel (never beyond it toward the toes) and aligned directly to the center of their foot. This is a difficult transition for students with tight hips, the typical result being the inward (medial) splaying of the front knee (and risk to the knee ligaments), outward (lateral) splaying of the front hip (and undue pressure on the ligaments and bursas in the hip joint), and excessive forward rotation of the pelvis (and added pressure to the lumbar spine).

- In beginning-level classes, sequence standing balance asanas toward the early part of the standing pose sequence, when students' legs are less likely to be fatigued.

- In beginning and intermediate-level classes, teach externally rotated-hip standing balance asanas (such as Vrksasana [Tree Pose]) before or amid the larger sequence of externally rotated-hip standing asanas.

- Teach Garudasana (Eagle Pose) immediately before a larger sequence of internally rotated-hip standing asanas in order to help stretch out the external rotators that, when tight, limit internal rotation.

- Prepare for twisting standing asanas by first practicing twist-free standing asanas that generate more general warming and stretch the hamstrings, hips, spine, and shoulder girdle.

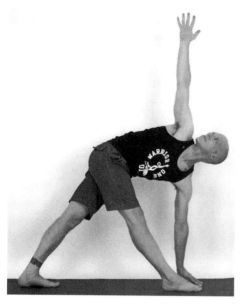

Parivrtta Trikonasana

- Introduce twisting standing asanas in a sequence that embodies the principle of moving from simple to complex, thereby allowing the gradual rotational opening of the spine (e.g., place Parivrtta Utkatasana [Revolved Chair Pose] earlier in the sequence than Parivrtta Ashta Chandrasana [Revolved Crescent Pose], place Parivrtta Ashta Chandrasana before Parivrtta Trikonasana, and place Parivrtta Trikonasana before Parivrtta Parsvakonasana [Revolved Extended Side Angle Pose]). "Before" does not mean immediately before, but earlier in the sequence.

- Twisting standing asanas are excellent preparation for back bends, especially those that open the hip flexors. Aside from standing asanas that inherently involve rotating the spine, explore the creative introduction of twisting variations to a variety of standing asanas in intermediate and advanced classes with a back bend theme or peak.

- In classes with an arm balance peak or theme, creatively integrate shoulder openers (e.g., the arm positioning from Gomukhasana [Cow Face Pose], Garudasana, Prasarita Padottanasana Variation C, and reverse *namaste*) into the standing asana sequence, particularly in Anjaneyasana, Ashta Chandrasana, Virabhadrasana I, and Virabhadrasana II. In doing so, counsel more awareness of pelvic neutrality in relation to the lumbar spine and lifting out of the pelvis to help protect the lower back.

- In intermediate and advanced classes, offer arm balances as transitions out of related standing asanas (e.g., from the wrapped variation of Parsvakonasana to Eka Pada Koundinyasana A [Two-Leg Sage Koundinya's Pose] to Chaturanga Dandasana [Four-Limbed Staff Pose]).

- In classes with a back bending focus, explore more deeply in the standing asanas that stretch the hip flexors (Anjaneyasana, Virabhadrasana I and Virabhadrasana II) and shoulder girdle as well as twisting standing asanas.

- Never transition from internal to external or external to internal rotation in standing balance asanas (such as Ardha Chandrasana [Half Moon Pose] to Parivrtta Ardha Chandrasana [Revolved Half Moon Pose]) because the extreme downward pressure of the entire weight of the body onto the femoral head can severely injure the femoral head, neck, labrum, and overall hip joint.[2] This risk is significantly increased when this movement is done repetitively (such as when making the same movement in practically every class), although strain or injury can occur even when not done repetitively.

- Except with very experienced and physically adept students, do not do more than three to five sustained standing asanas in a linked sequence on one side. In beginning-level classes, limit this to two asanas on one side (such as Virabhadrasana II and Parsvakonasana).

- Uttanasana (Standing Forward Bend Pose), Padangusthasana (Big Toe Pose), and Pada Hastasana (Hand to Foot Pose) are excellent energetically neutralizing asanas following a series of Surya Namaskara or other sustained standing asana sequences.

- Uttanasana is a good place to do other wrist therapy movements after any wrist-intensive asanas (see the sidebar on wrist therapy).

- Standing asanas can be related mostly to the *muladhara, manipura,* and *svadhisthana* chakras. Do note that chakra awakening is primarily about the consciousness we bring into the practice, not specific physical stimulation or location (see Chapter Thirteen).

Core Awakening

In popular fitness culture, the ideal core is often symbolized by "six-pack abs," the most superficial of the abdominal core muscles. Yet when so overdeveloped and tight, this rectus abdominis muscle is a source of compressed tension as well as spinal and breathing problems, compromising the grace and ease, poise and elegance, comfort and stability that come from a refined core. As yoga teacher Ana Forrest has long emphasized, we want to relieve emotional and physical constipation, restriction, and anxiety, not seal it in. Reminding students that yoga is largely about creating space, we want to guide students into cultivating a strong yet supple core, learning along

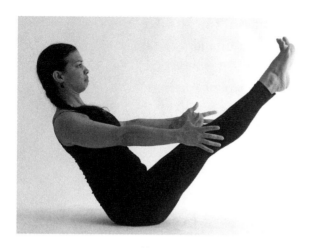

Navasana

the way to radiate outward while drawing awareness deep into the core of the body. As the core is strengthened, opened, and refined, it becomes a source of balance, stability, ease, and levity.

Taking an expanded view of the core, offer students a visual that extends from the medial arches of the feet, up the inseams of the legs to the floor of the pelvis, up through the spine, and out through the crown of the head. Throughout the asana practice, encourage students to draw energetically in toward the medial line while radiating out from it to create space. Refer to pada bandha and *mula bandha* as key energetic actions for awakening this energetic awareness. This in itself will help to strengthen and refine the muscles that are at the heart of core refinement and make the more specific core awakening practices more accessible and sustainable.

Here we will focus on asanas and dynamic movements designed to strengthen muscles in the front and center body that give support and mobility to the lower torso in its relationship to the pelvis and spine. (Contraction back bends and a variety of dynamic movements in and out of asanas will strengthen the muscles giving essential support to the spine from the back body.) Deep and sustained core awakening practices are largely contraindicated for pregnant students and should be approached very gingerly by students with lower-back issues.[3]

In Sequencing Core Awakening …

- Core awakening practices generally warm the body while bringing more targeted warming to the spine, pelvis, belly, and back.
- Give balanced awakening to all major abdominal core muscles: rectus abdominis, internal and external obliques, transversus abdominis, and the iliopsoas.
- Core awakening is ideally explored just before arm balances, creating an awakened source of levity in asanas such as Bakasana (Crane Pose) and stability in poses such as Adho Mukha Vrksasana (Handstand).

- Focus more on awakening the rectus abdominis and iliopsoas in preparation for Bakasana, Urdhva Kukkutasana (Upward Rooster Pose), Galavasana (Flying Crow Pose), and other arm balances in which the pelvis is being lifted higher than the shoulders.

- Focus more on awakening the transverse abdominis and oblique muscles in preparation for Parsva Bakasana (Side Crane Pose), Astavakrasana (Eight-Angle Pose), and other arms balances in which the torso is being twisted.

- After working intensively with the iliopsoas in asanas such as Paripurna Navasana (Full Boat Pose), stretch it out before exploring Adho Mukha Vrksasana in order to minimize anterior rotation of the pelvis.

- Never sequence deep back bends immediately following deep abdominal core strengthening practices. If core work is done prior to back bends, first neutralize the core through a sequence of simple twists.

- Core abdominal work is excellent for bringing support to the lumbar spine following back bends.

- In a sustained core sequence, do Leg Lifts and Pelvic Tilts before Tolasana (Scales Pose), and do Tolasana before Lolasana (Dangling Earring Pose) to gradually bring awareness more deeply into the abdominal core.

Arm Support Asanas

Balancing the entire body on the hands requires absolute focus, bringing students deeper into the meditative quality of dharana in their asana practice. Arm balances also bring students closer to a deeply held and perfectly rational fear of falling, a fear that is inextricably interwoven with the ego and the desire at least to appear in control. This makes arm balances the perfect asana family for cultivating self-confidence and humility. Because most students will find at least some arm balances very challenging, these asanas are also a wonderful place to explore the practice with a sense of humor and playfulness. As with any asana, patience and practice make them more accessible and sustainable while impatience almost invariably leads to frustration or injury.

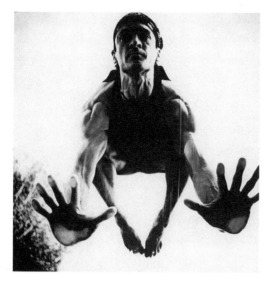
Bakasana

The wrists are at greatest risk in all arm support asanas. Students with acute wrists issues, including carpal tunnel syndrome, should not do full arm balances, while students with even mildly strained wrists are advised to minimize pressure on the wrists and use a wedged hand prop until they are free of pain. Whether interspersing support asanas throughout a practice or teaching them as a cluster of asanas, it is important to offer students the wrist therapy exercises described in the Healthy Wrist Sequence. Students should have sufficient wrist extension to place their palms flat on the floor and move their forearms perpendicular to the floor without strain or pain before attempting any arm balances. Students with weak, unstable, or impinged shoulders are advised to do the Healthy Shoulder Sequence until developing sufficient stability and flexibility in the shoulder girdle to hold Adho Mukha Svanasana for two minutes free of pain before attempting more shoulder-intense arm balances. Limited shoulder flexion is also the primary cause of a banana shape to the spine in Adho Mukha Svanasana and Pincha Mayurasana (Feathered Peacock Pose, or Forearm Balance).

Healthy Wrist Sequence

Students experiencing mild wrist pain can benefit from warming up their fingers, hands, arms, and shoulders before beginning their practice. Wrist and forearm massage is also effective in helping reduce pain. So long as the pain is mild, the following exercises can be healing:

1. *Tadasana wrist therapy:* Gently rotate the wrists through their full range of circular motion, repeatedly changing direction, then gently shake out the wrists for around thirty seconds. This can be incorporated in brief form into every Surya Namaskara.

2. *Uttanasana wrist pratikriyasana:* Whenever folding into Uttanasana amid Surya Namaskara, place the backs of the wrists toward or onto the floor and make an easy fist. This is less intense on the wrists than Pada

Hastasana (also, more students can do it, and it can easily be done with the exhale into Uttanasana).

3. *Wrist pumps:* Holding the fingers of one hand with the fingers of the other hand, move the wrist forward and back while resisting the movement with the opposing hand. Repeat for one to two minutes if pain-free.

4. *Anjali mudra:* Press the palms and fingers (from the knuckles to the fingertips) firmly together at the chest in a prayer position for one to two minutes. This is also known as reverse Phalen maneuver; if there is a burning sensation inside the wrist joint within thirty seconds, this could indicate carpal tunnel syndrome. Reverse the position of the hands, placing the backs of the wrists and hands together, and press firmly for up to a minute (Phalen maneuver).

5. *Hand dance:* Kneeling comfortably, place the hands down on the floor with the fingers pointed forward, then turn the palms up, then down with the fingers out, up with the fingers in, down with the fingers back, up with the fingers back, continuing in this fashion with every permutation of palms up and down with the fingers pointed forward, back, in, and out.

Persistent wrist tenderness or strain usually benefits from ice, splints worn during sleep, anti-inflammatory agents (including turmeric and ginger), acupuncture, and other alternative treatments. Encourage students to explore all possible measures and to consult a doctor for additional guidance.

Healthy Shoulder Sequence

The key to healthy shoulders is balanced strength and flexibility. If imbalance is creating instability or impingement, first avoid painful activities and refrain from unstable movements in which the elbow is lifted above the shoulder, especially with any whipping motion such as throwing a ball. Treat persistent pain with ice and anti-inflammatory agents. To develop healthy range of motion and strength, explore the following asanas and exercises:

1. Lying prone on a table with the arm dangling down, simply swing it forward and back in Codman's pendulum-swing exercise and around in small circles.

2. Stretch the rhomboids with Garudasana arms; use one arm to pull the other gently across the chest in horizontal adduction if unable to get into the Garudasana position.

3. Use Gomukhasana arms to stretch the triceps, latissimus dorsi, infraspinatus, teres minor, and pectoralis major of the upper arm and the pectoralis major, biceps, serratus anterior, and trapezius of the lower arm.

4. Use Parsvottanasana arms to stretch the infraspinatus, teres minor, serratus anterior, anterior deltoids, and pectorals.

5. Use Prasarita Padottanasana C arms to stretch the pectorals and anterior deltoids.

6. Stabilize the scapula by strengthening and stretching the serratus anterior and rhomboid muscles: on all fours and keeping the arms straight, slowly alternate between lowering the chest toward and away from the floor; when easy, do this in Phalakasana (Plank Pose) and progress to moving slowly back and forth between Phalakasana and Chaturanga.

7. To strengthen the rotator cuff muscles: supraspinatus through abduction of the arms into Virabhadrasana II; infraspinatus and teres minor through external rotation of the arms in Adho Mukha Svanasana; subscapularis through isometric contraction in Parsvottanasana.

8. If free of pain, explore further strengthening of the shoulders by keeping the arms overhead in flexion in Salabhasana C (Locust Pose) and Virabhadrasana III. If still pain-free after these asanas, explore holding Adho Mukha Svanasana for up to one minute, eventually working up to five minutes. If still pain-free, explore Adho Mukha Vrksasana, eventually holding for up to two minutes.

Along with strength and stability in the wrists, arms, and shoulders, arm balances require and awaken the abdominal core muscles. As discussed above, abdominal work prior to arm balances helps students create a feeling of lifting and radiating out from their core. Yet arm balances also require suppleness in the core, not gripping or bearing down. Finding this balance between active engagement and spreading through the core is one of the key elements to balancing the body on the hands. This is most evident in Adho Mukha Vrksasana, where strong core muscles stabilize the center of the body, but where tight core muscles, especially in the psoas and rectus abdominis muscles, limit full extension of the hips and spine in relation to the pelvis, exacerbating the forward rotation of the pelvis and the banana shape in a student's lower back.

In Sequencing Arm Balances …

- Students should practice Phalakasana, Chaturanga Dandasana, and Adho Mukha Svanasana for at least one year to strengthen the wrists, arms, and shoulders in preparation for bringing more weight onto their hands.
- Sequence arm balances following the warming effects of Surya Namaskara, standing asanas, core awakening, or inversions.
- Core awakening helps students to better activate the abdominal engagement that lends to levity and stability in arm balances.
- When introducing arm balances to students new to them, teach one arm balance asana only and provide detailed, step-by-step explanation and demonstration of positioning and movement into it. Provide ample time for students to attempt the asana at least three times.
- Introductory-level arm balances include Bakasana, Vasisthasana (Side Plank Pose, or Side Arm Balance), Bhujapidasana (Shoulder-Squeezing Pose), and Adho Mukha Vrksasana Prep.
- Introduce Adho Mukha Vrksasana by reviewing Adho Mukha Svanasana, and then do the two-stage Handstand Introduction Sequence at a wall to get students more comfortable in placing greater weight on their wrists, arms, and shoulders.
- Introduce Pincha Mayurasana by reviewing Shishulasana (Dolphin Pose) and then proceed as for the Handstand Introduction at the wall.
- When introducing or exploring more than one arm balance in an intermediate level class, select asanas that are closely related in form and action while moving from simple to complex (e.g., Adho Mukha Vrksasana and Pincha Mayurasana; Bakasana, Bhujapidasana, and Tittibhasana [Firefly Pose]; Parsva Bakasana and Dwi Pada Koundinyasana).

- In intermediate to advanced classes you can interweave arm balances with standing asanas, applying the intelligence and opening developed in successive standing asanas to the foundation of each arm balance as follows:
  - Utthita Trikonasana, Prasarita Padottanasana, Utkatasana (Chair Pose), and Malasana (Garland Pose) in preparation for Bakasana and Tittibhasana. Use Malasana or Utkatasana's classical form as the initial foundational position for cuing students into Bakasana.
  - Uttanasana, Malasana, and Prasarita Padottanasana in preparation for Bhujapidasana. Use Prasarita Padottanasana A as the initial foundational position for cuing students into Malasana, or in more experienced classes, begin in Adho Mukha Svanasana and leap from the feet around the arms to set up the foundation for Bhujapidasana.
  - Utthita Trikonasana and Utthita Parsvakonasana in preparation for Eka Pada Koundinyasana A.
  - Parivrtta Trikonasana, Parivrtta Parsvakonasana, and Parivrtta Utkatasana in preparation for Parsva Bakasana and Eka Pada Koundinyasana B.
- In intermediate to advanced flow-style classes, transition from the wrapped variation of Utthita Parsvakonasana to Eka Pada Koundinyasana A to Astavakrasana to Eka Pada Koundinyasana A to Chaturanga Dandasana.
- In intermediate to advanced flow-style classes, incorporate Adho Mukha Vrksasana into transitions to Chaturanga Dandasana (e.g., from Uttanasana, Virabhadrasana III, or Parivrtta Ardha Chandrasana).
- In advanced classes, use Sirsasana II (Headstand II, sometimes called Tripod Headstand) as the foundational asana for arm balance vinyasas, as follows:
  - Sirsasana II to Bakasana to Sirsasana II to either Balasana (Child's Pose) or Chaturanga Dandasana (or move several times from Sirsasana II to Bakasana to Sirsasana II, holding Bakasana for five to eight breaths each time).

- Sirsasana II to Parsva Bakasana to Dwi Pada Koundinyasana to Eka Pada Koundinyasana B to Sirsasana II to the other side to either Balasana or Chaturanga Dandasana, holding each arm balance for five to eight breaths.
- Sirsasana II to Urdhva Kukkutasana or Parsva Kukkutasana to Sirsasana II (if Parsva, do the other side) to either Balasana or Chaturanga Dandasana.

- Arm balances generally warm the body and are thus good preparation for back bends. Depending on which arm balances are in the pre–back bend sequence, stretch the related shoulder muscles before doing the back bends.
- Adho Mukha Vrksasana and Pincha Mayurasana are excellent preparation for shoulder flexion back bends such as Urdhva Dhanurasana (Upward-Facing Bow Pose) and Natarajasana (King Dancer Pose). They are also the foundational asanas for Vrschikasana (Scorpion Pose), which is best explored at a wall.

Always offer a variety of wrist therapy stretches following sustained arm balance sequences.

Back Bends

With deep stretching across the entire front of the body, especially through the heart center, belly, and groin, back bends stimulate a passionate response among students. The passion tends to go toward either unbridled effort or fearful withdrawal, offering students another opportunity for cultivating equanimity amid these emotional poles. The primary physical purpose of back bends is to open to the full movement of breath and energy in the front of the body, not to go into the most gloriously deep stretch of the front of the body. You can guide students into finding a sense of sustainable effort in playing the edge in their back bend practice by emphasizing the heart-opening qualities of this practice: feeling compassion toward oneself in feeling one's way toward the edge, opening to a sense of innate inner harmony as a source of aparigraha, sensing a healing presence within the breath that reinforces a sense of assessment rather than judgment, and recognizing pure love in the heart as the glue that holds everything together in the unending

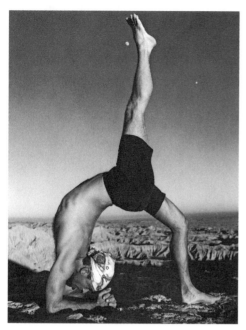
Eka Pada Urdhva Dhanurasana

process of change. Encourage back bends as a practice of equanimity, not attainment, and purification for the purpose of freedom, not perfection, focusing on opening the heart.

Asanas in the back bend family can be usefully categorized into contraction, traction, and leverage back bends, each of which has important distinctions and actions:

- *Contraction back bends:* Muscles along the back of the body concentrically contract to overcome gravity (e.g., lifting up into Salabhasana A).
- *Traction back bends:* Muscles in the front of the body eccentrically contract to overcome gravity (e.g., lowering back into Ustrasana [Camel Pose]).
- *Leverage back bends:* The arms and/or legs press against a stable object (floor, wall, or another part of the body) to stretch the front of the body (e.g., Dhanurasana [Bow Pose] or Urdhva Dhanurasana).

Within each of these categories of back bends the humerus can either be in extension or flexion. It is in extension in asanas such as Salabhasana A, Ustrasana, or Setu Bandha Sarvangasana (Bridge Pose); it is in flexion in asanas such as Salabhasana C, Kapotasana (Pigeon Pose, not to be confused with the asymmetrical hip opener Eka Pada Raj Kapotasana popularly given this name), or Viparita Dandasana (Inverted Staff Pose). These different arm positions require different areas of engagement and release through the shoulder girdle, as follows:

- *Shoulder extension back bends:* Extension of the arms requires the scapulae to be stabilized by the rhomboids, lower trapeziuses, and serratus anterior muscles while the pectoralis majors and minors must release.
- *Shoulder flexion back bends:* Flexion requires the rhomboids, latissimi dorsi, pectoralis majors, and triceps to release.

In Sequencing Back Bends ...

- Back bends are naturally integrated into Surya Namaskara as part of the warming and initiating practice. It is important to emphasize light and gradual exploration of back bends in these initial flowing sequences.

- Move gradually into successively deeper back bends only as the warmth and openness of the body invites without straining.

- Deep and sustained back bends should be sequenced at the peak of a practice when the body is warmest and most prepared for these relatively complex asanas.

- Never sequence a deep or sustained back bend practice immediately following a deep or sustained core awakening practice because tightened core muscles inhibit elongation and extension of the spine.

- Surya Namaskara, standing asanas, arm balances, and inversions all generate the warmth required for safe and deep back bends.

- Back bends that require active use of spinal erector muscles (i.e., contraction back bends such as Salabhasana A) should be sequenced before back bends in which the arms, legs, or a wall leverage the asana in order to further warm and awaken muscles along the spine and thereby enable them to more easily soften in leveraged back bends.

- Use standing asana sequences to open the quadriceps, hip flexors, and groin muscles, allowing greater hip extension.

- Anjaneyasana, Ashta Chandrasana, and Virabhadrasana I provide excellent preparation for all back bends as they open the hip flexors and help to teach pelvic neutrality in relation to extension of the spine.

- Use Virasana (Hero Pose) to teach internal rotation of the femurs in preparation for exploring Supta Virasana (Reclined Hero Pose), which for most students is a back bend in itself and excellent preparation for deeper back bends as it stretches the thighs, hip flexors, and groin muscles.

- Use shoulder flexion openers (opening the latissimi dorsi, pectoralis majors, and rhomboids) to prepare the shoulders for safe flexion in back bends: Adho Mukha Svanasana, Gomukhasana arms, and Garudasana arms.

- Supta Baddha Konasana (Reclined Bound Angle Pose) and Anjaneyasana, both of which have mild back bend elements, offer excellent opening of the hips and thighs in preparation for back bends. Both asanas can incorporate shoulder flexion stretches for greater ease in shoulder flexion back bends.

- Use asanas like Prasarita Padottanasana C to open the shoulders for shoulder extension in Setu Bandha Sarvangasana. Also explore this same arm position and shoulder stretch folding forward in Ashta Chandrasana.

- Do not alternate back and forth between back bends and forward bend. Amid a back bending sequence, do not draw the knees into the chest or do other forward bending positioning of the spine until the sequence is complete—stay in a back bending or neutral spinal position until the back-bending practice is completed.

- In exploring prone back bends such as Dhanurasana, move dynamically in and out of a successively deeper Salabhasana A to give targeted warming and awakening to the muscles on the back of the body.

- In exploring supine back bends such as Setu Bandha Sarvangasana, first do a series of Bridge Rolls by gradually lifting the hips up toward the Bridge while sweeping the arms overhead to the floor, then lifting the heels to tuck the tailbone further under and create space in the lower back while releasing one vertebra at a time back to the floor before releasing the arms back to the starting position on the floor by one's sides.

- Place symmetrical foundation back bends (in which the feet, legs, and pelvis are in the same position on the left and right sides) before asymmetrical foundation back bends.

- Introduce *eka pada* (one-leg) variations of Setu Bandha Sarvangasana, Urdhva Dhanurasana, and Viparita Dandasana only when students display steadiness and ease in the basic forms of these asanas.

- Use Virabhadrasana I to teach internal rotation of the back leg from a position of relative pelvic neutrality and symmetry in preparation for asymmetrical back bends such as Eka Pada Raj Kapotasana (One-Leg King Pigeon Pose), Hanumanasana (Divine Monkey Pose), and Natarajasana. Use this rotation to (1) minimize pressure in the sacroiliac joint and (2) maximize movement of the hips to an even positioning that minimizes any twisting in the lumbar spine. In practicing Eka Pada Raj Kapotasana and Hanumanasana, ensure that the pelvis is stable and has level grounding on both sides. This will require the use of a prop for most students.

- In preparation for the asymmetrical standing balancing back bend of Natarajasana, include the foundational asana of Virabhadrasana III. Strongly encourage use of a strap in order to help maintain the relative symmetry of the pelvis, torso, and shoulder girdle.

- The essential preparation—a long-term strengthening practice—for dropping back from Tadasana to Urdhva Dhanurasana and for transitioning from Urdhva Dhanurasana up to Tadasana is in the dynamic practice of Laghu Vajrasana (Little Thunderbolt Pose), moving slowly up and down from Ustrasana toward Kapotasana only as far as one feels steady and at ease. Students should drop back only as far as they can come back up without straining, gradually

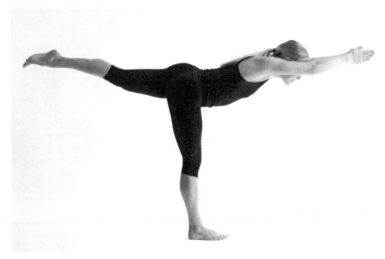

Virabhadrasana III

developing the strength to drop back to Kapotasana with their palms in anjali mudra (prayer position, or reverence seal).

- Introduce drop-backs from Tadasana to Urdhva Dhanurasana only when a student displays steadiness and ease in Urdhva Dhanurasana along with alignment of the wrists under the shoulders, straight arms, feet parallel and hip distance apart, knees aligned with the hips, and the top front pelvic bones (anterior superior iliac spine or ASIS) level with the lower ribs.

- The pratikriyasana practice for back bends starts with relaxation of the spine in a neutral position. Simple options differ depending on whether one completes the back bends standing, prone, or supine. If standing, come to either a prone or supine position, or alternately stretch and relax the spine in Adho Mukha Svanasana while being attentive to keeping the lumbar spine in neutral extension (if necessary bending the knees).

- In some intermediate and advanced classes, back bends might be sequenced as one in a series of peak practices. This requires doing counterasanas that neutralize the spine and prepare the bodymind for the next pathway to a peak.

- From a prone position, transition to a modified form of Balasana with the toes together and feet wide apart, thus allowing easier release through the hips and thereby minimizing flexion of the lumbar spine. Students with more openness in the lower back can explore moving gently yet directly into the traditional form of Balasana. In intermediate classes one can transition from a prone position into Adho Mukha Svanasana, as described above.

- In transitioning from a supine position, place the feet as for Setu Bandha Sarvangasana but separated to the edges of the mat; let the knees rest together and the arms either drape down by one's sides or rest on the floor overhead. Other initial options for relaxing the spine include Ananda Balasana (Happy Baby Pose), Savasana, or Supta Baddha Konasana with or without a block placed under the sacrum. In the Savasana position, offer a bolster under the knees to further reduce pressure in the lower back.

- Use gentle twists—not deep twists—for initial release of tension, transitioning from side to side after relatively brief holds before moving into successively deeper and more sustained twists.

- Forward folding hip openers, particularly those like Gomukhasana that stretch the external rotators and piriformis muscles, will help release pressure in the lower back and sacroiliac joint and make more deeply relaxing forward bends more accessible. Give time for students to move slowly and deeply into these counterasanas, encouraging them to continue following their breath while enjoying the awakened energy and consciousness that back bends naturally stimulate.

- Core integration movements following back bends will help to stabilize the lower back. However, this is not advised when the overall sequence is moving toward cooling down or evening classes due to how back bends stimulate the sympathetic nervous system.

- Move gradually into deeper forward bends, including lateral stretches such as Parivrtta Janu Sirsasana (Revolved Head to Knee Pose) and deep forward bends like Paschimottanasana (West Stretching Pose, sometimes called Seated Forward Bend Pose).

- Offer Halasana (Plow Pose), Salamba Sarvangasana (Supported Shoulder Stand), Pindasana (Embryo Pose), and Karnapidasana (Ear-Squeezing Pose) along with the counterasanas for these asanas along the path to Savasana.

Twists

Twists delightfully penetrate deep into the body's core, stimulating and tonifying internal organs, particularly the kidneys and liver, while creating suppleness and freedom in the spine and opening the chest, shoulders, neck, and hips. Active supine twists, such as Jathara Parivartanasana (Revolving Twist Pose), strengthen the abdominal obliques, which are the most important group in many asanas involving rotational movement (such as Parsvakonasana or Astavakrasana). Regular twisting helps maintain the normal length and resilience of the spine's soft tissues and the health of the vertebral disks and facet joints of the spine, restoring the spine's natural range of motion.[4]

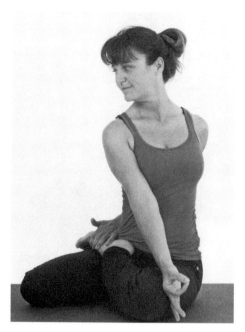

Bharadvajrasana

In a beautiful poetic irony, we find that in twisting our body more and more into a pretzel, we more easily unwind the accumulated physical and emotional tension contained inside. Along with this release of tension, twists tend to bring the bodymind to a more neutral, sattvic state. Thus, they are neither generally warming nor cooling, but both: warming if coming from a relatively cool condition, cooling if coming from a relatively warm condition. These qualities allow us to place twists in a variety of places in any given sequence.

In Sequencing Twists ...

- Always practice any given twist evenly on each side, promoting balance.
- Gradually introduce twists throughout the warming part of the practice as well as on the pathway to the peak as a means of reducing tension that may arise in doing asanas from other asana families.
- The dynamic twisting action of Jathara Parivartanasana is generally warming and can be done as part of relieving tension and maintaining warmth in the body on the pathway to the peak.
- Standing twists, which are excellent for teaching how to stabilize the pelvis and lengthen the spine, are ideally practiced in preparation for seated twists that call for these same qualities of stable grounding and lengthening. Teach Parivrtta Trikonasana from the stable base of Parsvottanasana in preparation for teaching seated twists such as Ardha Matsyendrasana (Half Lord of the Fishes Pose), Bharadvajrasana (Sage Bharadvaj's Pose), and Marichyasana C (Sage Marichi's Pose C).
- Releasing the large outer layers of the trunk muscles with forward bends, back bends, and side bends allows easier and fuller rotation at the deep level of the small spinal muscles.
- As neutralizing asanas, twists are excellent for calming anxiety and relieving lethargy.

- Twists will mildly stimulate the nervous system and reawaken energy following deeply relaxing sequences of forward bends and hip openers.
- Along with preparatory warming asanas from other asana families, twists are excellent preparation for back bends and excellent initial neutralizing asanas (including calming) following back bends.
- Twists are excellent for specifically neutralizing the spine after deep back bends and forward bends.
- Twists can be creatively explored in a variety of nontwisting asanas such as Utkatasana, Virasana, Gomukhasana (but without its arm component or forward fold), Ardha Prasarita Padottanasana (Half Spread-Leg Forward Fold Pose) and Utthita Hasta Padangusthasana (Extended Hand to Foot Pose).
- Twists done gently are cooling and should be explored in that way as part of the integrative pathway toward Savasana. However, prior to settling into Savasana, follow any twists with a symmetrical forward fold such as Paschimottanasana to further release tension in the spine and any sense of imbalance that have arisen in twisting one side and then the other.
- After an intensive twisting sequence, explore the following for pratikriyasana:
  - A symmetrical forward bend such as Upavista Konasana (Wide-Angle Forward Fold Pose) to realign the hips and legs.
  - Supta Baddha Konasana to further release through the hips and open up space around the diaphragm and through the heart center.
  - A simple back bend such as Setu Bandha Sarvangasana to further open the chest.

Forward Bends

Forward bends are deeply calming asanas that draw us into the inner mysteries and dynamics of our lives. The classic seated forward bend, Paschimottanasana, translates from Sanskrit as "west stretching pose," signifying the sunset of

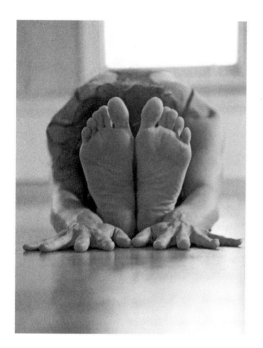

Paschimottanasana

a practice traditionally initiated facing the rising sun. Here, as we fold into ourselves, the asana naturally lends to deeper self-reflection, which can be emotionally nourishing or difficult depending on what comes up. Other forward bends like Balasana are deeply nurturing; we are in this position during nine months of gestation and naturally return to this fetal position to nurture or protect ourselves. In stimulating the pelvic and abdominal organs, the subtle energetic effects of forward bends are concentrated in the lower chakras, often revealing base emotions held deep in the body. Holding forward bends for at least a few minutes while refining the flow of the breath allows students to safely explore these feelings.

In folding forward we stretch and expose the vulnerable back side of our bodies, most of which we will never directly see. Just as there is often heightened fear in dropping back into the unknown in back bends such as Laghu Vajrasana, we tend to hold on with the back side muscles when folding forward. To fully release into forward bends, we must let go of an entire chain of muscles that start in the plantar fasciae of the feet and move through the Achilles tendons, gastrocnemii, and solei in the lower legs, hamstrings and adductors on the backs and insides of the thighs, gluteus maximi, piriformis and quadratus lumborum muscles around the back of the pelvis and into the lower back, and then the muscles across the entire back, primarily the spinal erectors, multifidi, and latissimi dorsi (Aldous 2004, 65). This release requires patience as the back side gradually releases and allows the graciousness of the forward bend to manifest. When pursued aggressively, injury to the hamstrings or lower back is likely. Students with disk injuries should explore forward bends with keen awareness and patience, staying with asanas in which they can focus the stretch in the hamstrings and hips, not the lower back, such as Dandasana (Staff Pose) and Supta Padangusthasana (Reclined Big Toe Pose).

In Sequencing Forward Bends ...

- All forward bends should be approached with conscious attention to a deep sense of sukham, beginning with the warming movements of Surya Namaskara when folding into Uttanasana.

- Although forward bends can be practiced at any time, they are most safely approached when the body is warm and awakened through other asanas, particularly through the lower back and hips.

- Supine forward bends such as Supta Padangusthasana are safest for the lower back and should be placed before other intense hamstring stretching asanas when working with new or relatively tight students. Encourage use of a strap if that is what it takes to keep the shoulders on the floor while clasping the big toe (clasping the strap instead).

- Seated forward bends are best initiated through the intelligence of Dandasana, which is the foundational asana for all other seated forward bends. Dandasana is a forward bend; if indicated, encourage students to sit onto a prop in order to establish pelvic neutrality and use a strap around the feet to deepen the stretch along the backs of the legs while working to rotate the pelvis forward as the source of any further forward folding.

- Hip openers like Gomukhasana and Kapotasana Prep that release the hip extensors and external rotators are excellent partial preparation for seated forward bends.

- Virasana is excellent for preparing the knees for seated forward bends. While sitting in Virasana, position the arms as for Garudasana to open the muscles in the mid to upper back (particularly the rhomboids and mid-trapezius muscles) that are asked to release in forward bends.

- A series of standing asanas will generally warm the body sufficiently for safe and deep forward bends. Parsvottanasana, Utthita Trikonasana, and Ardha Chandrasana are excellent for warming and releasing the hamstrings in preparation for deeper hamstring stretches in seated forward bends.

- As deeply calming asanas, a sustained sequence of forward bends is ideally sequenced as part of the "tha" practice following the practice's peak asana, especially for cooling down after doing back bends, arm balances, or stimulating inversions (particularly Sirsasana).

- If offering a class focused on reducing anxiety, do not alternate back and forth between forward bends and back bends or twists, which will be stimulating. (As noted earlier, do not alternate back and forth between sustained forward bends and back bends, regardless of energetics, as doing so can strain the back.)

- Following back bends or arm balances, Supta Padangusthasana will give a hip-opening and hamstring stretch that physically prepares your students for greater openness and ease in seated forward bends.

- From Dandasana, the foundational seated forward bend, gradually explore deeper symmetrical forward bends, starting with Paschimottanasana. Counsel light dynamic movement from Dandasana toward Paschimottanasana while keeping the sitting bones rooted, legs active, breath steady, and heart center lifted and spacious.

- Follow asymmetrical seated forward bends (in which the two legs are in different positions) with symmetrical forward bends to reestablish balance in the sacroiliac joint.

- Forward bending asanas can be interspersed with seated or supine hip openers and twists. The hip openers will tend to generate deeper calm, while the twists will be relatively stimulating.

- Use forward bends to create the opening and body intelligence for arm balances in which there is a similar positioning of the body, as follows:

  - Upavista Konasana and/or Kurmasana (Tortoise Pose) in preparation for Tittibhasana.
  - Both sides of Akarna Dandasana (Archer's Pose) in preparation for Astavakrasana.
  - Both sides of Marichyasana A in preparation for Bhujapidasana.
  - Both sides of Tiriang Mukha Eka Pada Paschimottanasana (Three Limbs Facing One Foot West Stretching Pose) in preparation for Eka Pada Bakasana (One-leg Crane Pose).

Following a deep forward bending practice, offer gentle back bends such as Setu Bandha Sarvangasana as a counterasana to reintegrate the hamstrings and simple twists to reintegrate the spine.

Hip Openers

While most standing asanas and all forward bends stretch the muscles in and around the pelvis, the purer family of hip openers is found in seated, supine, or prone positions. When stable and open, the hips are the key to our mobility in the world. Yet habitual sitting in chairs and participation in intense athletic activity can combine with genetics to make the hips one of the tightest parts of the body, resulting in limited range of motion and, potentially, strain in the lower back. Open hips are one of the key elements to practicing safe and deep back bends, forward bends, and in sitting effortlessly in Padmasana (Lotus Pose) or another crossed-legged position for meditation. In exploring hip openers, stay attuned to pressure in the knees; when the pelvis and feet are fixed in position, most positions that stretch hip-related muscles will put pressure in the knees and possibly sprain the knee ligaments or strain muscles attaching in and around the knees.

We can develop and maintain a healthy range of motion in the hips through a balanced practice that addresses each of the associated muscles, with a variety of benefits that will show up in standing, back bending, and forward bending asanas:

- *Hip flexors:* When the primary hip flexors—iliopsoas and rectus femoris—are tight, the pelvis is pulled into anterior rotation and the lower back tends to develop a lordosis. Tight hip flexors also limit back bends. While the standing asanas Anjaneyasana and Virabhadrasana I and II are very effective in stretching these muscles, classic hip openers like Supta Virasana and Eka Pada Raj Kapotasana Prep offer more targeted release of the hip flexors.

- *Hip extensors:* Tight hip extensors pull the sitting bones toward the backs of the knees, potentially flattening the lower back and leading to kyphosis in the thoracic spine. Tight hip extensors—especially the hamstrings and lower gluteus maximus fibers—limit forward bending; they are most directly stretched in straight-leg forward bends.

- *Hip abductors:* Tight abductors—especially gluteus medius—are a prime cause of the front knee splaying outward in standing lunge asanas (along with weak adductors), the nemesis of students attempting to cross their knees in Garudasana and Gomukhasana and a source of pressure on the sacroiliac joint. Again, the asanas in which their tightness most limits the range of motion also most stretch them, especially Gomukhasana.

- *Hip adductors:* Tight adductors (along with weak abductors) cause the front knee to splay inward in standing lunge asanas and make it more difficult to bring the legs apart in a variety of standing, arm balance, and seated asanas. (Relatively short femoral heads and/or iliofemoral ligaments will also limit range of motion often thought to be caused by tight adductors.) Upavista Konasana and Baddha Konasana (Bound Angle Pose) are the classic seated asanas for opening the adductors.

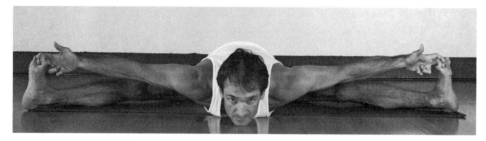

Upavista Konasana

- *Internal rotators:* Tightness in the internal rotators can cause the knees to splay toward each other when standing in Tadasana and limit opening into poses like Padmasana and Virabhadrasana II. Closely associated with the adductors, Upavista Konasana and Baddha Konasana are effective for stretching these muscles.

- *External rotators:* The most powerful muscles in the body, glutei maximi are the primary external rotator of the femurs. When tight or overused—as is the case with many dancers—the knees and feet tend to turn out, causing misalignment in many standing asanas and placing pressure on the sacroiliac joint. Gomukhasana and Supta Parivartanasana (Reclined Revolved Pose) effectively stretch these muscles.

In Sequencing Hip Openers ...

- In flow-style classes, Surya Namaskara initiates the journey into the hips through a series of forward bends, back bends, and standing poses that focus awareness in and around the pelvic girdle.

- Most standing asanas are hip openers that warm and open the lower body in effective preparation for deeper hip-opening requirements in many arm balances, back bends, and deep seated hip openers and forward bends. Use dynamic exploration of hip opening in preparation for more sustained hip-opening work when seated, supine, or prone.

- In Adho Mukha Svanasana, offer the option of extending one leg up and actively stretching the hip in a "scorpion tail" positioning.

- A supine hip opener like Eka Pada Raj Kapotasana Prep A is excellent for learning to isolate stretches through the hips while maintaining the natural curvature of the lumbar spine. Modifications like placing one foot on a block or wall make this asana accessible even to very tight students. Explore this pose in conjunction with Ananda Balasana to cultivate balanced opening of the external and internal rotators of the hips. Note that supine hip openers are more stimulating than prone hip openers.

- Thread the Needle is excellent preparation for Eka Pada Raj Kapotasana Prep B. If transitioning into Eka Pada Raj Kapotasana from a standing asana sequence, do Anjaneyasana and/or Virabhadrasana I to prepare for the challenge of internally rotating the back leg and moving toward symmetrical positioning of the pelvis. All of these asanas stretch the iliopsoas and thereby allow more freedom of movement between the trunk and the legs. Note that this is among the riskiest asanas for the knees. It is vitally important to have the hip of the front leg firmly grounded on the floor or a block while keeping the back leg extended straight back from the hip, knee pointed straight down, thigh internally rotating, and that side of the pelvis rotating forward.

- Moving more deeply into releasing the internal rotators and adductors (especially when sequencing toward Padmasana), explore

Baddha Konasana, Akarna Dandasana, and Agnistambhasana (Fire Log Pose).

- In moving from simple to complex in seated cross-legged positions, start with a simple crossed-legged Sukhasana (Simple Pose) and progress gradually to Ardha Padmasana (Half Lotus Pose) before attempting full Padmasana.

- Specific hip openers can be intelligently sequenced in preparation for many arm balances that require open, awakened, activated hip flexors or adductors. See the section above on arm balances for these relationships.

- Hip openers can be creatively adapted to include shoulder openers in preparation for arm balances and back bends. For example, in Virasana, the arms can be positioned as for Garudasana to focus the stretch in the center of the back, or as for Gomukhasana to stretch the latissimi dorsi, deltoids, pectoralis majors, and triceps.

- In the "tha" part of the practice, sustained hip openers are deeply calming and allow deeper integration of strong sequences of standing asanas, arm balances, back bends, and inversions.

- Hip openers are naturally combined energetically with forward bends, side bends, and gentle twists along the path toward Savasana.

Inversions

When we go upside down, the world appears to be inverted. Here even the simplest of movements can be confusing as we experience this opposite and unfamiliar relationship to gravity. This shift in perspective and neuromuscular awareness creates an opportunity to further expand our sense of being in the world while reversing the effects of gravity in the body. The brain is flushed with nourishing blood, the mind clears, the nerves quiet down, and everything seems to become more still yet awake, offering a graceful invitation to meditation. With practice even what is at first the most challenging inversion—Salamba Sirsasana (Supported Headstand)—becomes as stable its opposite, Tadasana, allowing students to remain in this asana for several minutes at a time. Whether in Salamba Sirsasana or Salamba Sarvangasana, students develop more nuanced muscular coordination that adds stability and ease to a variety of other asanas, including in fluid movements into and out of Adho Mukha Vrksasana. (See Chapter Four for detailed instructions.)

Students who are not practicing Salamba Sirsasana I or Salamba Sarvangasana can receive most of the benefits of full inversion in Viparita Karani (Active Reversal Pose, "the action or doing of reversing, turning upside down"), perhaps the most calming and deeply restorative asana, included below along with the other inversions. This is an excellent asana for all students, especially following a vigorous practice, stressful day, or when feeling energetically down.

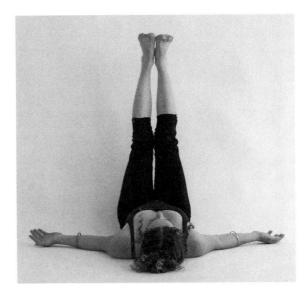

Viparita Karani

In Sequencing Inversions …

- Salamba Sirsasana I is an excellent warming asana that with proper preparation can be done early in intermediate and advanced classes.

- In sequencing for Salamba Sirsasana I toward the beginning of class, start the class standing on their feet in Tadasana, teaching students about grounding and the principle of roots and extension, which will directly apply later in Salamba Sirsasana I. Progressing further toward Salamba Sirsasana I, offer students Uttanasana, which stretches the back and gives a sense of what it is like breathing while inverted.

- To open the shoulder girdle in preparation for Salamba Sirsasana I, explore Adho Mukha Svanasana, Garudasana arms, and Gomukhasana arms. These stretches will create easier shoulder flexion in Salamba Sirsasana I.

- In intermediate and advanced classes, practice Shishulasana to further open the shoulder girdle and to learn to embody the actions required in drawing the shoulders away from the wrists.

- In preparation for a sustained Salamba Sirsasana I practice, especially when it includes variations, do more targeted warming and awakening by opening the hip flexors, the lower back, and the abdominal core.

- Give patient and methodical preparation to the base of Salamba Sirsasana I: fingers loosely interlaced to ensure rooting of the ulnar wrist point, firm grounding of the elbows, rooting of the scapulae against the back ribs while drawing the shoulders away from the wrists, steady rooting down through the crown of the head to stimulate the spinal erector muscles and thereby open space up through the spine.[5]

- Before releasing from Salamba Sirsasana I, offer intermediate and advanced students the pike variation, Urdhva Dandasana (Upward Staff Pose), in which, over time, the legs are lowered and held level with the floor before extending them back overhead and eventually releasing to Balasana.

- Salamba Sirsasana I can be sequenced as a peak asana and explored with numerous variations in leg position (scissors, bent as for Baddha Konasana, folded into Padmasana) and torso position (twisting, forward bending, and back bending).

- When placing Salamba Sirsasana I in a finishing sequence, do Salamba Sarvangasana after Sirsasana (not vice versa) to more deeply calm the bodymind.

- Intermediate and advanced students can explore transitioning from Salamba Sirsasana I to Viparita Dandasana, which is a deep back bend.

- Advanced students can explore several variations in arm position in Salamba Sirsasana (versions II–VI), eventually balancing free of the arms (Niralamba Sirsasana, "without support," a pure headstand).

- Salamba Sirsasana I is excellent preparation for Pincha Mayurasana.

- In releasing from Salamba Sirsasana I and after resting in Balasana, offer asanas to release tension in the neck, including Setu Bandha Sarvangasana, Halasana, or Salamba Sarvangasana.

- Halasana is both an inversion and a calming forward bend. Close in form to Salamba Sarvangasana, it is the basic foundational pose for transitioning into Salamba Sarvangasana.

- Prepare for Halasana by opening the chest with the arm extension back bend of Setu Bandha Sarvangasana, emphasizing grounding through the shoulders and arms to expand the chest and upper back while maintaining space under the neck. Encourage the use of blankets under the arms and shoulders to help create that space and to reduce flexion and pressure in the cervical spine.

- In contrast to Salamba Sirsasana I's stimulating effects, Salamba Sarvangasana is calming and cooling. Sequence it as part of the pratikriyasana path to Savasana.

- Prepare for Salamba Sarvangasana with Halasana.

- Variations in Salamba Sarvangasana include alternately releasing one leg toward or to the floor overhead, Baddha Konasana legs, Upavista Konasana legs (including revolving through the torso and hips), and releasing the legs forward into Setu Bandha Sarvangasana.

- From Salamba Sarvangasana, offer the option of Urdhva Padmasana and Pindasana to students who are stable and can safely fold their legs into Padmasana. Otherwise offer Halasana and Karnapidasana.

- Intermediate and advanced students can explore transitioning from Salamba Sarvangasana to Setu Bandha Sarvangasana (and vice versa).

- Advanced students whose bodies are fully extended with the ears, hips, knees, and ankles vertically aligned can explore placing the hands on the sides of the thighs in Niralamba Sarvangasana. This is contraindicated for anyone with neck issues.

- Prepare for Karnapidasana by first establishing all of the elements of Halasana, and then slowly release the knees toward the ears while attentive to sensation in the neck and lower back.

- Counterpose Halasana, Salamba Sarvangasana, and Karnapidasana with Matsyasana (Fish Pose) and Uttana Padasana (Extended Leg Pose). With Uttana Padasana, start with the modified form in which the elbows remain on the floor beneath the shoulders and the legs are extended forward on the floor.

- Viparita Karani is the simplest and most accessible inversion asana. It is deeply relaxing and cooling. Students who choose for whatever reason not to do a full inversion such as Sirsasana or Salamba Sarvangasana can receive most of the benefits of full inversion with this asana. Students with tight hamstrings and lower back issues should place a bolster under the sacrum and/or set up with their hips positioned farther away from the wall.

- Release from Viparita Karani by sliding the feet down the wall, either drawing the knees in toward the chest into Apanasana (Wind-relieving Pose) or away from each other into a modified Supta Baddha Konasana.

Savasana

Savasana (from *sava*, "corpse") is the ultimate asana for reintegration after practicing other asanas and pranayama. Ask students to lie onto their backs and spread out as comfortably as possible with their arms draped onto the floor and palms facing up. If they feel any discomfort in their lower back, suggest placing a rolled blanket under their knees. Lift the chest a little to let the shoulder blades relax slightly toward each other, then lie back down with more spaciousness across the heart center. Take one last deep inhale, then with the exhalation, let everything go, starting with allowing the breath to flow however it naturally will. Give minimal guidance in cuing students to scan and release tension all through their bodies. There is finally no need for the muscles to do anything at all. Encourage students simply to watch what is happening. Suggest a sense of all the muscles and bones letting go of each other, a sense of detachment all through the body. Similarly, as naturally as thoughts come and go, encourage letting the thoughts flow, interested without

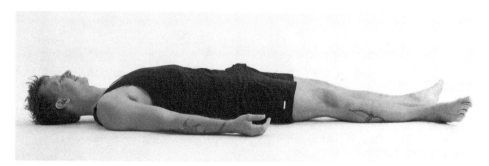

Savasana

being attached, becoming stiller, quieter, and clearer—breath by effortless breath. Stay in Savasana for at least five minutes.

If students must leave class early, encourage them to rest in Savasana before leaving. Gently awaken the class from Savasana with a soft voice, bringing awareness back to the breath. Suggest feeling the simple rising and falling of the chest and belly, cuing the class to gradually breathe more deeply and consciously, using the breath to reawaken awareness in the body-mind while changing as little as possible. Suggest bringing small movements into the fingers, hands, toes, and feet. With a deep inhalation, suggest stretching the arms overhead before rolling onto the right side, curling up, and nurturing oneself for a few breaths before slowly coming up to sitting. Now is an ideal time to meditate.

Table 3.2. Basic Arc Template Applied to Different-Level Yoga Classes

	Level 1: 75 minutes	Level 2: 90 minutes	Level 3: 108 minutes
Seated meditation and ujjayi pranayama	2–3 minutes;Introduce ujjayi	3–5 minutes; Refine ujjayi	3–5 minutes; Expand ujjayi
Initial warming	Cat and Dog Tilts; Extended Cat and Dog; Puppy Dog; Balasana	Introduce kapalabhati, 1–3 rounds of 45 seconds; Cat and Dog Tilts; Adho Mukha Svanasana 1–2 minutes	Kapalabhati, 1–3 rounds of 1–2 minutes; Adho Mukha Svanasana 2–3 minutes
Surya Namaskara	3 Classical; 1–2 A's 1–2 B's	1–3 Classical; 2–3 A's 2–3 B's	3–5 A's 3–5 B's
Standing—external	From Prasarita stance: Virabhadrasana II; Utthita Parsvakonasana; Utthita Trikonasana; From Tadasana: Vrksasana Hold each asana 5–8 breaths before changing sides.	From Prasarita stance or in fluid transition from Virabhadrasana I: Virabhadrasana II to Utthita Parsvakonasana on each side, then transition to: Tadasana to Vrksasana or Utthita Hasta Padangusthasana Utthita Trikonasana to Ardha Chandrasana.	From Virabhadrasana I: Virabhadrasana II to Utthita Parsvakonasana; Optional transition to Chaturanga through Eka Pada Koundinyasana I; Utthita Trikonasana; Ardha Chandrasana. Hold each 1–2 minutes; offer variations.

Sequencing Within and Across Asana Families

	Level 1: 75 minutes	Level 2: 90 minutes	Level 3: 108 minutes
Standing—internal	Prasarita Padottanasana A; Parsvottanasana; Ashta Chandrasana	Prasarita Padottanasana A and C; Parsvottanasana; Parivrtta Trikonasana.	Prasarita Padottanasana A (with Bakasana option), then variation C; Parsvottanasana; Parivrtta Trikonasana to Parivrtta Ardha
	Hold each 5–8 breaths.	From Down Dog: Ashta Chandrasana to Parivrtta Parsvakonasana Prep Pose Hold each 5–8 breaths.	From Down Dog: Ashta Chandrasana to Virabhadrasana III to Parivrtta Hasta Padangusthasana to Virabhadrasana III to Adho Mukha Vrksasana to Chaturanga.
			Virabhadrasana I to Parivrtta Parsvakonasana; optional transition to Chaturanga through Eka Pada Koundinyasana II.
Abdominals	Paripurna Navasana Prep 3 times; Yogic Bicycles 1 minute	Paripurna Navasana to Ardha Navasana 2–3 times); Yogic Bicycles 1–2 minutes; Jathara Parivartanasana 3–5 times; Leg lifts.	Paripurna Navasana to Ardha Navasana to Tolasana 3–5 times; Tolasana to Lolasana 3–5 times, holding 5–10 breaths; Yogic Bicycles 2–3 minutes; Jathara Parivartanasana 5–10 times); Kapalabhati Pranayama concluding with Bahya Kumbhaka and Uddiyana Bandha.
Arm balances	Adho Mukha Vrksasana Prep 1 at wall; Forearm Balance Prep 2 at wall. Wrist and shoulder stretches.	Bakasana; Bhujapidasana; Adho Mukha Vrksasana Prep 1 and 2 at wall; optional Adho Mukha Vrksasana at wall. Pincha Mayurasana Prep 1 and 2 at wall; optional Pincha Mayurasana at wall. Wrist and shoulder stretches.	Adho Mukha Vrksasana, Pincha Mayurasana; Sirsasana II Arm Balance vinyasa (options: Bakasana, Tittibhasana; Parsva Bakasana, Eka Pada Koundinyasana, Urdhva Kukkutasana). Astavakrasana, Galavasana, Uttana Prasithasana.

	Level 1: 75 minutes	Level 2: 90 minutes	Level 3: 108 minutes
Back bends	Salabhasana A 3 times; Setu Bandha Sarvangasana 1–3 times.	Prep: Anjaneyasana with shoulder stretches. Salabhasana A 1–3 times; Salabhasana C Prep 1–3 times; Setu Bandha Sarvangasana 1–3 times; or Dhanurasana 1–3 times Optional Urdhva Dhanurasana 1–3 times	Optional Urdhva Dhanurasana 1–3 times Prep: Anjaneyasana, Virasana and shoulder stretches. Salabhasana A 5 breaths to Chaturanga vinyasa to Salabhasana B 5 breaths to Chaturanga vinyasa to Salabhasana C 5 breaths to Chaturanga vinyasa to Dhanurasana 1–3 times to Chaturanga vinyasa to Urdhva Dhanurasana 1–3 times to Viparita Dandasana 1–3 times Optional Eka Pada in Urdhva Dhanurasana and Viparita Dandasana; optional drop-backs.
Twists	Jathara Parivartanasana with both knees bent; Bharadvajrasana I; Marichyasana C Prep. Hold each 1–2 minutes.	Jathara Parivartanasana; Ardha Matsyendrasana Prep; Marichyasana C; Swastikasana. Hold each 1–2 minutes.	Jathara Parivartanasana; Ardha Matsyendrasana; Marichyasana C; Bharadvajrasana II; Marichyasana D; Swastikasana. Hold each 1–2 minutes.
Forward bends and hip openers	Dandasana; Paschimottanasana; Baddha Konasana; Upavista Konasana.	Dandasana; Paschimottanasana; Janu Sirsasana A; Parivrtta Janu Sirsasana; Baddha Konasana; Upavista Konasana.	Dandasana; Paschimottanasana; Janu Sirsasana A; Baddha Konasana; Tiriang Mukha Eka Pada Paschimottanasana; Krounchasana; Parighasana; Upavista Konasana; Kurmasana
Inversions	Viparita Karani; Salamba Sarvangasana Prep	Viparita Karani, or Sirsasana I; Balasana; Halasana; Salamba Sarvangasana; Karnapidasana; Uttana Padasana.	Sirsasana I (or I–6); Halasana, Salamba Sarvangasana; Urdhva Padmasana; Matsyasana; Uttana Padasana. Add optional Tolasana with kapalabhati for 1 minute, then vinyasa.
Savasana	5 minutes or longer.	5 minutes or longer.	5 minutes or longer.
Meditation	Up to a few minutes.	Several minutes.	As long as possible.

The Next Step in Sequencing

Considering the general properties of asanas within and across asana families covered above, one is close to having the basic tools and insights for crafting classes. The next step in the process is to more closely and specifically identify the constituent elements of individual asanas and what this suggests about their interrelationships and sequencing. Appendix B provides an overview of these elements and relationships that we will draw upon in the design of a variety of classes. Before taking that next step into designing classes, we will look at one final aspect of sequencing in the next chapter: how to sequence your guidance of the asanas, including the order of actions in the asanas and the related instructional cues.

Chapter Four

Sequencing Asana Instructions

The existing phrasebooks are inadequate. They are
well enough as far as they go, but when you fall down
and skin your leg they don't tell you what to say.
—MARK TWAIN

The central irony and challenge of teaching yoga is that the essence and mechanisms of yoga asana practice are primarily internal and largely invisible to you as a teacher. How a student feels in an asana is his or her principal source of instruction and refinement. What he or she does in an asana to explore that refinement ultimately relies on internal mechanisms of feeling, reflection, and action, including intention, attention, the breath, and the body, with its many springs and levers of movement. Thus one's role as a teacher is somewhat limited, relying as it does on your ability to give clear instructions about the breath, alignment, energetic actions, variations, modifications, use of props, risks, and techniques for finding greater ease and stability in each asana and transition. Since every student is different, our effectiveness depends on our ability to give both general guidance to a class and individualized suggestions that address the unique experiences of different students. Your ability to see and hear students in their practice—including challenges to their alignment, the qualities of their stability and ease, their attentiveness—and then to relate to them meaningfully and appropriately based on your perception and understanding are the keys to your effectiveness in sequentially instructing the asana practice.

Teaching What You Know

Working with this reality, it is important to teach asanas sensitively and systematically. This begins with acknowledging your own personal abilities and limitations, and then committing yourself to teaching what you know from experience. Before instructing an asana, you should know what you will teach and how you will teach it, including at least the basic alignment principles and energetic actions, stage-by-stage verbal cues that clearly guide students into and out of the asana, methods of demonstration, alternative forms of the asana, physical cues, and the use of props to support students in most safely and deeply exploring the asana. Your years of practice, intensive study, teacher training, apprenticing, and practice teaching now all come together, fully incorporated into your personal practice and transferred from there onto your teaching palette.

Before teaching an asana to your class, teach it to yourself first. Do the asana over and over, testing what you think you know and playing around with what you understand as its basic principles. Then do the same for a sequence of asanas, experimenting with the effects of different sequences and ways of transitioning. Put together the sequences into an entire class, then do the class on your own, giving yourself silent verbal cues throughout to develop and hone the narrative overlay to your class. Go through each of these steps teaching your friends or family, practicing again and again to refine your skills and knowledge. Reflect on what

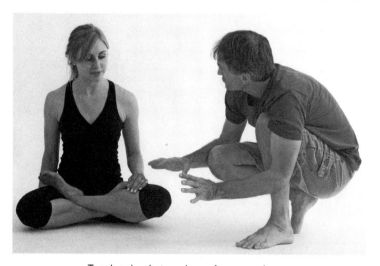
Teach only what you know from experience.

seems to flow easily and not so easily for you, gradually integrating more and more knowledge into your practice teaching. Focus more on the asanas you find most challenging in your own practice and those that seem most difficult to explain throughout your career as a teacher, continuously refining your knowledge and skills.

Before looking at the specific order of actions and related verbal cues in each asana family, we will first address the five essential steps in giving effective guidance.

Step One: Demonstrating Asanas

Demonstration is an essential part of the teaching and learning process, especially for more visually oriented students. With rare exception, you should generally begin your instruction of any asana by demonstrating it to students along with explaining its contraindications, foundational elements, alignment principles, energetic actions, and modifications. Here you are giving your students a clearer map of the path ahead. There are two basic types of demonstration:

In-the-flow demonstration: You or an assistant model what you are instructing as you are saying it, giving students a live example of what you are asking them to do as they are doing it. Ideally, you mirror the class, facing them from a place where they all see you and vice versa, then demonstrating as if they are looking into a mirror (i.e., your left foot turns out when you say, "Please turn your right foot out."). This is an essential skill for all flow-type classes and one that is useful in all styles of Hatha yoga, allowing your students to see what you are asking them to do without interrupting their practice.

Gather-around demonstration: You pause the flow of the class and ask students to gather around you or an assistant to observe an asana. This allows you to provide more detailed instruction and demonstration while students can more closely observe the various elements of an asana as you demonstrate and explain it to the class.

Generally, do in-the-flow demonstrations to cue the initial movement visually into each asana throughout the class. Depending on the nature of the class—primarily the steadiness of the flow and the students' level of proficiency with the asanas—you can devote more or less time to this initial visual cue. With beginning-level classes that deserve more elaborate guidance, give slower

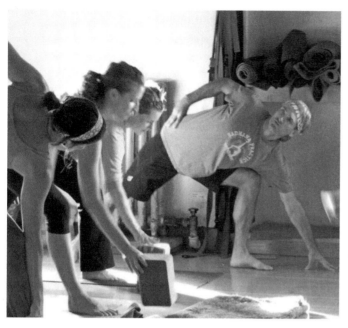
Demonstrating an asana

demonstrations that more fully highlight the alignment and risk-reduction elements of the asana, even when in the flow of the practice. With more advanced classes, you might give the visual demonstration in the span of a single breath, instructing the class to stay with the asana as you begin to move around, observe students in their practice, and give further guidance.

Try positioning yourself where everyone can most easily see you, initially on your mat but throughout the class wherever your visual line with the most students is most open (they can see you and you can see them). From the first asana, demonstrate exactly what you are asking your class to do. For example, say, "Stepping your feet together at the front of your mat, please draw your palms together at your heart." While saying these words, do exactly that in a slightly dramatic fashion that captures the students' attention and effectively conveys what you are asking them to do, matching verbal cues with your physical movements. As the class progresses into more complex asanas, continue to show how to move into each asana. Always emphasize how the breath initiates and guides the movement of the body.

While workshops are the likeliest place you will give elaborate gather-around demonstrations, it benefits students when you pause the flow from time to time to focus on a single asana or small number of linked asanas.[1] When using the gather-around method, do the following:

- Position yourself in the middle of the room, and ask everyone to gather in to see you.
- Encourage the class to move around during the demonstration so that they can observe from different vantage points.
- Explain what you are about to do, and very briefly demonstrate the final pose or the short sequence while explaining what you are

doing and noting any significant risks. For example, if demonstrating Bakasana (Crane Pose) from Salamba Sirsasana II (Tripod Headstand), come to all fours (explain wrist placement and energetic actions), place your head down on the floor (discuss placement and alignment of the head, neck, and shoulders), slide your feet in (discuss changes in the foundation and spine), extend your legs overhead into Salamba Sirsasana II (show alternatives, including one leg up at a time, bent knees to chest, and piking up with both legs together), draw your knees to your shoulders (explain core activation as the primary source of levity), elevate into Bakasana (highlight shifting the weight, pada bandha, and mula bandha), release your head back to the floor (reiterate neck alignment), return to Salamba Sirsasana II (address the lower back and neck), and return to all fours, Balasana (Child's Pose), or demonstrate moving from Salamba Sirsasana II to Chaturanga Dandasana (Four-Limbed Staff Pose).

- Repeat the same demonstration, this time pausing stage by stage to explain in detail the alignment, energetic actions, modifications, variations, and use of props for the asana. Speak as clearly as you can, staying with the essentials of the asanas and giving only three or four main points for each.
- If props are involved, ask students to have them in place.
- Be particularly clear about the gradual and successive movements of the body while transitioning into the asana, refining it, and transitioning out.
- After your demonstration, ask for questions. Ask the students if anything was unclear to them. Further prompt questions by asking about specific aspects of the asana, including transitions in and out.
- When students return to their mats, guide them through the same sequence of steps while moving around the room to offer individualized guidance and support.

Step Two: Transitioning into Asanas

Frequently reminding students to stay present, stay with their breath, and relax, begin your instruction of every asana by succinctly explaining its initial foundation and most essential elements. This includes the initial alignment of the body prior to coming into the asana, focusing on whatever is (a) most connected to the floor, (b) most immediately relevant to the spine, and (c) potentially most at risk of being strained. The foundation is about balanced grounding that lends to stability, ease, and the cultivation of space throughout the body, especially along the spine. While the most basic foundation is built through whatever is on the floor, in many asanas there are secondary sources of foundation that greatly affect how the full asana is ultimately expressed. For example, the feet and legs are the basic foundation for standing asanas, while the pelvis is the secondary foundation, the positioning of which will affect the spine, shoulders, arms, and breath. These secondary foundations are most often in the pelvic and shoulder girdles but may be elsewhere, as we will see later in this chapter when looking at sequencing cues within each asana family. Even though not the primary foundation, consider the secondary foundations as essential to the overall asana.

From the foundation, explain the other elements of the asana while guiding the class into it stage by stage. While specific instructions will vary depending on the specific asana, basic cues for transitioning should almost invariably begin with "staying grounded" or some similar statement that emphasizes the foundation of the asana.

In the same breath that you are cuing students to stay grounded, begin every specific movement cue by saying "inhaling ...," "with the inhalation ...," or a similar statement that cues students to initiate the movement from the initial foundation while inhaling. In inhaling, students will create more space in their bodies. Depending on the specific asana, you can focus their attention on directing that space to wherever their sense of tension in the specific asana indicates. With some asanas, it will be helpful to cue the connection between the flow of the breath and the initiating actions more than once before making the full transitional movement, rehearsing the connection of breath and movement to better embody it before doing it.

For example, when preparing for Setu Bandha Sarvangasana (Bridge Pose), students will be lying supine with their feet placed parallel to each other and in line with their hips. Your initiating cues might go as follows:

- *As calm and relaxed as can be, please let your knees rest together for a moment and draw your palms to your heart and belly, feeling the natural movement in your body with the flow of the breath.*

- *Feel how, with each slow, deep full breath in, everything expands—your side and back ribs spread, your chest expands, your collarbones spread away from each other.*

- *As you slowly release the breath, feel how everything in your body releases. Fully completing the exhalations, feel how your belly naturally engages, your lower back presses toward the floor, and your tailbone starts to curl up off the floor.*

- *Staying with this, expanding the breath, keep allowing the natural pauses between the breaths.*

- *With the completion of the exhalation, feel your tailbone curling up and your pubic bone drawing back toward your belly. This is the action that you want to initiate your movement into back bends like Bridge Pose, Setu Bandha Sarvangasana.*

- *Staying with it, please separate your knees just above your heels and release your arms down by your sides.*

- *Staying with the breath, on your next few exhales feel your tailbone curl up and go with it a little more.*

- *Activating pada bandha to help rotate your inner thighs downward and help take pressure away from your sacrum, when you next exhale all the breath out and feel your tailbone start to curl up, with the inhalation keep rooting through your feet and let your tailbone lead the way up into your expression of Bridge Pose.*

Depending on the style of Hatha yoga and the level and intention of the class, the methods and details of transitional action will vary to some degree. For example, in some styles such as Iyengar yoga, standing asanas are generally approached from Tadasana (Mountain Pose) or Prasarita stance, while in flow-oriented classes such as Vinyasa Flow, most standing asanas are approached from Adho Mukha Svanasana (Downward-Facing Dog Pose) or directly from another standing asana. In some classes you will give more emphasis to subtle energetic actions such as mula bandha, while in others you will keep your cues focused on the most basic elements. But regardless of style, level, and other considerations, cue the initiation of movement into the asana with the inhalation, all the while rooting and expanding with stability and ease.

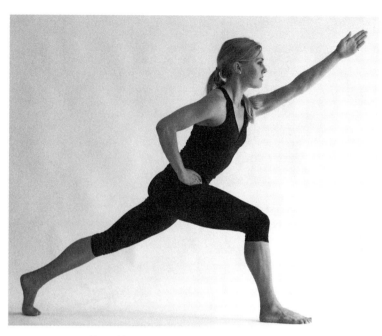

Transitioning into Parivrtta Parsvakonasana

How one transitions into an asana often determines what the asana will be like once in it. Ideally one transitions into asanas with clear transitional alignment. In moving from one body position to another the alignment elements change, as do the energetic actions. Thus it is important to give clear guidance to the alignment and energetic actions that help bring students into the asana in a way that helps ensure proper alignment, engagement, and release. With many asanas, if a student transitions into it out of alignment, not only will associated risks be exacerbated, the surest path to getting properly aligned might require starting over. For clarity let's look at cuing a class into Virabhadrasana II (Warrior II Pose) from Tadasana; these cues are for transitioning in, not refining the asana once there (which is the topic of the next section):

- *Preparing for Warrior II, please step or jump your feet about four feet apart facing this direction* (you are already standing in that direction and facing the entire class, your feet already positioned to demonstrate the transition into Virabhadrasana II).
- *Separate your feet the length of one of your legs plus one of your feet, positioning your feet parallel with each other* (appreciating that

cuing arbitrarily set distances is problematic given that students' physical proportions are typically widely varied).

- *Turn your right foot out ninety degrees and your left foot slightly in.* (You are demonstrating this.) *Please draw your hands to your hips, and position your hips where they feel level* (demonstrate this with exaggerated movement to make clear what you are asking). *Now move your pelvis forward and back a few times to find where it feels like your pelvis is neutral or level.*

- *Maintaining level hips and a neutral pelvis, please extend your arms out away from each other, turn your palms up for a moment, bend your elbows, root your shoulder blades down against your back ribs, and then keeping them there, stretch your arms back out away from other and turn your palms back toward the floor.*

- *Gazing over your right fingertips, radiating down through your legs while rooting your feet with pada bandha, draw in a deep inhale while extending up taller through your spine.*

- *Exhaling, slowly bend your right knee, guiding it to the center-line of your foot while keeping your back leg straight, strong, and grounded and your spine tall. If your knee travels beyond your heel, crawl your toes father forward so that no matter how deeply you bend your knee, it is aligned directly above your heel.*

- *Notice how in bending your knee there may be a tendency for your pelvis to rotate forward. Be more interested in maintaining pelvic neutrality than how deeply you bend your knee while over time exploring bending your knee until your thigh is level with the floor.*

Imagine for a moment simply asking a mixed-level class (which most are, despite class level distinctions) to come into Virabhadrasana II. Looking around, you will find that the front knee of many students has traveled beyond their heel, which can place potentially injurious pressure on the anterior cruciate ligaments when pressing back out of the asana. You will also likely find the front knee splayed in, which can cause twisting forces in the knee (which doesn't twist at all in this position) and outward (abduction) force in the hip (a major issue for students with bursitis or a replaced hip). The pelvis will likely be rotated forward, causing excessive lordosis in the lumbar spine and causing misalignment farther up the spine. And there is plenty more that could be awry, from the back foot and leg to the shoulders, neck, and arms. Clearly, guiding students in transitions matters.

Allowing ample time to guide your class clearly into each asana will help ensure that each student comprehends your instructions in their bodymind. Exercising patience and speaking with clarity will allow your students to feel more comfortable in gradually establishing the various elements of the asana. By encouraging more conscious transitioning into the asanas, students will more deeply appreciate the importance of paying attention to what they are doing and will move with more refined awareness. The effect of this more conscious transitioning will be the safer exploration and refinement of students' asana practices, and for those students interested in going farther, a surer path to a deeper, sustainable practice.

Step Three: Refining Asanas

Asanas are always alive and evolving with every breath. As students tune in to what they feel in an asana, they have the opportunity to explore the deepening of their experience in it—stretching more or less, applying more or less effort, cultivating simpler balance, involving different parts of their bodies in varying ways, refining the breath, consciously awakening and moving energy and opening to more subtle awareness. In a student's personal practice, he or she might fully and constantly be present to all these elements, fully present to the experience, and conscious in exploring.

As a teacher you can encourage and guide this process of self-reflection and refinement by suggesting attentiveness to these elements of refinement along with giving specific suggestions for modification and variation based on your observation. Indeed, your guidance on refinement, including modifications, begins when you initially guide students into an asana, your verbal cues ideally always deriving in part from what you are observing in the class. Once students are in an asana you will have plenty of new insight that informs further specific guidance. This starts with keen, appreciative, systematic observation. Beginning from the initial setting of the foundation of the asana, your verbal cues should increasingly reflect your observation of the entire class and individual students as you teach to the tendencies that you are observing rather than to a predetermined script of cues.[2]

After initially guiding students into an asana, pause and notice what they are actually doing. The relative attentiveness, understanding, body intelligence, muscle strength and flexibility, bone structure, and other factors will result in often tremendous variation in how different students appear in the asana. Looking closely, what do you see? Look at the student from her foundation to her spine to her breath to her face to her limbs, observing from different angles to notice what might be more or less obvious from the front, back, and different sides. Does she appear stable? Relaxed? How is her breath flowing? Does her face appear relaxed or tense? Are her eyes soft and focused or hard and shifting? Does she appear balanced? Is she making occasional large adjustments in position or smaller adjustments synchronized with her breath? What is your overall impression? What do you first notice, especially in relationship to what is most at risk in the asana? What one or two simple modifications do you think will most benefit the student's sense of stability, ease, balance, and happiness in the asana? Has she followed the initial alignment instructions? Does it appear that she is consciously grounding and radiating? What parts of her body appear actively involved in the asana? Do you see where she might benefit from applying more or less effort to create more stability, ease, and space? Does she appear ready to explore variations that take the asana in a more challenging direction?

Based on your observations, give more specific instructions. Be clear in directing instructions to the entire class rather than to an individual student or subset of students. For example, in Utthita Trikonasana (Extended Triangle Pose), some students will likely hyperextend the knee of their front leg. Instructing the entire class, you can say, "Rooting down strongly from the top of your legs and down through your feet, keep awakening the muscles in your legs, engaging your quadriceps and feeling your kneecaps lifting." Addressing those with hyperextension in their knee, continue by saying, "If you tend to hyperextend your front knee, try to microbend it and maintain that positioning while still trying to engage your quads." If you are addressing a single student with specific instructions, either go directly to that student to work with him or her (observe, give verbal cues, give hands-on cues, offer a prop) or say the person's name from a distance to ensure that it is clear the specific instruction is for that student only. Ideally you will give more individualized verbal cues quietly to just that student.

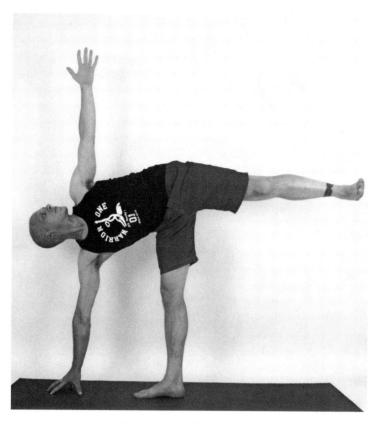

Refining Ardha Chandrasana

In giving refining cues, start by addressing whatever is most at risk in the asana. For instance, if the class has just arrived in Utthita Trikonasana with a cue to gaze up to the thumb tip, the neck is generally most at risk (unless a student has an injury or some condition that is placed at greater risk in the asana). The first verbal cue would then be something like, "If it troubles your neck holding your head up, completely relax your neck and let your head gently drop down." Similarly, if there is a pregnant student in the class and you are in an asana in which there are modifications for her stage or condition of pregnancy, cue the modification before moving to other areas of refinement.

Many students will arrive in an asana attempting to go much farther than they should, usually causing misalignment in their positioning and compromising the breath. In reiterating basic alignment cues, blend in verbal, hands-on, and demonstrative cues for modifying in ways that make the asana more accessible, including the use of props. Here you might also suggest that students make the breath more interesting than the asana, exploring the asanas around the integrity of the breath rather than trying to squeeze the breath into what they are attempting to do with their body.

To better guide students into alignment, offer balanced alignment cues that help them to better feel and understand how combining different energetic actions leads to greater stability and openness. Here are several examples of oppositional balances:

Table 4.1. Cueing Oppositional Actions

Oppositional Balances	Unifying Verbal Cues	Examples of Asanas
	Front–Back	
Feet	"Root down equally through your heels and the balls of your feet."	All standing asanas
Lower legs	"Draw your shins back while releasing your calves toward your heels."	All standing asanas
Knees	"Engage your quadriceps muscles, lifting your kneecaps while spreading the backs of your knees."	Tadasana
Thighs	"Press the tops of your thighs back while releasing evenly through your hamstrings."	Utthita Trikonasana
Pelvis	"Draw your pubic bone back and up while drawing your tailbone back and down."	Adho Mukha Svanasana
	"Lift the front of your hips away from your front leg while lightly drawing your lower belly and sacrum toward each other."	Virabhadrasana I
Spine	"Expand your lower back ribs while allowing your lower front ribs to soften in."	Virabhadrasana II
Shoulders	"Allow your shoulder blades to release down your back while spreading across your collarbones."	Tadasana
Neck/head	"Draw your chin very slightly forward, down, and in while spreading across the back of your neck."	Adho Mukha Svanasana
	Upper–Lower	
Pada/mula bandha	"Rooting evenly through your feet while lifting your inner arches, spiral your inner thighs back while drawing your sitting bones toward each other and lifting steadily from the front floor of your pelvis with mula bandha."	All standing asanas, inversions, and back bends
Feet/hips	"Root down from the tops of your femurs through your feet and into the earth while engaging pada bandha and drawing the muscular energy in your legs in and up."	Parsvottanasana
Pelvis/spine	"Maintaining a feeling of pelvic neutrality and mula bandha, energetically draw up tall through your spine."	Utkatasana
Shoulders/fingers	"Lightly hugging your shoulder blades to your back ribs, radiate out through your arms and fingertips."	Urdhva Hastasana
Mula bandha/palate	"Aware of mula bandha, feel a sense of energy drawing up through your spine and lending a quality of light lifting and spreading of your palate."	Padmasana

Table 4.1. Cueing Oppositional Actions (continued)

Oppositional Balances	Unifying Verbal Cues	Examples of Asanas
	Upper–Lower	
Mula bandha/ corona capitis	"Staying with mula bandha, lengthen from the base of your spine out through the crown of your head."	Dandasana
Pada bandha/ corona capitis	"Connecting with the earth, feel the awakening of your feet and inner arches as a source of energy up through the midline of your body and out through the crown of your head."	Tadasana
	Inside–Outside	
Feet	"While rooting the outer edge of your back foot, keep grounding through the ball of your foot."	Utthita Trikonasana
Ankles	"Bring the inner and outer ankle bones level and centered between the foot and leg."	All standing asanas
Knees	"Relaxing through your hips and inner thighs, bend your knees and draw your feet together while maintaining a sense of even pressure through the inside and outside of your knees."	Baddha Konasana
Legs	"Cultivating pada bandha, spiral your inner thighs back while energetically drawing your shins toward each other."	Tadasana
Pelvis	"Spiraling your inner thighs back to create spaciousness in your sacrum, draw the outside of your hips in toward the core of your body, feeling an accentuated lift of your perineum."	Tadasana Dandasana Urdhva Dhanurasana
Spine	"Engaging mula bandha, visualize and consciously feel energy drawing into the core of your spine while radiating out from your spine through the sides of your torso."	All asanas
Shoulders	"Drawing your shoulder blades in against your back ribs, spiral your shoulder blades out away from your spine."	Adho Mukha Svanasana
Arms	"Spiraling your inner forearms toward the floor while rooting firmly across the entire span of your palms and out through your fingers, spiral your shoulder blades out away from your spine as if to wrap the triceps side of your arms out and down toward the floor."	Adho Mukha Svanasana

Once basic alignment and safety are addressed, go back to the foundation of the asana to emphasize the relationship between roots and extension. Here are several ways to guide this relationship:

Table 4.2. Roots and Extension

Foundation	Principles and Verbal Cues	Asana Examples
Hands	• When the palms are on the floor, instruct students to spread their fingers as wide as they comfortably can, their thumbs not quite so wide (about one-third less than maximum) in order to prevent injury in the thenar space between the thumb and index finger. • Radiating out from the center of the palm through the knuckles and tips of each finger and thumb, students should root down firmly through all of their knuckles, the entire span of their palms, and through the entire length of each finger and thumb. • From this rootedness, ask students to create a feeling of drawing up energetically from the inner palm through the inner wrist and up through the arms and into the shoulders. • It is important to root the knuckles of the index fingers and thumbs in order to balance the pressure across the entire span of the palms and create a balanced foundation for stability and space through the wrists.	Adho Mukha Svanasana (Down Dog) Adho Mukha Vrksasana (Handstand) Chaturanga Dandasana (Four-Limbed Staff Pose)
Feet	• Balance the weight equally through the "four corners" of each foot. • Root more firmly down into the inner edge of the balls of the feet to more fully awaken and lift the inner arches and ankles. • Spread the toes wide and press them down without clinching.	All standing asanas
Sitting bones	• In all seated asanas, the primary initial action is to root down firmly into the sitting bones, emphasizing the front portion of the sitting bones rooting more firmly down as a means of cultivating a neutral pelvic tilt. • Do not pull the flesh of the buttocks away from the sitting bones. • Create a subtle feeling of drawing the sitting bones toward each other to stimulate the light contraction of the transverse perineal muscles and thereby awaken mula bandha. • Try to maintain the connection of the sitting bones into the floor when folding forward and/or twisting.	Tadasana (Mountain Pose) Paschimottanasana (Seated Forward Bend)
Legs	• When the legs are straight, run a strong line of energy from the tops of the thighbones down through the legs, ankles, and the center of the heels. Do this whether sitting or standing, whether with the legs together (as in Tadasana) or apart (as in Prasarita Padottanasana). • Create a feeling of drawing the musculature of the legs into the bones of the legs, while spiraling the inner thighs down (if sitting) or back (if standing in internally rotated standing asanas).	Dandasana (Staff Pose) Upavista Konasana (Wide-Angle Forward Bend Pose)

Table 4.2. Roots and Extension (continued)

Foundation	Principles and Verbal Cues	Asana Examples
Arms	• With the shoulder blades spiraling out away from the spine while rooted down against the back ribs, integrate the arms into the torso. • Extend strongly from the top of the arm bones down through the arms, elbows, and wrists into the hands and out through the fingertips. • Drawing the musculature of the arms evenly to the bone, energetically draw energy up through the arms.	Adho Mukha Svanasana (Down Dog) Adho Mukha Vrksasana (Handstand)
Head	• Maintaining the natural curvature of the cervical spine, press the top of the head (corona capitis) firmly into the floor without grinding the head down.	Sirsasana I (Headstand)

When holding an asana for a relatively long duration, you can introduce a variety of instructions to cue a deeper refinement or opportunity for further exploration. Here are a few examples, each of which assumes that the class is ready to go deeper and that individual student modifications have been addressed:

Table 4.3. Deeper Refining Cues

Tadasana (Mountain Pose)	"Maintaining pada bandha, feel the awakening of your inner thighs, slightly spiraling them back, and from there a feeling of lightly drawing your sitting bones toward each other, awakening a sense of mula bandha as you lift lightly and steadily from your perineum, energetically lifting from the floor of your pelvis up through your spine, expanding across your heart center and lengthening out through the crown of your head."
Uttanasana (Standing Forward Bend Pose)	"While rooting through your feet and feeling the rebounding effect as your legs engage, feel your sitting bones extending up. Now try to create a feeling of pitching your pubic bone more back and up while stretching your belly button toward your heart, your heart toward the earth."
Urdhva Mukha Svanasana (Upward-Facing Dog Pose)	"Inhaling into Upward-Facing Dog, create a feeling of pulling your spine through toward your chest, lifting and spreading across your collarbones while drawing your shoulder blades down and in against your back ribs; exhaling, engage from your belly to lift your hips up and back to Downward-Facing Dog, your pubic bone leading the way."
Adho Mukha Svanasana (Downward-Facing Dog Pose)	"While pressing firmly and evenly down through your palms and fingers, try to engage your legs more fully, pressing the tops of your thighbones strongly back to cultivate more length through your spine."

Table 4.3. Deeper Refining Cues (continued)

Virabhadrasana I (Warrior I Pose)	"Keeping the outer edge of your back foot firmly rooting down, try to maintain a feeling of pelvic neutrality while spiraling the inner thigh of your back leg strongly back. Feel from that strong foundation more openness in your lower back, breath by breath consciously lengthening up through your spine. Try to keep your lower front ribs softening in to help maintain the natural curvature of your spine while stretching strongly up and back through your arms and fingertips."
Virabhadrasana II (Warrior II Pose)	"Without moving either of your feet, imagine your mat is covered with warm honey and ghee. How would you maintain your stability? Bring more awareness into your feet. Without actually moving them, create an energetic action of drawing your feet toward each other. Feel this more fully awaken the muscles in the inside of your legs, and from there feel a more natural and full awakening of mula bandha, all the while breathing and creating more and more space through your spine and across your heart center as you run lines of energy out through your fingertips and the crown of your head."
Ardha Chandrasana (Revolved Half Moon Pose)	"Exploring wrapping, please either stay as you are or, being attentive to keeping your left hip revolved on top of your right hip, change as little as possible in reaching back with your left hand to clasp your left foot. Honoring your intention and your lower back, explore either pulling that foot back away from your hip or, if you have the flexibility in your hips and shoulder, explore placing your hand on your foot in a Bhekasana (Frog Pose) position, then press your left foot toward your left hip. See if you can clamp your left hip with that same hand. If that is easy and you feel stable, begin to explore clasping that foot with both hands and balance on just your standing leg."
Sirsasana I (Headstand I)	"Without gripping in your belly, feel the light, subtle engagement of your belly with each and every exhalation, feeling with it a sense of more stability yet spaciousness through your pelvis and spine. Maintaining that awareness, stability, and spaciousness, begin to explore slowly lowering your legs halfway down toward the floor while running lines of energy out through your legs and through the balls of your feet. Go only so far down as you feel stable and free of strain. Try to hold for up to five breaths before slowly extending your legs back up overhead, all the while extending from the crown of your rooted head up through your spine and out through your feet."

Step Four: Transitioning out of Asanas

The very idea of asana can exert a powerful effect on the awareness of teachers and students, especially when asanas are approached as something to be attained or mastered rather than as part of a process of self-discovery and transformation. One consequence is focusing so intently on getting into the deepest possible expression of an asana that little awareness is given to transitioning out. Considerable anecdotal evidence based on years of observation indicates that more students are injured coming out of an asana than either transitioning into it or holding and exploring it. As Desikachar (1995, 27) says, "It is not enough to climb the tree; we must be able to get back down too."

Guiding students out of asanas involves applying your understanding of what is at risk in the transitional movement and giving specific physical actions students can apply in their own movement. Just as the extent of risk will vary depending on the asana and the students, your instructions should be tailored to address this varied situation. In most asana transitions this begins with bringing awareness back to the foundation of the asana and reestablishing a feeling of stable grounding. Encouraging students to keep the spine and other potentially vulnerable joints in mind, your verbal cues should guide them through sequential releasing actions in which the stable foundation of the asana is maintained. In most asanas this involves bringing greater effort into a specific line of energy that, when activated, relieves potential pressure on vulnerable joints.

For example, in transitioning a class from Utthita Trikonasana back to standing upright, many students—especially those with the idea that asanas are poses disconnected from how one approaches and releases from them—will lackadaisically, unconsciously, or quickly draw right back up. This way of transitioning will cause some students to experience stress in the lower back or to strain the hamstrings of the front leg. To cue actions to minimize these risks, you can say, "Completing your exhale, root down more firmly from the top of your back hip into your back foot. Maintaining that steady energetic action, inhaling, slowly draw your torso back up to standing across the span of that entire inhalation."

In a variety of other standing asanas in which the torso is extended laterally or folded forward, you can use a similar cue along with emphasizing the natural engagement of the abdominal muscles as the breath flows out, then cueing the class to maintain the light engagement of their core while inhaling back up. For example, in transitioning out of Parsvottanasana (Intense Extended Side Stretch Pose), the full weight of the upper body is suspended forward and down from the pelvis, requiring the hip extensors and muscles along the low back to strongly contract in bringing the torso back up to vertical, which for many students places undue stress on their lower back. With the last exhalation in this asana, you want students to maintain the activation of their abdominal muscles and then ground more strongly down through their legs and feet while leading with their heart in drawing all the way up, their belly giving added support to their lower back.

Many transitions out of asanas involve moving part of the body toward the earth rather than away, in which case the risk is in losing control and either straining a stabilizing muscle due to stretch reflex or falling to the floor. This includes many standing balance asanas, arm balances, and inversions. For instance, in lowering the feet to the floor from Sirsasana I (Headstand I), the tendency is for the legs to drop quickly without much awareness, often causing a shift in the foundation of the asana (impacting the neck) and stretch reflex in muscles that are eccentrically contracting across the back of the body. Here again it is important to reiterate grounding actions, core abdominal support, and slow movement in order to have a more conscious, simpler, and safer release. You can also offer transitional options, starting with bending the knees, drawing the heels toward the hips, and then slowly releasing the thighs toward the chest as part of an easier path to getting the feet and legs back to the floor.

As appropriate for the level of experience among students in your class, give a visual demonstration of how to safely transition out of these asanas prior to guiding students into them. Once you have guided the class into the asana, give clear cues on transitioning out a few breaths prior to asking them to release out or down. When releasing from inverted asanas, encourage students not to suddenly spring fully upright, as this can cause light-headedness and fainting.

A common thread in these examples is that in all asana transitions, it is important to emphasize a gradual release connected with the breath, allowing students to feel what starts to happen as they initiate the transitional movement. This allows the gradual relaxation of muscles that were active in supporting the asana while bringing more awareness to the muscles being newly activated when transitioning out. To the extent that the exiting transition is smooth and graceful, students can remain more attuned to the subtle energetic effects of the asana, which will then carry over more fully and naturally into the next asana.

Step Five: Absorbing and Integrating the Effects of Asanas

Every asana has an effect on the bodymind. Yet we often move so quickly from one asana to the next that many of the more subtle (and often not so subtle) effects are seemingly lost. As discussed in Chapter Two, the pratikriyasana practice is one important way of most fully absorbing and integrating the effects of asanas. So is simple rest, allowing or encouraging students to pause, especially after particularly intense asanas or sequences, and soak in the energetic sensations pulsating through them. Refer back to the sidebar in Chapter Two on *Deepening the Integration of Asana* for several ways to create space for this exploration.

Sequencing Cues Within Asana Families

We can now look more specifically at the order of cues in each asana family. The suggestions presented here should be approached in the broader context

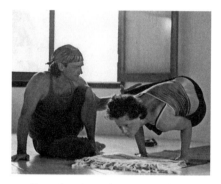

Be patient in cueing your students.

of the five-step process presented above for guiding students in all asanas. Clearly, there is potentially a lot to say, and all those words can get in the way of students being in the inner experience of their practice. With time and practice, you will find brevity in your cues by being more succinct with efficient and clear language. To help refine your verbal guidance, record yourself teaching once a month for the first year of teaching, every three months in the next few years, and at least once a year after ten years of teaching—and listen to your recordings.

Sequencing Cues for Standing Asanas

Using Tadasana as the foundational asana, instruct from the ground up, as follows:

- Give instructions for pada bandha and teach the importance of balancing the weight equally between the front, back, inside, and outside of each foot.

- With pada bandha active, instruct the contraction of the quadriceps along with the slight internal rotation of the femurs while pressing the femurs back, emphasizing how the internal rotation eases discovery of pelvic neutrality while broadening the space between the sitting bones.

- Note that most students tend to tilt their pelvis anteriorly, which compresses the lower back and can lead to vertebral disk problems. A practice of opening and strengthening of the hip flexors, hip extensors, and abdominal core will help students move into stable pelvic neutrality.

- Guide students into feeling the connection between pada bandha and mula bandha, encouraging them to maintain mula bandha throughout their asana practice.

- With pelvic neutrality, the spine will come into its natural curvature (neutral extension) in most students unless there is significant muscular imbalance or a pathological condition such as scoliosis, kyphosis, or leg length discrepancy.

- Guide students into the light abdominal engagement that occurs naturally with complete exhalations, emphasizing how this helps to stabilize and lengthen the lumbar spine. The belly should be supple and stable.

- Cue the further lengthening of the spine by encouraging lifting the lower rim of the ribs up and away from the upper rim of the pelvis while allowing the floating ribs to soften naturally into the body.

- Cue students to lift and broaden the sternum from inside while allowing the shoulder blades to draw lightly down and against the back ribs, further accentuating an expansive heart center while stabilizing the shoulders and creating ease in the neck.

- Instruct the broadening of the collarbones by first lifting the shoulders toward the ears, then drawing them back and down without losing the alignment in the lower- and mid-thoracic areas of the spine.

- Refine the positioning of the neck and head by instructing students to feel the positioning of their ears in line with their shoulders, then to draw the chin very slightly forward and down, lengthening the back of the neck while lifting through the throat.

- Finally, cue opening the crown of the head to the sky.

Sequencing Cues for Arm Support Asanas

In introducing arm balances, start with simple preparatory practices as described later for each asana. Offer students an opportunity to practice each arm balance two to three times. Ask them to pay close attention to what happens in each attempt: Where did they feel their weight? Where is their gaze? How is the breath flowing? What caused or led them to come out of the asana? What are they thinking about? What are they feeling? Encourage students to keep reflecting on what happens each time they try the asanas, gradually refining what they are doing to make the asanas simpler, more stable, and more fun.

- Explain the foundation, which is either through the hands or the forearms and hands.
- With the hands, emphasize spreading the fingers wide part but the thumbs not so wide apart so that the nerves and ligaments in the thenar space between the base of the thumb and the metatarsal of the index finger are not strained.
- Teach balanced rooting across the entire span of the palms, including firmly rooting down through the knuckles of the index fingers in order to create a balanced foundation and to equalize pressure through the wrist joints. This action is accentuated by creating a feeling of spiraling the inner forearms down (while rotating the shoulders out broadly away from the spine).
- Cue the relationship between firmly rooting the hands and lifting out through the wrists, arms, and shoulders.
- Keep the gaze focused on a single point, usually between the thumbs, without straining the neck.
- Encourage a feeling of stable buoyancy in the shoulders, sufficiently engaged to maintain stability while sufficiently mobile to refine positioning and reduce pressure in the shoulder joints.
- Emphasize steady engagement of the abdominal core (light mula bandha and *uddiyana bandha*) to create more stability in asanas such as Adho Mukha Vrksasana (Handstand) in which drawing energy to the center of the body lends to balance and to levity in asanas such as Bakasana in which a sustained abdominal lift contributes to elevating the pelvis above the shoulders.

In arm support asanas in which the feet or legs are together, encourage students to commit to keeping them together as a source of stability.

Down Dog as the Foundational Arm Support Asana

Following the basic principles of sequencing instructions, guide the building of full Adho Mukha Svanasana (Downward-Facing Dog Pose) from the ground up and from what is at most risk of strain or injury: the wrists, shoulders, and hamstrings. We will look alternatively at the upper body (from the hands up) and lower body (from the feet up). Adho Mukha Svanasana is an excellent asana for learning and embodying the principle of roots and extension. Encourage students to press firmly down into the entire span of their hands and length of their fingers, paying close attention to rooting the knuckle of the index finger as a way of balancing pressure in the wrist joint. This rooting action should originate at the top of the arms. With it, ask students to feel the "rebounce" effect of this rooting action in the natural lengthening through their wrist, elbow, and shoulder joints.

The fingers should be spread wide apart, the thumbs only about two-thirds of the way in order to protect the ligaments in the thenar space between the thumb and index finger. Generally, the middle fingers should be parallel and in line with the shoulders. Look to see if the student's arms are parallel; this will indicate if their hands are in line with their shoulders. The alignment of the wrists with the shoulders allows the proper external rotation of the shoulders, which activates and strength-

ens the teres minor and infraspinatus muscles (two of the four principal rotator cuff muscles), stabilizes the shoulder joint by drawing the scapula firmly against the back ribs, creates more space across the upper back, and thereby allows the neck to relax more easily. If a student has difficulty straightening his or her arms, play with asking that person to turn his or her hands slightly out; if a student tends to hyperextend his or her elbows, have that person turn the palms slightly in.

Tight or weak shoulders create specific risks to the neck, back, elbows, wrists, and shoulders themselves in Adho Mukha Svanasana. In either case, moderate effort in this asana develops both strength and flexibility, opening the shoulders to full flexion while developing deeper, more balanced strength. The shoulder blades should be rooted against the back ribs while spreading the shoulder blades

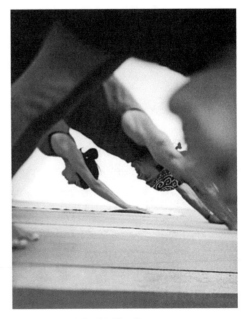

Adho Mukha Svanasana

out away from the spine. Note that externally rotating the shoulders tends to cause the inner palms to lift. This can be countered by internally rotating the forearms.

The roots-and-extension principle applies equally to the lower body. Rooting into the balls of the feet will contribute to lifting the inner arches, which is one effect of pada bandha. This will help to stimulate the awakening of mula bandha. The feet should be placed hip distance apart or wider, with the outer edges of the feet parallel. Firming the thighs and pressing the tops of the femur bones strongly back is a key action (along with rooted hands) in lengthening the spine in this asana. While firming the thighs, encourage students to slightly spiral the inner thighs back to soften pressure in the sacrum, all the while drawing the pubic bone back and up, the tailbone back and slightly down. The first few times in this asana in any given practice, it can feel good and help the body in gently opening to "bicycle" the legs, twisting and sashaying alternately into each hip and stretching long through the sides of the body while exploring the hamstrings, lower back, shoulders, ankles, and feet.

Very flexible students tend to hyperextend their knees in Adho Mukha Svanasana. Guide them to bend their knees slightly. Students with tight hips and hamstrings will find it difficult, painful, or impossible to straighten their legs. Encourage them to separate their feet wider apart (even as wide as their yoga mat) to ease the anterior rotation of the pelvis and the natural curvature of the lumbar spine. Let them know that it is okay to keep their knees bent while holding this asana, very gradually moving into deepening the flexibility of their hamstrings and hip extensors.

With regular practice, the neck will become sufficiently strong and supple to support holding the head between the upper arms (with the ears in line with the arms). Until that strength is developed, encourage students to let their neck relax and head hang. With each and every exhalation, students will feel the light and natural engagement of their abdominal muscles. Encourage them to maintain that light and subtle engagement in their belly while inhaling, without gripping or bearing down in their belly. Keep bringing students' awareness back to the balanced ujjayi pranayama, to roots-and-extension, to a steady gaze, and to the cultivation of steadiness and ease.

Sequencing Cues for Back Bends

- Relax. This is by far the most effective way to go into the deepest, safest back bend.

- Establish the foundation. The mental preparation for back bends draws awareness to the spine and heart center. While this is where we do want to ultimately draw awareness in back bends, the stability of the foundation will allow students to move more safely into their deepest possible back bend.

- Rotate the thighs internally. This internal rotation is most effectively instructed and felt using a block between the thighs in Tadasana, then in Setu Bandha Sarvangasana, and drawing the block back (in Tadasana) or down (in Setu Bandha Sarvangasana). When the bottoms of the feet are on the floor, apply pada bandha to accentuate this action.

- Never deliberately squeeze the buttocks. Instead, cue students to try to soften the upper (more horizontal) fibers of the glutei maximi, which, if contacting, will externally rotate and abduct the thighs, thereby adding pressure to the sacroiliac joint at the base of the spine.

- Posteriorly tilt the pelvis. This action will draw more length into the lumbar spine, reduce pressure on the lower intervertebral disks, and help share the back bend up the spine. Further cue this by asking students to bring the anterior superior iliac spine (ASIS bones) toward their lower front ribs.

- Create length through the spine to allow greater spinal extension (i.e., a deeper back bend). After relaxing along the spine, elongate the spine as much as possible before creating extension.

- Focus the back bend in the thoracic spine. The attachment of ribs (and muscles) to the thoracic spine, combined with the structure of the thoracic vertebrae, limits the extension of the spine and leads to excessive bending in the lumbar and cervical spine segments.

- Add extension of the cervical spine last. Allow the cervical spine to remain neutral or bring it into extension only after maximizing the back bend through the thoracic spine.

- Draw the lower tips of the shoulder blades in and up toward the heart. This deepens the thoracic center of the back bend and further opens the heart center.
- Lift the sternum up. This adds more expansiveness to the heart center.
- Keep the breath steady and soft. Breathe as if through the heart and into areas of tension.

Sequencing Cues for Twists

- Breathing deeply, rooting down, and lengthening up are the keys to deeper twisting.
- When twisting, the vertebrae are naturally drawn closer together, compressing the rib cage and lungs, which makes it more difficult to fully inhale and slowly exhale. While emphasizing roots and extension, give even more emphasis to deepening the inhalation and slowing the exhalation.
- As with other asanas the key to lengthening is rooting, especially in seated twists. Instruct students to firmly root down through their sitting bones and pelvis in all seated twists in order to maintain length and stability in the lower back.
- If one foot is on the floor, as in Ardha Matsyendrasana (Half Lord of the Fishes Pose), cue students to press it down as though standing on it to accentuate the roots-extension relationship.
- Whether seated or supine, guide students to bring more elongation through the spine with each inhale, creating more space to allow a deeper twist as the breath flows out.
- Encouraging students to explore this process dynamically, cue them to back slightly out of the twist with each inhale, thereby finding more ease in lengthening and further rotation on the following exhale, continuing in this way until releasing out of the twist.
- In asymmetrical seated twists, ask students to try to keep their sitting bones even and pelvis neutral; the tendency is for the sitting bone and the side of the pelvis that one is twisting toward to shift back, which creates the illusion of a deeper twist while tending to

draw the twist more into the lumbar spine, and for the pelvis to slump back.

- In supine twists, invite students to be more interested in keeping their shoulder on the floor rather than getting the knee to the floor on the opposite side; this will help to keep the twist more in the thoracic spine rather than in the lower back.
- The neck can be held evenly or added to the twist if comfortable; students can add space and comfort to the neck when twisting by drawing the shoulder blades down the back and spreading across the collarbones.
- In all twists, guide students to initiate movement from the mid-thoracic spine, creating the twist up and down the spine from there.
- Counsel caution and comfort in leveraging twists.
- Twist evenly on both sides. If a student is seated on an elevated prop, arrange the prop to be the same thickness under each sitting bone, thereby promoting the development of equal sitting amid the challenge of drawing the higher sitting bone down.

Sequencing Cues for Forward Bends

- Before folding forward, draw awareness to the breath and through the breath to the entire length of the spine, focusing on relaxing and elongating the spine.
- In all seated forward bends, make the grounding of the sitting bones the primary action. This is best conveyed in Dandasana; rooting down through the sitting bones naturally awakens lines of energy up through the spine and out through the legs, creating the foundation for a safe and deep forward fold.
- Assess students' posture when they are sitting in Dandasana; if they are unable to attain pelvic neutrality (with the sacrum tilted slightly forward), they should sit sufficiently high on a firm prop to ease into that neutrality and work there to elongate the spine.
- Initiate and maximize the forward fold through the anterior rotation of the pelvis while maximizing the neutral extension of the spine. For many students, this will mean remaining in an upright position when exploring most seated forward bends.

- Supine forward bends such as Apanasana (Wind-relieving Pose) and Supta Padangusthasana (Reclined Big Toe Pose) are easiest on the lower back and hamstrings.
- In seated forward bends in which one or both legs are straight (e.g., Dandasana or Paschimottanasana [West Stretching Pose]), internally rotate the thighs while pressing them down to ease the anterior rotation of the pelvis and thereby maintain space in the lower back.

Sequencing Cues for Inversions

The greatest physical risk in inversions is to the neck (this does not apply to Viparita Karani [Active Reversal Pose]). It is very important to give students clear and methodical guidance in setting up for inversions in a way that minimizes this risk. Students with cervical spine issues are advised not to practice any asanas that further strain their neck. Here we will closely look at setting up for the two most commonly taught inversions—Salamba Sirsasana I and Salamba Sarvangasana (Supported Shoulder Stand)—before discussing other inversions. For Salamba Sirsasana I:

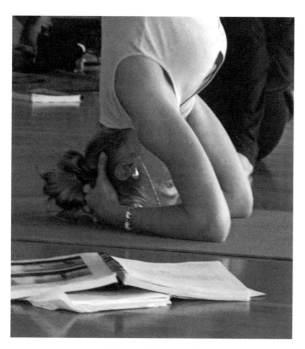

Salamba Sirsasana I

- If students are new to this asana, have them practice it next to a wall.
- Instruct two basic roots: the forearms and top (crown) of the head, starting with the positioning of the arms with the elbows shoulder distance apart.
- Begin with the knees and forearms on the floor. In interlacing the fingers, instruct students to keep the palms wide open and their fingers sufficiently loose to be able to firmly root down from the ulnar side of the wrists to the elbows.
- The top of the head should be placed directly down on the floor with the back of the head braced lightly against the base of the thumbs.

- Ask students to slowly straighten their legs while pressing firmly down through their forearms and drawing their shoulder blades down against their back ribs, their shoulders drawing away from their wrists.

- Maintaining this position, guide students to walk their feet in toward their elbows until bringing their hips as high as possible over their shoulders; encourage students to keep the spine long in this transition. Encourage steady ujjayi pranayama and dristana.

- Rooting down more firmly through the elbows, ask students to try to draw their knees in toward the chest and the heels toward their hips, and then to rotate the pelvis up and slowly extend the legs straight up toward the sky.

- Once upside down, bring awareness back to the roots in the forearms, and cue students to create a feeling of pulling the elbows toward each other without actually moving them; this will broaden the shoulders, activate the latissimi dorsi, and add stability.

- Now accentuate the other source of rooting: press the top of the head fairly firmly down, thereby triggering the roots-and-extension effect, activating the spinal erector and multifidus muscles close to the spine. This will relieve pressure in the neck, elongate the entire spine, and create a feeling of grounded levity.

- Finally, instruct students to bring their ankles together, strongly flex their feet (toes toward their shins), and energetically extend out through their heels before pointing their feet and spreading their toes like lotus petals.

- In releasing from Sirsasana, the easiest method is to bend the knees and draw them toward the chest, slowly lowering into Balasana.

In practicing Salamba Sarvangasana, most students' necks will press into the floor. Over time, with openness and strength in the upper back, shoulders, arms, and chest, their neck will not press into the floor. Until that develops, instruct students to set up a platform using folded blankets, then lie down with their shoulders about three inches in from the edge of the blankets. Once

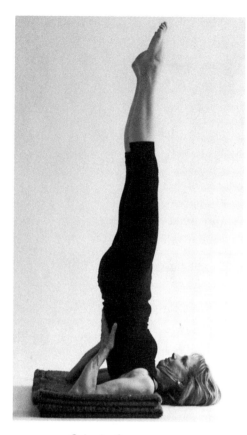

Salamba Sarvangasana

their legs are brought overhead, their shoulders should remain on the platform, their neck free, and their head on the floor. From there, instruct as follows:

- With the arms down by the sides, exhale, pressing into the palms and slowly drawing the legs overhead into Halasana (Plow Pose).

- If the feet do not reach the floor, either prop the hips with the hands and elbows in Ardha Salamba Sarvangasana or come down and practice with a chair or wall overhead for the feet.

- With the feet on the floor overhead, interlace the fingers behind the back and slightly shrug the shoulders under to bring the weight of the body more onto the shoulders.

- Press the feet firmly down into the floor to activate the legs, pressing the tops of the femurs up to help rotate the pelvis anteriorly and thereby draw more length through the lumbar spine. If possible, do this with the feet pointed in plantar flexion; if necessary, keep the toes curled under and consider placing them on a block, chair, or wall.

- Now place the hands on the back as close to the floor as possible (supporting the back) and slowly extend the legs up toward the sky (the easiest method is with the knees bent and using one leg at a time, then, over time, with straight legs moving up together).

Part Two

Designing Beginning,
Intermediate, and
Advanced Classes

Chapter Five

Surya Namaskara—
Sun Salutations

Here comes the sun, and I say / It's all right.
—GEORGE HARRISON

Surya Namaskara (Sun Salutations), which first came into yoga asana practice through the innovative work of K. V. Iyer and T. Krishnamacharya in the 1930s,[1] are an excellent way to begin most yoga asana practices. With modifications and variations, most students can do them. In a group class, they help to unify the class as everyone breathes and moves largely in unison. They warm and awaken the entire body, soften the muscles, open the joints, and stimulate the neurological, circulatory, and subtle energetic pathways, initiating conscious awareness and synchronization of movement in the breath, body, mind, and spirit. With innovation they are a foundation for a variety of creative sequences across all families of asanas.

There are numerous variations and adaptations of Surya Namaskara. In her book *Sun Yoga* (2001), Janita Stenhouse describes twenty-five different variations of Sun Salutations. Here we will focus on three forms: Classical

Surya Namaskara and Surya Namaskara A and B forms. Within each form, there are many variations and modifications that enable teachers to accommodate the varying abilities, special needs, and conditions of different students.

Table 5.1. Twelve Asanas in the Surya Namaskara Family

Asana	Salutation Form
1. Tadasana (Mountain Pose)	Classical, A, B
2. Urdhva Hastasana (Upward Hand Pose)	Classical, A
3. Uttanasana (Standing Forward Bend Pose)	Classical, A, B
4. Ardha Uttanasana (Half Standing Forward Bend Pose)	Classical, A, B
5. Anjaneyasana (Low Lunge Pose)	Classical
6. Phalakasana (Plank Pose)	Classical (A/B option)

Table 5.1. Twelve Asanas in the Surya Namaskara Family (continued)

Asana		Salutation Form
7. Chaturanga Dandasana (Four-Limbed Staff Pose)		A, B
8. Salabhasana B (Locust Pose or "Easy Cobra")		Classical (A/B option)
9. Utkatasana (Chair Pose)		B
10. Urdhva Mukha Svanasana (Upward-Facing Dog Pose)		A, B
11. Adho Mukha Svanasana (Downward-Facing Dog Pose)		Classical, A, B
12. Virabhadrasana I (Warrior I Pose)		B

General Properties of Surya Namaskara

- Excellent for initiating the conscious connection of the breath to movement in the body.
- Excellent for warming the entire body and preparing for all other asanas.
- Classical Surya Namaskara offers a gentler sequence of asanas appropriate for beginning-level and early morning classes.

- Excellent dynamic awakening of the spiral erector muscles, hip flexors, and shoulder girdle.
- In beginning classes, consider preparing for Surya Namaskara with Cat and Dog Tilts, supine hamstring stretches, and basic shoulder openers.
- Surya Namaskara A more deeply warms and awakens the entire body than the classical sequence.
- Surya Namaskara B is a strong sequence appropriate for more experienced students and offers a deeper exploration of the hip flexors and the relationship between pelvic neutrality and spinal extension.
- Dynamic movement of the arms and shoulders in the flowing phases plus shoulder flexion in Urdhva Hastasana (Upward Hands Pose), Utkatasana (Chair Pose), Anjaneyasana (Low Lunge Pose), and Virabhadrasana I (Warrior I Pose) are excellent preparation for back bends and inversions.
- Stretching the hamstrings prepares the body for deeper forward bends and standing asanas.
- Creative flow sequences such as Dancing Warrior can be designed to focus on specific areas of opening in preparation for a specific peak asana.

Classical Surya Namaskara

Classical Surya Namaskaras are an excellent way to begin any yoga practice. This integrated series of asanas sequentially highlights several essential physical qualities of asana practice:

- Roots, extension, and equanimity in Tadasana (Mountain Pose) or Samasthihi (Balanced Standing Pose).
- Spinal integrity and lengthening in Urdhva Hastasana.
- Calming stretch of the back body in Uttanasana (Standing Forward Bend Pose).
- Grounded spinal extension and heart awakening in Ardha Uttanasana (Half Standing Forward Bend Pose).

- Awakened stretching of the hip flexors, quadriceps and shoulder girdle in Anjaneyasana.
- Strengthening of the arms, shoulders, core and legs in Phalakasana (Plank Pose).
- Strengthening the spinal erectors and hip extensors in a modified form of Salabhasana B (Locust Pose B).
- Strengthening and stretching of the entire body in Adho Mukha Svanasana (Downward-Facing Dog Pose).

Classical Surya Namaskara moves fluidly through the asanas shown in Sequence One, each of which is held for just the length of the natural pauses between breaths. Refer to Table 5.2 for sequencing your cues to help students synchronize the phases of the breath with movements in and out of the asanas. For elaborate details on guiding students in these movements and asanas, see Stephens (2010, 159–67) and www.markstephensyoga.com/resources.

Table 5.2. Sequencing Cues for Breath and Movement in Classical Surya Namaskara

Inhaling	Exhaling
1. Reach the arms out and up from Samasthihi to Urdhva Hastasana;	2. Fold forward and down into Uttanasana;
3. Extend the spine and heart center forward into Ardha Uttanasana;	4. Step the right foot back, knee down to the floor, toes back;
5. Draw the torso and arms up into Anjaneyasana;	6. Swan-dive the palms to the floor;
7. Step back to Phalakasana;	8. Slowly release the knees-chest-chin sequentially to the floor;
9. Root into the palms and lift the chest to Salabhasana B (with feet rooting down);	10. Press to all fours or directly up and back to Adho Mukha Svanasana;
11. Step the right foot forward and rise into Anjaneyasana;	12. Swan-dive the palms to the floor;
13. Extend the spine and heart center forward into Ardha Uttanasana;	14. Fold into Uttanasana;
15. "Swan dive" up to Urdhva Hastasana;	16. Grow taller while drawing the palms back to the heart, Samasthihi.

Sequence 1: Classical Surya Namaskara

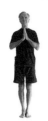

1. Samasthihi
1–5 minutes. Welcome, set intention, begin guiding.

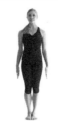

2. Tadasana
Exhale.

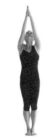

3. Urdhva Hastasana
Inhaling, sweep the arms out and up overhead.

4. Uttanasana
Exhaling slowly swan dive forward and down.

5. Ardha Uttanasana
Inhaling, lift the heart toward the horizon.

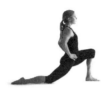

6. Anjaneyasana Prep
Exhaling, step the right foot back, knee down, toes back.

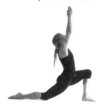

7. Anjaneyasana
Inhaling, sweep the arms out and up overhead.

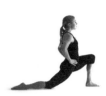

8. Anjaneyasana Prep
Exhaling, release the hands back to the floor.

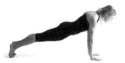

9. Phalakasana
Inhaling, step to back into plank position.

10. Ashtanga Pranam
Exhaling, release the knees, chest, and chin to the floor.

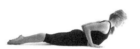

11. Salabhasana B
Inhaling, root the hands while lifting the shoulders level with the elbows and shrugging them down the back.

12. Bidalasana
Exhaling, press to all fours or …

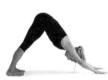

13. Adho Mukha Svanasana
… directly into Downward Facing Dog.

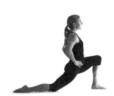

14. Anjaneyasana Prep
Empty of breath, step the right foot forward.

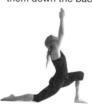

15. Anjaneyasana
Inhaling, sweep the arms out and up overhead.

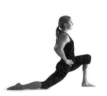

16. Anjaneyasana Prep
Exhaling, release the fingertips to the floor.

17. Ardha Uttanasana
Inhaling, lift and lengthen the heart toward the horizon.

18. Uttanasana
Exhaling, fold down.

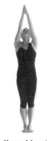

19. Urdhva Hastasana
Inhaling, swan dive up sweeping the arms out and overhead.

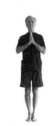

20. Samasthihi
Exhaling, release the palms to the heart.

Surya Namaskara A

Surya Namaskara A begins and ends the same as in Classical Surya Namaskara, with Samasthihi, Urdhva Hastasana, Uttanasana, and Ardha Uttanasana. It introduces four new elements: Chaturanga Dandasana (Four-Limbed Staff Pose), Urdhva Mukha Svanasana (Upward-Facing Dog Pose), "floating," and holding Adho Mukha Svanasana for five or more breaths. In combination, these new elements make this sequence considerably more challenging and tapas-oriented than the Classical form.

Sequence your instructions as with the Classical Surya Namaskara until arriving in Ardha Uttanasana. In instructing the first Surya Namaskara A, ask the entire class to step back from Ardha Uttanasana to Phalakasana. Explain the various aspects of Phalakasana as described above for Classical Surya Namaskara. Emphasize that the *danda* (staff or stick) aspects of Phalakasana are essential in the transition down to Chaturanga Dandasana. When instructing the movement from Phalakasana to Chaturanga, emphasize the following five energetic actions: (1) active legs (firm thighs, inner thighs spiral up), (2) heel pressing back, (3) active core (belly drawing lightly to the spine with the exhalation), (4) shoulder blades down the back, and (5) sternum toward the horizon. Suggest (and demonstrate) the option of lowering all the way down to the floor with "knees-chest-chin" as in Classical Surya Namaskara as an alternative to lowering to Chaturanga Dandasana. If a student is lowering with "knees-chest-chin," encourage him or her to stay with Salabhasana B rather than Urdhva Mukha Svanasana. As the elbows bend, they track directly behind the shoulders without squeezing into the sides or splaying out. While lowering down, encourage students to press firmly across the entire span of their palms and to keep the knuckles of their index fingers rooting down; these actions in the hands will help balance pressure in the wrists and thus reduce the incidence of repetitive stress in this vulnerable joint. The gaze is down so the neck is in its natural curvature, or over time and with practice, stability, and ease in the neck, the gaze is toward the horizon.

The flowing quality of Surya Namaskara often results in a very sloppy (and thus potentially injurious) Chaturanga Dandasana or the virtual disappearance of this asana altogether. Remind students that Chaturanga Dandasana is an asana that should be held for that brief natural pause in the breath between the exhalation and the inhalation that initiates movement into Urdhva Mukha

Svanasana. In guiding students into Chaturanga, emphasize that the front of the shoulders should lower just to the level of the elbows while continuing to root the shoulder blades down the back and in against the back ribs for greater stability. This is the essential preparation for transitioning into Urdhva Mukha Svanasana, as described below. When the shoulders go lower than the elbows in Chaturanga, excessive pressure is placed on the labrum of the shoulder joint. This positioning also collapses the chest and leads to an Urdhva Mukha Svanasana in which the shoulders tend to scrunch up toward the ears, creating undue pressure in the neck and compromising the expansiveness of the heart center. If students lack the strength to keep their shoulders from going lower than their elbows when lowering to Chaturanga, encourage them to keep their knees on the floor in this transition.

As students develop the strength to stably and comfortably lower into Chaturanga from Phalakasana, introduce them to the more fluid movement of floating from Ardha Uttanasana directly to Chaturanga Dandasana (or to the floor). Many students have learned to jump back to Phalakasana, which is problematic for two reasons: (1) the jarring impact on the lumbar spine, and (2) disruption of the synchronized connection of the breath to movement into Chaturanga (due to exhaling the breath completely out when jumping back). Teach the floating movement from Ardha Uttanasana by instructing students to bend their knees deeply enough to firmly root their palms into the floor while pulling their chest forward through the window of their arms on the inhale. Then guide students to bend their elbows while simultaneously jumping the feet back and extending the chest forward directly into Chaturanga (or to the floor). Encourage students to keep this movement simple; with time and practice, they might float up into Adho Mukha Vrksasana (Handstand) along the way to Chaturanga. When introducing the floating technique, hold Ardha Uttanasana for a few breaths while highlighting how the belly naturally engages when exhaling, stimulating the light uddiyana bandha that creates greater levity.

Urdhva Mukha Svanasana is an intense and powerfully awakening back-bending asana. It is set up through the alignment qualities of Chaturanga Dandasana described above. Always offer students the option of Salabhasana B as an alternative in the following conditions: lower-back pain or insufficient arm, shoulder, or leg strength to suspend their body on the hands and feet. In learning Urdhva Mukha Svanasana, it is helpful to first practice Salabhasana B, which strengthens the lower back and teaches the leg activation that is important in this asana. Emphasize active and aligned legs: the feet are extending back and pressing firmly down while legs are firm with the inner thighs spiraling up. Encourage students to press the tops of their feet firmly down and create a sense of extending their toes straight back. In rooting the feet down, the legs become more active. From this base in the feet, instruct students to pull their pelvis forward, away from their ankles, press their tailbone back toward their heels, and keep their buttocks soft while allowing the weight of the pelvis to provide traction on the lower back. Do not instruct squeezing the gluteal muscles, which causes the femurs to externally rotate and compresses the sacroiliac joint.

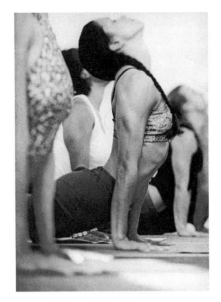

Urdhva Mukha Svanasana

Guide students into the full expression of the asana by asking them to press firmly into their hands, lift their chest, and create a feeling of focusing the back bend in their heart center. Rooting firmly into the knuckles of the index fingers helps to ensure balanced pressure across the hands and wrist joints, thereby reducing the likelihood of strain in the wrists. Strong and balanced rooting of the hands also leads to greater lengthening through the arms and lifting and spreading of the chest, which is essential in creating the length in the spine required for deepening the back bend. The wrists should be aligned directly beneath the shoulders in Urdhva Mukha Svanasana. If the wrists are positioned forward of the shoulders, students will feel excessive pressure in their lower back; if positioned farther back than the shoulders, they will hyperextend their wrists. The movement of the feet in the transition from Chaturanga determines where the shoulders end up relative to the wrists. Keeping the tiptoes fixed and rolling over them will bring the hips and shoulders farther forward; extending the feet back while pressing the arms straight will result in the shoulders being farther back. There is no correct method. Rather, the unique (and changing) geometry of each student's body—length of the arms, legs, feet, and torso, plus the degree of their back-bending arc—determines how much to emphasize rolling over the toes versus extending the feet back. Demonstrating these alternatives, highlight the effect on the lower back, wrists, and overall integrity of Urdhva Mukha Svanasana.

Ask students to draw the curve of the back bend up their spine consciously and to create a sense of pulling the lower tips of their shoulder blades in and up as if into their heart center. Students with weak shoulders will tend to hang in their shoulders. This tends to strain the neck, close the heart center, compromise the breath, and exacerbate the tendency to dump into the lower back. Encourage these students to more actively press into their hands (wrists allowing) in order to better draw the shoulders down away from the ears. The head can be held level; with practice, ease, and stability, the final action of the asana can be releasing the head back. While pressing the palms firmly down, encourage students to energetically spiral the palms out to create more space across the heart center and pull the spine through, toward the heart, to deepen the back bend.

The transition from Urdhva Mukha Svanasana to Adho Mukha Svanasana is initiated with the exhalation. After feeling the fullness of Urdhva Mukha Svanasana at the crest of the inhale, cue students to feel their belly naturally engaging with their exhale, using the gradual engagement of their abdominal core to help lift their hips up and back. In an effort to find pelvic neutrality in Adho Mukha Svanasana, guide students to create a feeling of their pubic bone leading the way in pulling the hips up and back. Over time this movement involves rolling over the toes of both feet simultaneously. Newer students and those with tender toes or feet can "step" over first one foot and then the other. The arms should remain straight (but not hyperextended) and strong in this transition, with the shoulder blades spiraling out broadly away from the spine. Newer students and those whose strength is very challenged in this transition can bring their knees to the floor, tuck their toes under, and then press to Adho Mukha Svanasana. Experienced students with strong and stable shoulders can build additional strength by first lowering back to Chaturanga and then pressing back to Adho Mukha Svanasana.

Move from Adho Mukha Svanasana to Ardha Uttanasana by either walking the feet forward or "floating" the feet to the hands. Encourage new students and those with lower back or wrist issues to walk forward. The floating technique is best introduced by asking students to practice springing from their legs as high as they can, keeping their arms and shoulders strong and stable, and landing where their feet started in Adho Mukha Svanasana. Repeating this exercise several times, encourage them to fully straighten their legs as soon as they spring off the floor, aiming to elevate their shoulders over

Sequence 2: Surya Namaskara A

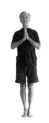

1. Samasthihi
1–5 minutes. Welcome, set intention, begin guiding.

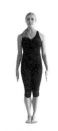

2. Tadasana
Same as Classical Surya Namaskara.

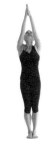

3. Urdhva Hastasana
Same as Classical Surya Namaskara.

4. Uttanasana
Same as Classical Surya Namaskara.

5. Ardha Uttanasana
Same as Classical Surya Namaskara.

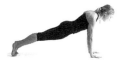

6. Phalakasana
Option 1: Step by to plank position to lower down.

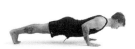

7. Chaturanga Dandasana
Option 2: Float directly into Chaturanga.

8. Urdhva Mukha Svanasana
Inhale into Urdhva Mukha Svanasana.

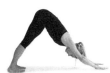

9. Adho Mukha Svanasana
Exhale to Adho Mukha Svanasana; hold for 5 breaths to 2 minutes.

10. Ardha Uttanasana
Option 1: Step forward.

11. Floating Forward
Option 2: Float to Ardha Uttanasana.

12. Piking Forward
Option 3: Pike and land lightly in Ardha Uttanasana.

13. Uttanasana
Same as Classical Surya Namaskara.

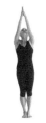

14. Urdhva Hastasana
Same as Classical Surya Namaskara.

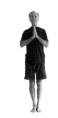

15. Samasthihi
Same as Classical Surya Namaskara.

the wrists, hips over their shoulders, and legs level with the floor in a pike position. Students will find greater ease and levity by keeping their palms rooted and arms strong; they will feel even more levity by completing the exhale and cultivating a very light uddiyana bandha just before launching their feet off the floor. After practicing this several times, instruct your students to once again spring as high as they can with the inhale, this time allowing their feet to release down to the floor as close to their hands as they can, with their torso already extended forward and spine long in Ardha Uttanasana at the crest of their inhale.

When exhaling down into Uttanasana in Surya Namaskara A or B, encourage students to place the back of the hands on the floor for just that moment of exhale as a means of counterposing tension in the wrists that might arise from all the Chaturanga–Up Dog–Down Dog–floating movements. They can also draw their fingers into a light fist to further stretch the back of their wrists. From here the path back to Samasthihi is the same as in the Classical Surya Namaskara. Over time, encourage students to build up to doing five continuous Surya Namaskara A cycles.

Surya Namaskara B

Surya Namaskara B introduces two more asanas to the Surya Namaskara family: Utkatasana and Virabhadrasana I. The sequence is initiated through a fluid movement from Samasthihi to Utkatasana. In instructing the first Utkatasana, ask students to place their hands into the creases of the groin, bend their knees deeply, push the femoral heads toward the heels, and then rotate their pelvis forward and back a few times to find where it feels like their spine is drawing naturally out of their pelvis. Maintaining this pelvic neutrality, instruct them to release their arms down by the sides, turn their palms strongly out, and feel their chest expanding as their shoulder blades draw down and in and against their back ribs. Cue the class to reach their arms out and up overhead with an inhalation, keeping their shoulder blades rooting down as they stretch up through their chest and arms. Students can keep their arms shoulder distance apart and their gaze slightly down or, with ease in the neck, toward the horizon. If they can keep their arms straight, invite them to draw their palms together and gaze up to their thumbs. Play around with guiding your classes from Samasthihi to Utkatasana and back to Samasthihi several times, emphasizing the connection of breath to movement, pada bandha to mula bandha, roots to extension up through the spine and arms. In the regular flow of Surya Namaskara B, transition from Utkatasana to Uttanasana by exhaling the legs straight while swan-diving forward and down. From Uttanasana, follow the same sequence from Surya Namaskara A to Adho Mukha Svanasana.

In transitioning from Adho Mukha Svanasana to Virabhadrasana I, there are two basic techniques. In traditional Ashtanga Vinyasa yoga the left heel is turned in about halfway and rooted down before stepping the right foot forward. In many Vinyasa Flow classes the right leg is first extended back and up while inhaling, then when exhaling the foot is drawn forward and placed next to the right hand. When using either method, consider first instructing Ashta Chandrasana (Crescent Pose) rather than Virabhadrasana I as a way of introducing high lunge poses and offering the space in which to gently awaken the hip flexors and groin while ensuring that students understand the important alignment principle of knee-over-heel. In further preparation for either the first Ashta Chandrasana or Virabhadrasana I, ask students to come high onto their fingertips, draw their shoulder blades down their back, and extend their sternum forward to draw more length through their spine and create more space around their neck.

In either the Ashta Chandrasana or Virabhadrasana I, ask students to straighten their front leg all the way while drawing their torso all the way up into a vertical position, place their hands on their hips, and bring their pelvis to a place of neutrality while pressing the back leg straight and strong. If starting with Ashta Chandrasana, next cue students to draw their back heel in and down to the floor to establish the foundation there for Virabhadrasana I: cultivate pada bandha, rotate the back hip forward, the inner thigh of the back leg rotating back and the pelvis level. With the hands still on the hips, ask students to try to maintain as much pelvic neutrality as they can—space between their hip and front thigh—while slowing bending their front leg and consciously guiding their knee toward the little-toe side of the foot. It is very important to ensure that the front knee does not travel out beyond the heel; allowing the knee to go farther forward places excessive pressure on the anterior cruciate ligament (ACL). If a student feels pressure in the back knee or lower back when bending the front knee into Virabhadrasana I, guide that person to back out of the lunge or explore bending the knee less deeply. Keeping the back heel lifted straight up in the Ashta Chandrasana positioning will also reduce or eliminate the pressure in the back knee and lower back. In either asana, once students are up in the lunge

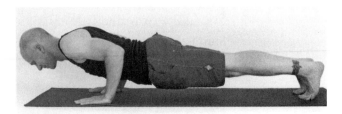

Chaturanga Dandasana

position, ask them to release their arms down by their sides, turn their palms out to feel the external rotation of their arms at the shoulder joint, and then reach their arms out and up overhead while keeping the shoulder blades rooted down and in against their back ribs. Cue the class to look down for a moment and draw their lower front ribs slightly in, then try to maintain that positioning while bringing the gaze forward and the arms back. This will help students to develop neutral extension of the spine with greater shoulder flexion, which is intrinsically beneficial and helpful in creating the body intelligence for asanas such as Adho Mukha Vrksasana. Encourage students who can keep their arms straight to draw their palms together overhead, and if it is okay with the neck, to gaze up to the tips of their thumbs.

To deepen the experience of Virabhadrasana I, emphasize the steady grounding of the feet, internal rotation of the back leg while pressing the shin firmly back to further ground the back heel, pada bandha in both feet, mula bandha and steady energetic lifting through the spine, through the heart center, and out through the fingertips. Suggest lifting the lower rim of the ribs up and away from the upper rims of the hips to create more space and ease in the lower back. The breath should be steady and even, the eyes soft, the heart open. Virabhadrasana I is an excellent asana in which to teach multiple lines of energy, the relationship between roots and extension, and the balance of sthira and sukham. In the transition from Virabhadrasana I to Chaturanga Dandasana, encourage students to keep the movement simple, fluid, and connected to their breath. You will observe many students, especially advancing beginners, keeping one foot off the floor all the way into and even through Chaturanga Dandasana. This undermines the stable foundation of Chaturanga Dandasana; the integrity of Four-Limbed Staff Pose is lost to an asymmetrical three-limb variation that compromises the balanced movement into Urdhva Mukha Svanasana. Done repetitively, this can destabilize the sacroiliac joint and lead to potentially chronic lower-back problems. After repeating Virabhadrasana I on the other side, transition from Adho Mukha Svanasana to Ardha Uttanasana to Uttanasana to Utkatasana and back to Samasthihi, completing the sequence. In subsequent sequences, guide the class to flow continuously with the breath through this sequence of asanas. Over time, encourage students to build up to doing five continuous Surya Namaskara B cycles.

Sequence 3: Surya Namaskara B

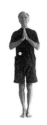

1. Samasthihi
1–5 minutes. Welcome, set intention, begin guiding.

2. Utkatasana
Inhaling, sweep the arms overhead while bending the knees deeply.

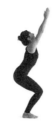

3. Uttanasana
Exhaling, expand and fold forward and down.

4. Ardha Uttanasana
Same as Classical Surya Namaskara.

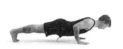

5. Chaturanga Dandasana
Same as Surya Namaskara A.

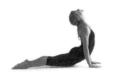

6. Urdhva Mukha Svanasana
Same as Surya Namaskara A.

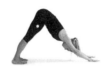

7. Adho Mukha Svanasana
Same as Surya Namaskara A.

8. Virabhadrasana I
Option 1: Stepping the right foot forward, inhale into Warrior I.

9. Tail of the Dog
Option 2a: Inhaling, extend the right leg up.

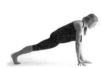

10. Warrior Prep
Option 2b: Exhaling, step the right foot forward.

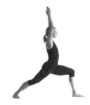

11. Virabhadrasana I
Option 2c: Inhale into Warrior I.

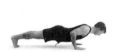

12. Chaturanga Dandasana
Exhale to Chaturanga.

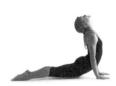

13. Urdhva Mukha Svanasana
Same as Surya Namaskara A.

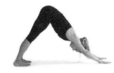

14. Adho Mukha Svanasana
Exhale completely in preparation for the other side. Repeat asana 8–13 on the other side, returning to Adho Mukha Svanasana and holding for 5 breaths.

15. Ardha Uttanasana
Same as Surya Namaskara A.

16. Uttanasana
Exhaling, fold.

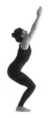

17. Utkatasana
Inhaling, bend the knees while sweeping the arms out and up overhead.

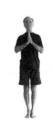

18. Samasthihi
Exhale to standing.

Dancing Warrior

Dance and yoga likely have a long and rich interrelated history dating at least to the rise of tantra in the latter part of the first millennium of the Common Era. There are well-known dances ascribed to various deities and mythological figures in Indian culture, most notably Shiva and Parvati. There is also considerable evidence that a variety of dance forms, including harmonial gymnastics and esoteric dance forms, that developed in Europe and the United States in the nineteenth century were significant sources of the creative innovations in modern yoga asana practice in the early twentieth century in India (Singleton 2010, 143–60). This trend continues in the present, with perhaps the most popular expression known as "Dancing Warrior," developed by Shiva Rea in part through her study of yoga and dance in the World Arts and Cultures Department at UCLA in the 1990s. This beautiful flowing sequence warms the entire body and is excellent preparation for a variety of asanas in intermediate and advanced classes.

Starting in Down Dog, inhaling, extend the right leg back and up. Exhaling, step the right foot forward and draw the left heel in and down for Warrior I. Inhale up into Warrior I. Exhale, open into Warrior II attentive to the alignment of the front knee above that heel (emphasize keeping the knee from splaying in and that hip from splaying out). On the next inhalation slide the left hand down the left leg into a Side Warrior while stretching the right arm overhead, making it a side stretch rather than a back bend and attentive to not press down onto the back knee. Then with the exhalation keep circling the right arm to compete a 360 degree circle while bringing the torso forward into the Extended Side Angle Pose. With the next inhalation keep circling the right arm forward and around in another 360 degree circle in transitioning back into Warrior II. On the exhalation transition through Chaturanga Dandasana and Up Dog on the way to Down Dog. Repeat on the other side. Keep flowing in this way for up to five full cycles of Dancing Warrior. Offer alternatives such Ashtanga Pranam. Encourage students to make it more of a breathing practice, stretching the breath to stretch their practice and allowing a sense of the asanas and transitions to find expression through the integrity of the breath rather than trying to squeeze the breath into what they are doing with their body. Intermediate and advanced students can play with integrating Eka Pada Koundinyasana I and Astavakrasana into the transition to Chaturanga.

Sequence 4: Dancing Warrior

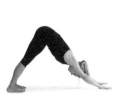

1. Adho Mukha Svanasana
Exhale completely.

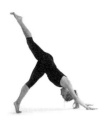

2. Tail of the Dog
Inhaling, extend the right leg up.

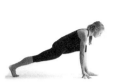

3. Warrior Prep
Exhaling, step the right foot forward to Warrior Prep.

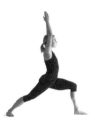

4. Virabhadrasana I
Inhaling, draw up into Warrior I.

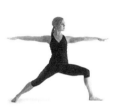

5. Virabhadrasana II
Exhaling, revolve the left hip open while extending the arms out away from each other.

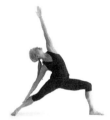

6. Parsva Virabhadrasana
Inhaling, slide the left hand down the left leg while stretching the right arm overhead.

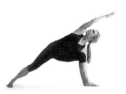

7. Utthita Parsvakonasana
Exhaling, extend the torso forward while stretching the right arm overhead.

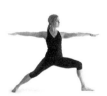

8. Virabhadrasana II
Inhaling, circle the right arm forward and around 360 degrees to come back into Warrior II.

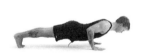

9. Chaturanga Dandasana
Exhale to Chaturanga.

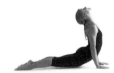

10. Urdhva Mukha Svanasana
Inhale into Urdhva Mukha Svanasana.

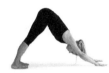

11. Adho Mukha Svanasana
Exhale to Adho Mukha Svanasana. Repeat asanas 2–10 on the other side, then continue 3–5 times.

Chapter Six

Introductory and Beginning-Level Classes

And the day came when the risk to remain tight
in a bud was more painful than the risk it took
to blossom.
—ANAÏS NIN

People first come to yoga with a variety of conditions and motivations. Most have previously participated in exercise classes and may have high body intelligence. But very few have experienced a physical practice in which they are invited to move and explore in the specific ways asked of them in yoga: consciously connecting breath-body-mind amid increasingly complex and challenging positioning of the body. With most new students starting off in regularly scheduled classes rather than introductory workshops, they find themselves diving into a flowing stream surrounded by unfamiliar words, techniques, and challenges. Yoga teacher Max Strom (1995) recalls being "completely confused" and feeling "anger and despair" when taking his first yoga class in 1991. Add a spiritual dimension—even chanting *aum*—and many new students put up such defenses that complicate their experience.

Beginning-level yoga is the first stage in practice. Irrespective of age or condition, here the practice is about creating an initial awakening of awareness and energy throughout the bodymind, what in Ashtanga Vinyasa is called yoga chikitsa, or "yoga therapy." The body's energy pathways are gradually opening and prana is beginning to flow more simply and fully throughout the body, helping rid it of toxins and relaxing the nervous system. Doing this safely and sustainably involves learning to move with the breath, to use the breath as a guide in exploring the asanas, learning proper alignment and how to refine that positioning to gradually move into deeper stability and ease. Along the way, one encounters obstacles and difficulties as accumulated tension and habitual forms of posture and breathing continue to manifest, leading to either frustration or self-acceptance (or both). Practice by practice, one strengthens and stretches the entire body, releasing chronic tension, discovering simpler sources of balance and openness while cultivating yoga as a step-by-step process of self-discovery and self-transformation.

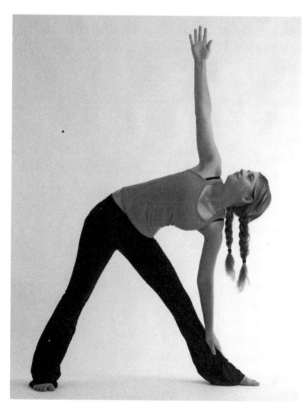

A new student in Utthita Trikonasana

Teaching new students is an opportunity to deepen our own practice of "beginner's mind" and to encourage it among others in class. In this mind-set, we open ourselves to whatever we are doing as if it is the first time. Although the bodymind knows from prior experience where it is going and what to expect, the idea is to soften that preconditioned mind-set in order to feel what is happening more freshly and relatively free of preconceptions. When we do this as teachers, it allows us to have a more empathetic understanding of new students' experiences, thereby making it easier to give them the guidance and support it takes for them to do the most they can. This is actually far more challenging than teaching highly complex asanas to advanced students, so, inevitably, teaching new students deepens your skill as a teacher.

All new students deserve an individualized welcome from their teacher. Along with asking about prior experience, injuries, and intentions, this initial contact is essential in helping new students feel more comfortable in class. It is important to tell them explicitly that in yoga we are interested in *how* we go, not how *far* we go; that it is a process of consciously connecting breath-body-mind while exploring the development of strength, flexibility, and balance as part of a long-term sustainable practice of holistic integration. In yoga perhaps more than in any other physical activity or discipline, change comes slowly, often over years, as sustained practice undoes habits set over a lifetime. This change, moreover, is rarely linear. Emphasize the importance of steadiness and ease, show them Balasana (Child's Pose), and encourage them to rest in that or any other asana whenever they feel the need. Whether or not they think they need props, ask them to have a block, strap, and two blankets or a bolster next to their mat since is it likely they will benefit from using some or all of them during class. If possible, group new students close to one another so you can more easily give demonstrations and more specific guidance to them while remaining attentive to the larger class. Also try to position them behind more experienced students whom you can count on to stay with the basic asanas (rather than behind a show-off student whose fancy variations will be confusing and possibly lead the new student beyond a safe practice).

Use the presence of new students in class to review the basics of ujjayi pranayama and the foundational elements of each asana; all experienced students will benefit from the review, including those students whose patience this might test. During Surya Namaskara, position yourself immediately next to new students to demonstrate more closely and explain each asana and transition. While the rest of the class is holding Adho Mukha Svanasana (Downward-Facing Dog Pose), bring new students back into Surya Namaskara (Sun Salutation) asanas in which they seemed confused or especially challenged, giving them more elaborate guidance and modification options.

Table 6.1. When and to Whom to Teach Pranayama

Pranayama	When	Whom
Natural breathing	Excellent way to initiate all classes.	All students.
Ujjayi	Teach at the beginning of every class.	All students.
Sama-vritti	Teach in conjunction with natural breathing and ujjayi.	All students.
Vishama-vritti	Teach in conjunction with natural breathing and ujjayi.	All students.
Antara kumbhaka	Teach in conjunction with ujjayi as a means of expanding and refining breath capacity	Intermediate students at ease with ujjayi and experienced with bandhas; not when pregnant, experiencing eye or ear complaints, or with high blood pressure.
Bahya kumbhaka	After developing ease with antara kumbhaka.	Intermediate students at ease with ujjayi and experienced with bandhas; not when pregnant, experiencing eye or ear complaints, or with high blood pressure.
Viloma	Teach in conjunction with ujjayi as a means of expanding and refining breath capacity	All students, especially when experiencing fatigue or anxiety.
Kapalabhati	At beginning of class to stimulate energy, awaken the breath, and more quickly warm the body; during asana sequences, especially as part of core awakening. If during asanas, teach with students either sitting (ideally in Virasana) or in Dolphin Plank Pose.	Intermediate students; not when pregnant, experiencing eye or ear complaints, or with high blood pressure.
Bhastrika	Pranayama class or as final energizing practice immediately before Savasana.	Intermediate students; not when pregnant, experiencing eye or ear complaints, or with high blood pressure.
Sitali	For cooling down.	All students.
Anuloma	Pranayama classes.	Students familiar and comfortable with ujjayi.
Pratiloma	Pranayama classes.	Students familiar and comfortable with ujjayi.
Suryabheda	Teach in conjunction with ujjayi.	All students.
Chandrabheda	Traditionally practiced on alternate days from suryabheda.	All students.
Nadi shodhana 1: Basic	Beginning of class.	Intermediate students.
Nadi shodhana 2: with viloma	When comfortable with Technique 1.	Intermediate students.
Nadi shodhana 3: with kumbhakas	When comfortable, steady, and at ease with Technique 2.	Intermediate students at ease with ujjayi and experienced with bandhas; not when pregnant, experiencing eye or ear complaints, or with high blood pressure.

Table 6.1. When and to Whom to Teach Pranayama (continued)

Pranayama	When	Whom
Nadi shodhana 4: with vilomas and kumbhakas	When comfortable with Technique 3.	Same as above
Nadi shodhana 5: with kapalabhati	When comfortable with Technique 4.	Same as above.

For detailed guidance on teaching and practicing these pranayamas, see Stephens (2010, 237–62).

Creating and Teaching Beginning-Level Sequences

- Introduce ujjayi pranayama in every class.
- Teach the relationship between breath and movement even within the relative stillness of a held asana. Start this exploration in a simple seated position, and then explore it with greater movement by doing Cat and Dog Tilts on all fours.[1]
- Teach *vritti pranayamas (sama-vritti* and *vishama-vritti)* as a means of gradually developing stronger control and easier freedom in all breathing practices.
- Teach the importance of dristana, in which the eyes are focused on a single point in each asana, helping to harness the mind to the breath and body.
- Teach the relationship between roots and extension, between actively grounding and creating more space. First teach this when sitting, then on all fours, then standing in Tadasana (Mountain Pose).
- Emphasize the importance of playing the edge to stay significantly engaged in the practice without straining.
- Remind students of the importance of rest. Teach Balasana.
- Keep the asana practice simple, offering modifications to make the path to the full expression of asanas simpler and more accessible. Do not offer variations that take basic asanas into more complex forms.
- Offer a slow warm-up involving asanas that will make Surya Namaskara more accessible.

- In exploring standing asanas, do one or two asanas on one side before changing sides, and then move on to another asana.
- Allow time for gradual and graceful transitions.
- Separately sequence external- and internal-rotation hip standing asanas.
- Limit standing balance asanas to Vrksasana (Tree Pose) and Garudasana (Eagle Pose).
- Use Adho Mukha Svanasana as the foundational asana that prepares the body for the introduction to arm balances in intermediate-level classes.
- Start back bends with dynamic movement in and out of Salabhasana A (Locust Pose A) before holding the asana for up to five cycles of breath; repeat two to three times. Continue back bends with Setu Bandha Sarvangasana (Bridge Pose), again exploring dynamically before holding for up to five breaths. Repeat two to three times.
- Offer a gentle release of the spine following back bends, starting with an easy Supta Parivartanasana (Reclined Revolved Pose) with both knees bent and together to take it easier on the lower back.
- Explore several simple forward bends and hip openers to further calm the nervous system and to release accumulated tension.
- Introduce Halasana (Plow Pose) and Salamba Sarvangasana (Supported Shoulder Stand) using blankets to elevate the shoulders and a wall or chair to support the feet. Offer Viparita Karani (Active Reversal Pose) as an alternative for students with cervical-spine issues.
- Allow at least five minutes for Savasana (Corpse Pose).
- Allow a few minutes after Savasana for sitting quietly and absorbing one's awareness in the awakened yet calm energy students will feel in their bodymind.

Beginning Class Sequences

Sequence 5: Basic Introduction to Yoga Class

1. Sukhasana
1–3 minutes. Welcome, set intention, begin guiding.

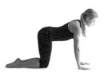

2. Bidalasana
5 Cat and Dog Tilts.

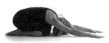

3. Utthita Balasana
5 breaths. Caution sensitivity to the knees and lower back.

4. Balasana
5 breaths.

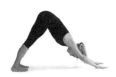

5. Adho Mukha Svanasana
30 seconds. Briefly alignment energetic action.

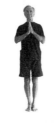

6. Samasthihi
Walk forward from Adho Mukha Svanasana and slowly roll up to standing. Teach Tadasana.

7. Classical Surya Namaskara
2 times. On the first time, pause in each asana to give refined instruction.

8. Surya Namaskara A
1 time, breaking down Plank–Chaturanga–Up Dog–Down Dog. Offer the alternative of knees-chest-chin and Salabhasana B as an alternative dynamic movement.

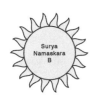

9. Surya Namaskara B
2 times. The first time, explain Utkatasana and Virabhadrasana I in detail.

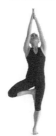

10. Vrksasana
30 seconds on each side.

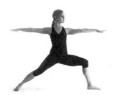

11. Virabhadrasana II
Prepare in a wide Prasarita stance. 5–10 breaths on each side.

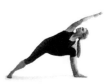

12. Utthita Parsvakonasana
Prepare in Warrior II. 5–10 breaths on each side.

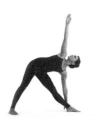

13. Utthita Trikonasana
5–10 breaths on each side.

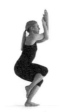

14. Garudasana
30 seconds on each side.

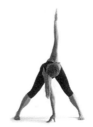

15. Parivrtta Ardha Padottanasana
5 breaths on each side, then step to Tadasana at the front of the mat.

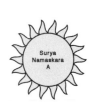

16. Surya Namaskara A
1 time.

Sequence 5: Basic Introduction to Yoga Class (continued)

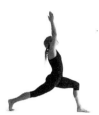

17. Ashta Chandrasana
5–10 breaths.

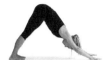

18. Adho Mukha Svanasana
Either step back to Adho Mukha Svanasana or transition through Chaturanga and Urdhva Mukha Svanasana.

19. Balasana
1 minute. Suggest positioning the knees wide apart to take it easier on the knees, hips, and lower back.

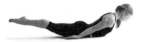

20. Salabhasana A
3 times for 3, 5, and 7 breaths, respectively. YS83 21. Setu Bandha Sarvangasana
2 times, 5–10 breaths each time.

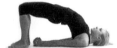

21. Setu Bandha Sarvangasana
2 times, 5–10 breaths each time.

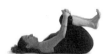

22. Apanasana
Guide gentle rotation of the knees in circles.

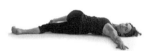

23. Supta Parivartanasana
2 times, 5–10 breaths on each side.

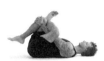

24. Eka Pada Raj Kapotasana Prep
1–2 minutes on each side.

25. Dandasana
1 minute. Explain grounding through the sit bones as the primary action in this and all other seated asanas.

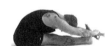

26. Paschimottanasana
1 minute.

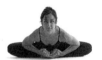
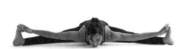

27. Upavista Konasana
1 minute.

28. Baddha Konasana
1 minute.

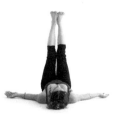

29. Viparita Karani
2 minutes.

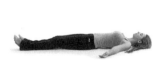

30. Savasana
5 minutes or longer.

31. Sukhasana
Meditation.

Sequence 6: Introduction to Yoga Workshop for More Physically Fit Students

1. Sukhasana
1–3 minutes. Welcome, set intention, begin guiding.

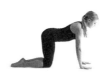

2. Bidalasana
5 times of Cat and Dog Tilts, warming the spine and refining the connection of breath to movement. Release to Utthita Balasana.

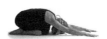

3. Utthita Balasana
5 breaths. Explain shoulder rotation as for Adho Mukha Svanasana. Caution sensitivity to the knees and lower back.

4. Balasana
5 breaths. Encourage students to visit Balasana as they please.

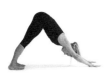

5. Adho Mukha Svanasana
1 minute. Briefly highlight arm and leg alignment, roots and extension, and actions in the arms, shoulders, and legs.

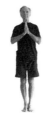

6. Samasthihi
Walk forward from Adho Mukha Svanasana and slowly roll up to standing. Teach Tadasana. Both sides.

7. Classical Surya Namaskara
3 times. On the first time, pause in each asana to give refined instruction.

8. Surya Namaskara A
1 time, breaking down Plank–Chaturanga–Up Dog–Down Dog. Offer the alternative of knees-chest-chin and Salabhasana B. Dog–Down Dog. Offer the alternative of

9. Surya Namaskara B
2 times. On the first time, explain Utkatasana and Virabhadrasana I in detail.

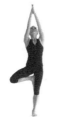

10. Vrksasana
30 seconds on each side.

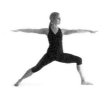

11. Virabhadrasana II
Prepare in a wide Prasarita stance. 5–10 breaths on each side.

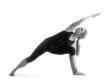

12. Utthita Parsvakonasana
Prepare in Warrior II. 5–10 breaths on each side.

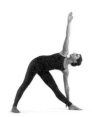

13. Utthita Trikonasana
Prepare in Prasarita stance. 5–10 breaths on each side.

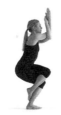

14. Garudasana
30 seconds on each side.

15. Parsvottanasana
Prepare in Prasarita stance. 5 breaths on each side, then step to the front of the mat for Tadasana.

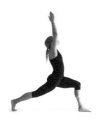

16. Ashta Chandrasana
Do a Sun Salutation to Adho Mukha Svanasana, then transition to Ashta Chandrasana. 5–10 breaths.

Sequence 6: Introduction to Yoga Workshop for More Physically Fit Students (continued)

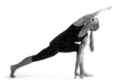

17. Parivrtta Ashta Chandrasana
Transition directly from Ashta Chandrasana. 5–10 breaths.

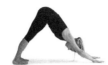

18. Adho Mukha Svanasana
Either step back or vinyasa to Adho Mukha Svanasana. Offer rest in Balasana.

19. Balasana
1 minute.

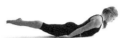

20. Salabhasana A
3 times for 3, 5, and 7 breaths, respectively. Offer the hand clasp on the third time.

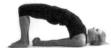

21. Setu Bandha Sarvangasana
3 times for 5–10 breaths each time.

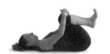

22. Apanasana
Guide gentle rotation of the knees to release tension in the lower back.

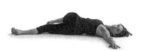

23. Supta Parivartanasana
5–10 breaths.

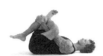

24. Eka Pada Raj Kapotasana Prep A
1–2 minutes on each side.

25. Dandasana
1 minute.

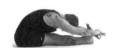

26. Paschimottanasana
1 minute.

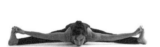

27. Upavista Konasana
1 minute.

28. Baddha Konasana
1 minute.

29. Gomukhasana
1 minute on each side.

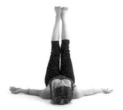

30. Viparita Karani
2 minutes.

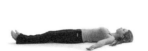

31. Savasana
5 minutes or longer.

32. Sukhasana
Meditation, setting intention, sealing in the practice.

Sequence 7: Beginning Level—Focus on Back Bends

1. Sukhasana
1–3 minutes. Welcome, set intention, begin guiding.

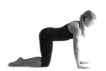

2. Bidalasana
5 times of Cat and Dog Tilts. Release to Utthita Balasana.

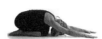

3. Utthita Balasana
5 breaths. Explain shoulder rotation as for Adho Mukha Svanasana. Caution sensitivity to the knees and lower back.

4. Balasana
5 breaths. Encourage students to visit Balasana as they please.

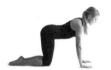

5. Bidalasana
1 breath in transition to Anahatasana.

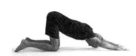

6. Anahatasana
1 minute. Cue external rotation of the shoulders.

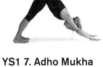

YS1 7. Adho Mukha Svanasana
1 minute. Briefly highlight arm and leg alignment, roots and extension, and actions in the arms, shoulders, and legs, then come to Tadasana.

8. Tadasana
1 minute. Teach pada bandha.

9. Classical Surya Namaskara
3 times.

10. Surya Namaskara A
2 times.

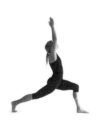

11. Ashta Chandrasana
Move in and out of the lunge 5 times, then hold 5 breaths.

12. Surya Namaskara B
2 times. Explain Utkatasana and Virabhadrasana I in detail the first time.

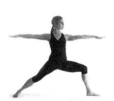

13. Virabhadrasana II
Prepare in a wide Prasarita stance. 10 breaths on each side.

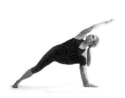

14. Utthita Parsvakonasana
10 breaths on each side.

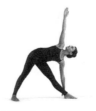

15. Utthita Trikonasana
10 breaths on each side.

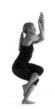

16. Garudasana
1 minute on each side.

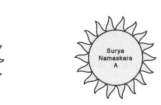

Introductory and Beginning-Level Classes   153

Sequence 7: Beginning Level—Focus on Back Bends (continued)

17. Prasarita Padottanasana C
1 minute.

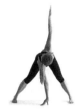

18. Parivrtta Ardha Prasarita
5–10 breaths on each side.

19. Classical Surya Namaskara
1 time, then transition to Adho Mukha Svanasana.

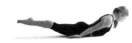

21. Salabhasana A
3 times for 3, 5, and 7 breaths, respectively. Offer the hand-clasp on the third time.

22. Bhujangasana
3 times for 5 breaths each time.

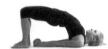

23. Setu Bandha Sarvangasana
Move dynamically in and out 3–5 times. Come up 2–3 more times for 5–10 breaths.

24. Apanasana
Guide gentle rotation of the knees in circles to release tension in the lower back.

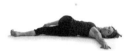

25. Supta Parivartanasana
5–10 breaths on each side.

26. Ananda Balasana
10 breaths.

27. Dandasana
1 minute.

28. Bharadvajrasana I
1 minute on each side, then return to Staff Pose.

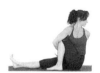

29. Marichyasana C
1 minute on each side.

30. Gomukhasana
1 minute on each side, then come to Dandasana.

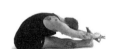

31. Paschimottanasana
1–2 minutes. Emphasize patient release of the back body.

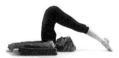

32. Halasana
Offer variations: feet on a wall, chair, or block; hips in hands in jackknifed position; or toes curled under.

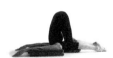

33. Karnapidasana
5 breaths. Emphasize awareness of sensation in the neck and lower back.

Sequence 7: Beginning Level—Focus on Back Bends (continued)

34. Uttana Padasana Prep
5 breaths. Counsel taking it easy on the neck in exploring extension of the head back and down.

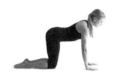

35. Supta Parivartanasana
5 breaths on each side.

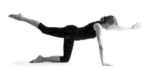

36. Savasana
5–10 minutes.

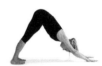

37. Sukhasana
Meditation, setting intention, sealing in the practice.

Sequence 8: Beginning Level—Focus on Hip Opening

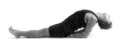

1. Sukhasana
1–3 minutes. Welcome, set intention, begin guiding.

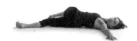

2. Bidalasana
5 times of Cat and Dog Tilts. Release to Utthita Balasana.

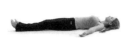

3. All Fours Arms/Legs Out
5 breaths on each side.

4. Adho Mukha Svanasana
1 minute. Teach the basic alignment and energetic actions.

5. Balasana
5 breaths. Remind students to rest here as they please.

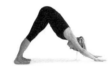

6. Adho Mukha Svanasana
5 breaths, then walk forward.

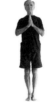

7. Samasthihi
Teach pada bandha, roots and extension, steady breath.

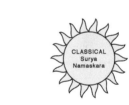

8. Classical Surya Namaskara
3 times. Pause each time in Anjaneyasana to explore dynamic movement, then hold Anjaneyasana each time for 5 breaths.

9. Surya Namaskara B
3 times. On the first time, move dynamically from Tadasana to Utkatasana to Tadasana 5 times, then hold Utkatasana 5 breaths. The first time in Ashta Chandrasana, move dynamically in and out 5 times. Introduce Virabhadrasana I the next 2 times.

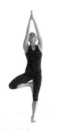

10. Vrksasana
Cue keeping the hips level and even to emphasize hips opening on the side of the lifted leg. 1 minute on each side.

11. Virabhadrasana II
Prepare in a wide Prasarita stance. 10 breaths.

Sequence 8: Beginning Level—Focus on Hip Opening (continined)

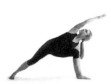

12. Utthita Parsvakonasana
Prepare in Warrior II. 10 breaths.

13. Utthita Trikonasana
Prepare in Prasarita stance. 10 breaths.

14. Garudasana
1 minute on each side, or modify with the next asana.

15. Garudasana Prep
Offer this prep position for those unable to cross their knees.

16. Parsvottanasana
Prepare in Prasarita stance. 10 breaths, then step to the front of the mat for Tadasana.

17. Surya Namaskara A
Hold Adho Mukha Svanasana 1 minute.

18. Balasana
5 breaths.

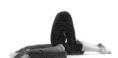

19. Dandasana
5 breaths.

20. Bharadvajrasana A
1 minute on each side, then return to Staff Pose.

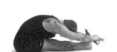

21. Paschimottanasana
1–2 minutes. Emphasize patient release of the back body.

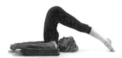

22. Halasana
5 breaths. Offer variations: feet on a wall, chair or block; hips in hands in jackknifed position; or Viparita Karani.

23. Karnapidasana
5 breaths. Emphasize awareness of sensation in the neck and lower back.

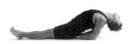

24. Uttana Padasana Prep
5 breaths. Counsel taking it easy on the neck in exploring extension of the head back and down.

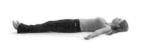

25. Savasana
5 minutes.

26. Sukhasana
Meditation, setting intention, sealing in the practice.

Sequence 9: Beginning Level—Focus on Twisting

1. Sukhasana
1–3 minutes. Welcome, set intention, begin guiding.

2. Parivrtta Sukhasana
Encourage dynamic exploration, twisting on each side for up to 1 minute. Explain roots and extension and playing the edge.

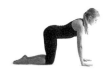

3. Bidalasana
5 times of Cat and Dog Tilts.

4. Urdhva Mukha Pasasana A
1 minute on each side, then return to Bidalasana to transition to the next asana.

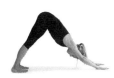

5. Adho Mukha Svanasana
5 breaths. Release to Balasana; repeat 4 times, then come to standing in Tadasana.

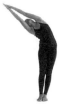

6. Parsva Urdhva Hastasana
5 breaths. Both sides.

7. Classical Surya Namaskara
3 times.

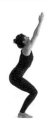

8. Utkatasana
1 minute. Emphasize pelvic neutrality in relation to the lower back.

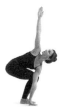

9. Parivrtta Utkatasana
5 breaths on each side, then come to Tadasana.

10. Surya Namaskara B
2 times. Offer Ashta Chandrasana in place of Virabhadrasana I. On the second time, move from Ashta Chandrasana to Parivrtta Ardha Chandrasana.

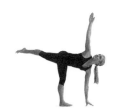

11. Parivrtta Ardha Chandrasana
5 breaths on each side, then complete Surya Namaskara B.

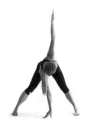

12. Parivrtta Ardha Prasarita
1 minute on each side.

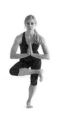

13. Garudasana Prep
1 minute on each side.

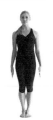

14. Tadasana
5 breaths. Anjali mudra, reaffirming intention.

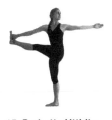

15. Parivrtta Utthita Hasta Padangusthasana
10 breaths on each side. Keep the lifted knee bent 90 degrees.

16. Classical Surya Namaskara
1 time, then rest in Balasana.

Introductory and Beginning-Level Classes

Sequence 9: Beginning Level—Focus on Twisting (continued)

17. Balasana
30 seconds.

18. Bharadvajrasana
10 breaths on each side.

19. Dandasana
5 breaths. Focus on grounding the sit bones and extending the legs and spine.

20. Ardha Matsyendrasana
10 breaths on each side.

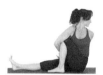

21. Marichyasana C
5 breaths on each side. Keep the back hand on the floor to help extend the spine.

22. Dandasana
5 breaths.

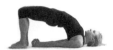

23. Setu Bandha Sarvangasana
3 times. Hold 5 breaths.

24. Apanasana
5 breaths.

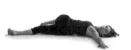

25. Supta Parivartanasana
10 breaths on each side.

26. Dandasana
5 breaths.

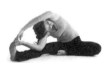

27. Parivrtta Janu Sirsasana
10 breaths on each side.

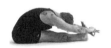

28. Paschimottanasana
1 minute.

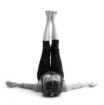

29. Viparita Karani
2 minutes.

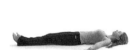

30. Savasana
5–8 minutes.

31. Sukhasana
Meditation, setting intention, aum.

Sequence 10: Beginning Level—Focus on Standing Balance

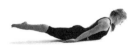

1. Sukhasana
1–3 minutes. Welcome, set intention, begin guiding.

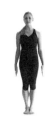

2. Tadasana
Workshop the pose, giving detailed guidance on pada bandha.

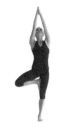

3. Vrksasana
1 minute on each side.

4. Classical Surya Namaskara
3 times.

5. Surya Namaskara A
2 times. The second time, introduce Tail of the Dog in transition to Ashta Chandrasana.

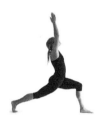

6. Ashta Chandrasana
Move dynamically in and out then hold for up to 1 minute on each side. Complete the Sun Salutation, returning to Tadasana.

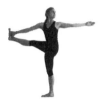

7. Parivrtta Hasta Padangusthasana
10 breaths on each side.

8. Prasarita Padottanasana A
10 breaths, equally balancing through the feet.

9. Prasarita Padottanasana C
5 breaths.

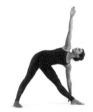

10. Utthita Trikonasana
Set up from Prasarita stance (at a wall, if available). Do each side twice, holding each time for up to 1 minute.

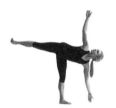

11. Ardha Chandrasana
5 breaths on each side. Introduce at a wall and with a chair or block for the grounding hand. Repeat up to 3 times.

12. Balasana
Rest for 1 minute.

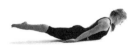

13. Salabhasana A
3 times for 3, 5, then 7 breaths, respectively. Offer the hand-clasp on the third time and hold 5–10 breaths.

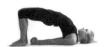

14. Setu Bandha Sarvangasana
3 times, holding 5 breaths each time.

15. Apanasana
5 breaths.

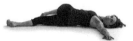

16. Supta Parivartanasana
10 breaths on each side.

Sequence 10: Beginning Level—Focus on Standing Balance (continued)

17. Virasana
1 minute. Encourage sitting on a block.

18. Ardha Matsyendrasana
5 breaths on each side.

19. Dandasana
5 breaths.

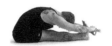

20. Paschimottanasana
10–15 breaths.

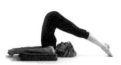

21. Halasana
5 breaths.

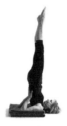

22. Salamba Sarvangasana
1–3 minutes.

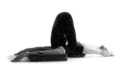

23. Karnapidasana
5 breaths.

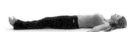

24. Savasana
5 minutes.

25. Sukhasana
Meditation, setting intention, sealing in the practice.

Sequence 11: Beginning Level—Focus on Arm Support

1. Sukhasana
1–3 minutes. Welcome, set intention, begin guiding.

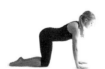

2. Bidalasana
5 times of Cat and Dog Tilts, warming the spine and refining the connection of breath to movement. Release to Utthita Balasana.

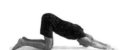

3. Anahatasana
10 breaths. Explain shoulder rotation as for Adho Mukha Svanasana.

4. Adho Mukha Svanasana
1 minute. Briefly highlight arm and leg alignment, roots and extension, and actions in the arms, shoulders, and legs. Come to standing.

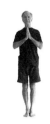

5. Samasthihi
1 minute. Teach pada bandha, roots and extension.

6. Classical Surya Namaskara
2 times. On the first time, pause in each asana to give refined instruction.

7. Surya Namaskara A
2 times. Hold Phal-akasana up to 1 minute each time.

8. Surya Namaskara B
2 times. The first time, explain Utkatasana and Virabhadrasana I.

9. Wrist Therapy.
See the sidebar on page 64 for details.

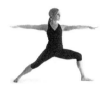

10. Virabhadrasana II
Prepare in a wide Prasarita stance. 10 breaths on each side.

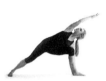

11. Utthita Parsvakonasana
Prepare in Warrior II. 10 breaths on each side.

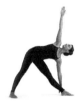

12. Utthita Trikonasana
Prepare in Prasarita stance. Hold each side 10 breaths.

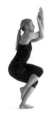

13. Garudasana
1 minute on each side. The following asana is an easier alternative.

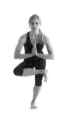

14. Garudasana Prep
1 minute on each side.

15. Prasarita Padottanasana C
1 minute, then transition to Tadasana.

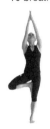

16. Vrksasana
1 minute on each side.

17. Surya Namaskara A
Hold Adho Mukha Svana-sana 1 minute.

18. Balasana
5 breaths.

19. Vajrasana
1 minute while teacher demonstrates preparatory forms of Vasisthasana.

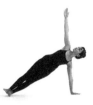

20. Vasisthasana Prep A
5–10 breaths, then switch sides. Do wrist therapy.

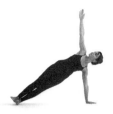

21. Vasisthasana Prep B
Hold for 5–10 breaths,
then switch sides.
Do wrist therapy.

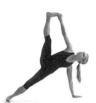

22. Vasisthasana
Hold for 5–10 breaths,
then switch sides.
Do wrist therapy.

23. Balasana
Hold for 1 minute.

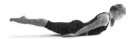

24. Salabhasana A
3 times for 3, 5, then 7
breaths, respectively. Offer
the hand-clasp on the
third time and encourage
students to stay as long as
they are at ease.

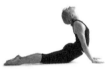

25. Bhujangasana
Emphasize anchoring in
the legs and pelvis as a
source of space in the
lower back while focus-
ing the arch in the mid-
thoracic spine. Do 2 times
for 5–10 breaths.

26. Dhanurasana
2 times for 5 breaths.

27. Balasana
Hold for 1 minute.

28. Bharadvajrasana I
5 breaths on each side.

**29. Ardha
Matsyendrasana**
10 breaths on each side.

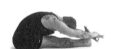

30. Paschimottanasana
Hold 1 minute.

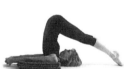

31. Halasana
Hold 1 minute.

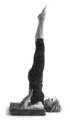

**32. Salamba
Sarvangasana**
Hold 2 minutes.

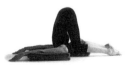

33. Karnapidasana
Hold 5 breaths.

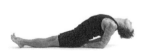

34. Uttana Padasana Prep
Hold 5 breaths.

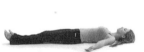

35. Savasana
5 minutes or longer.

36. Sukhasana
Meditation, setting intention,
sealing in the practice.

Sequence 12: Beginning Level—Focus on Forward Bends

1. Sukhasana
1–5 minutes. Welcome, set intention, begin guiding.

2. Parivrtta Sukhasana
Encourage dynamic exploration, twisting on each side up to 1 minute. Explain roots and extension and playing the edge.

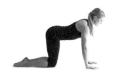

3. Bidalasana
5 rounds of Cat and Dog Tilts.

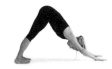

4. Adho Mukha Svanasana
Hold 30 seconds and release to Balasana; repeat 4 times.

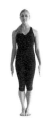

5. Tadasana
Emphasize pada bandha and roots and extension.

6. Classical Surya Namaskara
3 times. Hold Ardha Uttanasana 5 breaths each time, alternately bending and possibly straightening the legs.

7. Surya Namaskara A
2 times. Hold Ardha Uttanasana for 5 breaths each time, alternately bending and possibly straightening the legs. Hold Adho Mukha Svanasana 1 minute each time.

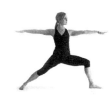

8. Virabhadrasana II
Prepare in a wide Prasarita stance. Hold each side 10 breaths.

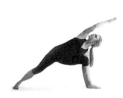

9. Utthita Parsvakonasana
Prepare in Warrior II. Hold each side for 5 breaths.

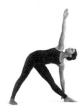

10. Utthita Trikonasana
Prepare in Prasarita stance. Hold each side 10–15 breaths.

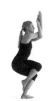

11. Garudasana
Hold each side 1 minute.

12. Garudasana Prep
Offer this prep position for those unable to cross their knees.

13. Prasarita Padottanasana A
Hold 1 minute.

14. Parsvottanasana
Prepare facing a wall, and use the wall to support the hands at hip height. Hold each side 10 breaths, then step to the front of the mat for Tadasana.

15. Surya Namaskara A
Hold Adho Mukha Svanasana for 1 minute.

16. Balasana
1 minute.

Sequence 12: Beginning Level—Focus on Forward Bends (continued)

7. Dandasana
2 minutes.

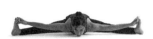

18. Upavista Konasana
2 minutes.

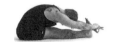

19. Paschimottanasana
2–3 minutes.

20. Apanasana
Move the knees in circles
for 1 minute.

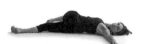

**21. Supta
Parivartanasana**
5–10 breaths on each side.
Repeat once on each side.

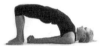

**22. Setu Bandha
Sarvangasana**
Hold for 10 breaths.
Repeat twice.

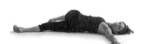

**23. Supta
Parivartanasana**
5–10 breaths on each side.

24. Viparita Karani
Hold 3 minutes.

25. Savasana
5 minutes or longer.

26. Sukhasana
Meditation, setting intention,
sealing in the practice.

Sequence 13: Beginning Level—Focus on Inversion

1. Sukhasana
1–5 minutes. Welcome, set intention, begin guiding.

2. Bidalasana
5 times of Cat and Dog Tilts, warming the spine and refining the connection of breath to movement. Release to Utthita Balasana.

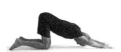

3. Anahatasana
10 breaths. Explain shoulder rotation as for Adho Mukha Svanasana.

4. Adho Mukha Svanasana
1 minute. Briefly highlight arm and leg alignment, roots and extension, and actions in the arms, shoulders, and legs.

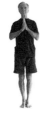

5. Samasthihi
Walk forward from Adho Mukha Svanasana and slowly roll up to standing. Teach Mountain Pose.

6. Classical Surya Namaskara
2 times. On the first time, pause in each asana to give refined instruction.

7. Surya Namaskara A
2 times, holding Adho Mukha Svanasana 1–2 minutes each time.

8. Balasana
1 minute.

9. Bharadvajrasana I
5 breaths on each side, then transition to Adho Mukha Svanasana and walk forward.

10. Ardha Uttanasana
10 breaths.

11. Uttanasana
Hold for 10 breaths.

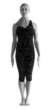

12. Tadasana
5 breaths.

13. Prasarita Padottanasana A
Hold for 2 minutes.

14. Prasarita Padottanasana C
Hold for 1 minute.

15. Surya Namaskara A
Hold Adho Mukha Svanasana for 1 minute. Release to a supine position.

16. Setu Bandha Sarvangasana
5 breaths. Repeat 3 times.

Sequence 13: Beginning Level—Focus on Inversion (continued)

17. Apanasana
5 breaths, moving the knees in circles.

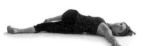

18. Supta Parivartanasana
5 breaths on each side.

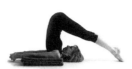

19. Halasana
Set up with blankets to bolster the shoulders and at a wall to support the feet. Hold 2 minutes. Release to lying supine or transition to the next asana.

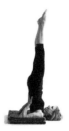

20. Salamba Sarvangasana
3 minutes.

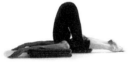

21. Karnapidasana
5 breaths.

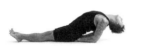

22. Uttana Padasana Prep
5 breaths.

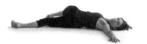

23. Supta Parivartanasana
5 breaths on each side.

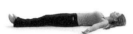

24. Savasana
5 minutes or longer.

25. Sukhasana
Meditation, setting intention, sealing in the practice.

Chapter Seven

Intermediate-Level Classes

A good traveler has no fixed plans and is not
intent on arriving.
—LAO TZU

Perhaps the greatest challenge in planning and teaching intermediate-level
classes is the sheer range of experience and ability among students in these
classes. While many studios maintain fairly clear class distinctions, most
have mixed-level classes (Level 1–2, 2–3, All Levels, etc.). Almost invariably,
students you might think are best served in a beginning-level class show up
in intermediate-level classes, whether because they think that is what is most
appropriate for them or because they have friends in intermediate classes and
want to share in the practice with them. With advanced students often looking
for an easier-going class in order to maintain their overall practice balance,
you are likely to have complete beginners mixed in with seriously advanced
students in the same class. Meanwhile, intermediate-level classes are not only
the most diverse; they tend to be the largest. This creates quite a challenge in
developing appropriate sequences for whoever is actually in a particular class.

There is no precise way to define an intermediate-level class. In Ashtanga Vinyasa the Intermediate Series clearly involves what for the vast preponderance of yoga students are very advanced positions. Indeed, in the Primary Series we find very complex asanas such as Marichyasana D (Sage Marichi's Pose D) and Setu Bandhasana (Supported Bridge or Charlie Chaplin Pose); the Intermediate Series has several complex asanas that by most standards are advanced, such as Dwi Pada Sirsasana (Two Legs behind Head Pose), in which the legs are positioned behind the back; Karandavasana (Duck Pose); and Vatayanasana (Horse Pose). While the Ashtanga Vinyasa approach emphasizes that the Intermediate Series, called nadi shodhana, meaning "nerve cleansing," is designed to further open and balance energy channels in and around the spine, the sheer complexity of its constituent asanas is likely to discourage many students or lead them to practice beyond the limits of sthira and sukham. As a result, many students end up with more, not less, nervous tension as they attempt to push their way through their practice. As David Swenson (1999, 129) suggests, "The depth of the asanas is not as important as the knowledge of how to approach them at a personal level."

In beginning level yoga we come into a more conscious relationship with ourselves. We learn the basics of breathing and moving in more conscious ways, and we learn some of the fundamental alignment principles and energetics in the asanas that make them more accessible and beneficial. Amid this we also increasingly encounter deep-seated emotional tension and other sensations that can be scary or just plain difficult to stay with. This marks the beginning of the opportunity to delve more deeply into how matters of consciousness are at play in doing yoga. Having established greater steadiness and ease in the basic asanas, in intermediate yoga we come to greater curiosity about the alchemy of yoga, the transformative potential contained in every breath when it is consciously connected to what is happening in the bodymind. With more strength and flexibility, we are able to hold asanas for longer and longer, thereby further strengthening the body while stimulating the deeper process of self-reflection that makes the asana practice more and more a meditative practice. The fruits are movement into emotional balance, a more stable and open mind, and a deepening sense of capacity as a conscious human being.

For our purposes here—designing classes that make sense for students where they presently are in their lives—it is helpful to have some criteria for differentiating intermediate classes from beginning classes. To begin, intermediate classes are ideally taught to students who can maintain steady ujjayi pranayama throughout a beginning level class without straining in the breath at all, and who can do an entire beginning-level practice without needing to rest. Second, a student should have an embodied understanding of the alignment principles, energetic actions and modifications for the asanas taught at the beginning level as well as the ability to do them without forcing anything or otherwise straining. They should be comfortable holding Adho Mukha Svanasana (Downward-Facing Dog Pose) and Phalakasana (Plank Pose) for at least one minute, and they should be able to hold Salamba Sarvangasana (Shoulder Stand) for two minutes (unless this asana is contraindicated due to cervical spine issues, high blood pressure, or retinal attachment issues). Rather than considering these as hard and fast tests of strength and flexibility that signifies one's preparation for doing intermediate level yoga, the idea is to use them as general guideposts for making decisions about where a student is best accommodated in cultivating their personal practice. It is therefore important to be prepared for a wide variety of students in these classes.

Before exploring how to address this challenge in planning and sequencing classes, let's consider another part of the normal experience among intermediate-level students: the plateau. In fitness culture, the concept of an "exercise plateau" refers to diminishing returns in relation to effort. Despite working just as hard or even harder than usual, it seems like nothing is changing, as though one is stuck in their practice. It is important for students to appreciate that they will encounter many plateaus along the lifelong path of their yoga practice. They will experience the most dramatic changes in their breath and bodymind in their first year of consistent practice, with the physical growth curve expanding less quickly and leveling off or even dropping from time to time thereafter. This is part of the practice, an absolutely essential part for those interested in going more deeply into the nonphysical aspects of yoga. Yet it is precisely here that many students burn out, give up, and abandon yoga for something that seems to resume

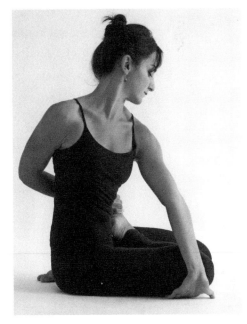

Bharadvajrasana

the experience of immediate results. It may well be that the body is asking for a break, even if only in the types of sequences one is doing or the setting. It is important to play with this, to explore whether a different path might make sense for at least a while or to explore a different approach on the same path, such as trying a different teacher or style. But before taking a different path, it is best to pause and reflect; the plateau may be an invitation to take the practice deeper by staying on the plateau but with a different attitude, opening to the possibility that by staying with it one might be close to a breakthrough that awakens the practice in amazing and altogether unexpected ways.

All of the asanas listed in the previous chapter as beginning level are part of the repertoire of intermediate-level classes. The difference is primarily in how they are approached and sequenced. In approaching them, students should keep applying the principle of playing the edge in order to best discern how to explore in and around each asana. In sequencing them, you should stay with the basic principle of moving from simple to complex, even as what before was complex might now be simple in relation to where the class is and where it is headed.

Creating and Teaching Intermediate-Level Sequences

- Continue to teach ujjayi pranayama at the beginning of each class even if as review, either when students are sitting, standing in Tadasana (Mountain Pose), or in Adho Mukha Svanasana.

- Separately introduce kapalabhati pranayama and nadi shodhana pranayama once students exhibit steadiness and ease with ujjayi throughout their asana practice.

- Introduce *antara kumbhaka* and *bahya kumbhaka* practices in conjunction with vritti pranayama practices.

- Introduce *anuloma* and *pratiloma* pranayamas once students are comfortable with basic vritti practices.

- Teach *viloma* pranayama after establishing comfort with combined vritti and kumbhaka practices.

- Introduce *suryabheda* and *chandrabheda* pranayamas.

- Introduce mula bandha, uddiyana bandha (only with retention of the exhalation), and *jalandhara bandha* in conjunction with pranayama practices.
- Give more detailed guidance to pada bandha an essential part of the entire asana practice.
- Continue offering a preparatory warming prior to doing Surya Namaskaras (Sun Salutations), especially in classes with students who are new to you or clearly at more of a beginning level.
- Intermediate-level classes can start with Surya Namaskara. Generally limit this dynamic warm-up to three Surya Namaskara A and three Surya Namaskara B sequences.
- Introduce variations in the Surya Namaskaras: extending one leg back and up when in Adho Mukha Svanasana; drawing the shoulders over the wrists while arching the spine and drawing one knee and the forehead toward each other; and arm variations in Virabhadrasana I to help open the back and shoulder girdle for arm balances and back bends.
- Integrate wrist therapy into the Surya Namaskaras by encouraging students to turn their palms up toward the ceiling whenever folding into Uttanasana (Standing Forward Bend Pose). They can go a bit farther with this by making small fists and moving their wrists around in circles.
- Begin linking more asanas together in standing sequences, up to five on each side before transitioning to the other side. If doing more than two asanas on each side, consider moving through Chaturanga–Up Dog–Down Dog between sides to help integrate the practice along the way. Give greater emphasis to all of the elements of Up Dog and Down Dog especially.
- Generally sequence externally rotated-hip standing asanas together and before internally rotated-hip standing asanas.
- Begin introducing more complex variations in the standing asanas, including wrapping in Utthita Parsvakonasana (Extended Side Angle Pose) and transitioning from that variation to Eka Pada Koundinyasana A (One-Leg Sage Koundinya's Pose) to Astavakrasana

(Eight-Angle Pose) to Chaturanga Dandasana (Four-Limbed Staff Pose).

- Do five to seven minutes of focused core awakening in partial preparation for arm balances. Key the specific core awakening to the most active abdominal muscles in specific arm balances, as discussed in Chapter Three.

- Open the hip flexors and shoulder girdle prior to doing arm balances or back bends in which the arms are positioned overhead in flexion.

- Introduce Adho Mukha Vrksasana (Handstand) and Pincha Mayurasana (Feathered Peacock Pose, or Forearm Balance) at the wall, offering ample time for students to explore coming into each asana two or more times.

- Introduce other arm balances with students on the mat away from the wall. Give these introductions focused attention prior to blending them into flowing sequences of arm balances.

- Significantly neutralize tension in the torso following core awakening before exploring back bends.

- Explore contraction and traction back bends prior to leveraged back bends.

- Continue offering Setu Bandha Sarvangasana (Bridge Pose) as the foundational supine back bend before introducing Urdhva Dhanurasana (Upward-Facing Bow Pose).

- In teaching Urdhva Dhanurasana, move slowly through each preparatory stage to cue proper alignment and energetic actions. Encourage staying with Setu Bandha Sarvangasana, Dhanurasana (Bow Pose), or Ustrasana (Camel Pose) as alternatives.

- Introduce *eka pada* (one-leg) variations of supine back bends only to students who are clearly stable and at ease in the basic forms of the asanas (Setu Bandha Sarvangasana, Urdhva Dhanurasana, Viparita Dandasana [Inverted Staff Pose]).

- Offer abdominal core strengthening movements as effective pratikriyasana following back bends.

- Do one to three brief twisting asanas to release tension along the spine following back bends.

- Explore a variety of calming forward bends and hip openers to stimulate the parasympathetic nervous system and further reduce tension along the path toward Savasana (Corpse Pose).
- Introduce Salamba Sirsasana I (Headstand) at the wall while encouraging students who are stable in this asana to gradually practice it farther away from the wall.
- Introduce variations in Salamba Sarvangasana, including various leg positions (apart, scissored, Baddha Kona, and Padma).
- Introduce Urdhva Padmasana (Upward Lotus Pose) and Pindasana (Embryo Pose) to students comfortable in Salamba Sarvangasana for at least three minutes.
- Introduce Karnapidasana (Ear-Squeezing Pose) to students practicing Halasana (Plow Pose).
- Introduce Uttana Padasana Prep (Extended Leg Pose) to students practicing Halasana.
- Introduce Matsyasana (Fish Pose) and full Uttana Padasana to students practicing Urdhva Padmasana and Pindasana.
- Explore nadi shodhana pranayama before releasing into Savasana.
- Allow at least five minutes for Savasana.
- Allow at least a few minutes after Savasana for sitting quietly and absorbing one's awareness in the awakened yet calm energy students will feel in their bodymind.

Intermediate Class Sequences

Sequence 14: Intermediate Level—Focus on Back Bends

1. Virasana
3–5 minutes. Welcome, set intention, begin guiding.

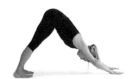

2. Adho Mukha Svanasana
Bicycle out the legs for 1 minute before coming to standing.

3. Classical Surya Namaskara
2 times, exploring Anjaneyasana with dynamic movement for 5 breaths each time in the asana. Hold Salabhasana B for 1 minute on the last time.

4. Surya Namaskara A
2 times, then Tail of the Dog in transition to the next asana.

Sequence 14: Intermediate Level—Focus on Back Bends (continued)

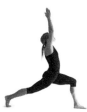

5. Ashta Chandrasana
Interlace the fingers behind the back, fold forward, holding for 1 minute before returning to Ashta Chandrasana and transitioning to Adho Mukha Svanasana. Switch sides.

6. Surya Namaskara B
3 times, holding Warrior I for 1 minute on the last time to further open the hip flexors.

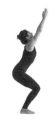

7. Utkatasana
Explore from Tadasana, moving in and out of the asana 5 times before holding 5 breaths.

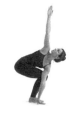

8. Parivrtta Utkatasana
5–10 breaths on each side, then transition to Surya Namaskara A and hold Adho Mukha Svanasana 1 minute.

9. Dancing Warrior
3 cycles, holding Warrior II for 1 minute on the last time on each side.

10. Balasana
5 breaths or rest in Adho Mukha Svanasana before transitioning to Tadasana.

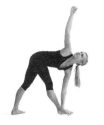

11. Utthita Trikonasana
Set up from Prasarita stance. 5 breaths on each side.

12. Prasarita Padottanasana A
10 breaths before coming up.

13. Prasarita Padottanasana C
10 breaths before coming up.

14. Parsvottanasana
5 breaths on each side.

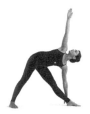

15. Parivrtta Trikonasana
10 breaths on each side, then come to Tadasana.

16. Surya Namaskara B
Substitute Ashta Chandrasana for Virabhadrasana and move dynamically in and out 5 times before holding for 5 breaths, repeating on the other side.

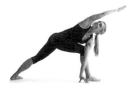

17. Parivrtta Parsvakonasana
Set up from Ashta Chandrasana, hold for 1 minute before transitioning to Chaturanga, Urdhva Mukha Svanasana, Adho Mukha Svanasana, repeating on the other side.

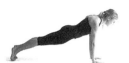

18. Phalakasana
5 breaths. Slowly release to the floor. 1 minute.

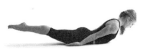

19. Salabhasana A
Hold 5 breaths, then rest or clasp hands behind the back for 5 breaths.

Sequence 14: Intermediate Level—Focus on Back Bends (continued)

20. Dhanurasana
3 times, holding for 5, 8, and 10-plus breaths.

21. Ustrasana
3 times, holding for 5, 8, and 10-plus breaths.

22. Laghu Vajrasana
Explore after 1–2 times in Ustrasana.

23. Balasana
1 minute with the knees wide apart to reduce pressure in the lower back.

24. Ardha Matsyendrasana
5–8 breaths on each side.

25. Ananda Balasana
10 breaths.

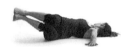

27. Jathara Parivartanasana
Move dynamically 5 times to each side.

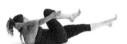

28. Yogic Bicycles
1–2 minutes.

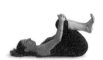

29. Apanasana
5 breaths, then rock and roll up to sitting.

30. Dandasana
5 breaths.

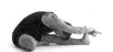

31. Janu Sirsasana A
1 minute on each side.

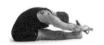

32. Paschimottanasana
2 minutes.

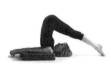

33. Halasana
5 breaths.

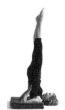

34. Salamba Sarvangasana
3–5 minutes.

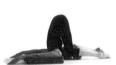

35. Karnapidasana
5 breaths.

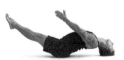

36. Uttana Padasana
5 breaths.

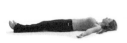

37. Savasana
5 minutes or longer.

38. Sukhasana
Meditation, setting intention, sealing in the practice.

Sequence 15: Intermediate Level—Focus on Back Bends II

1. Virasana
3–5 minutes. Welcome, set intention, begin guiding.

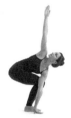

2. Adho Mukha Svanasana
Bicycle out the legs for 1 minute before coming to standing.

3. Classical Surya Namaskara
2 times, exploring Anjaneyas-ana with dynamic movement for 5 breaths each time in the asana.

4. Surya Namaskara A
3 times, holding Adho Mukha Svanasana for 1 minute each time.

5. Surya Namaskara B
3 times, holding Virabha-drasana I for 1 minute on the last time.

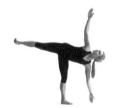

6. Parivrtta Utkatasana
5–10 breaths on each side. Release to Tadasana.

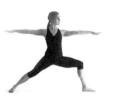

7. Virabhadrasana II
2 minutes on each side. Prepare in a wide Prasarita stance.

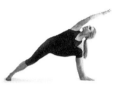

8. Utthita Parsvakonasana
2 minutes on each side. Give optional transitions: simple vinyasa or weave in Eka Pada Koundinyasana A to in transi-tion to Chaturanga.

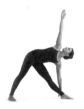

9. Utthita Trikonasana
Prepare in Prasarita stance 10 breaths. Transition into Ardha Chandrasana.

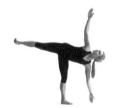

10. Ardha Chandrasana
5–10 breaths. Release to repeat this sequence on the other side.

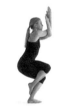

11. Garudasana
1 minute on each side.

12. Prasarita Padottanasana C
5–10 breaths.

13. Parsvottanasana
5 breaths. Transition to the next asana.

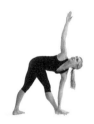

14. Parivrtta Trikonasana
5 breaths. Transition to the next asana.

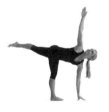

15. Parivrtta Ardha Chandrasana
5 breaths. Transition back to Parivrtta Trikonasana, then to Parsvottanasana. Switch sides and then step to Tadasana.

16. Surya Namaskara A
Flow to Adho Mukha Svanasana.

Sequence 15: Intermediate Level—Focus on Back Bends II (continued)

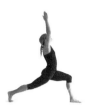

17. Ashta Chandrasana
1 minute. Transition to the next asana.

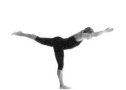

18. Virabhadrasana III
Hold 5 breaths, then transition to the next asana.

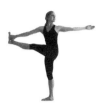

19. Parivrtta Hasta Padangusthasana
10 breaths. Transition back to Virabhadrasana III for 1 breath, then back to Ashta Chandrasana. Do a vinyasa and switch sides.

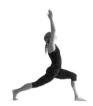

20. Ashta Chandrasana
5 breaths. Transition to the next asana.

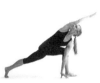

21. Parivrtta Ashta Chandrasana
5 breaths. Either return to Ashta Chandrasana and do a vinyasa or transition through Eka Pada Koundinyasana B to a vinyasa to Adho Mukha Svanasana.

22. Virasana
1 minute.

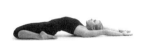

23. Supta Virasana
3 minutes with arms overhead in flexion. Transition through all fours to Adho Mukha Svanasana. Lie supine (if possible, float through the arms).

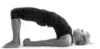

24. Setu Bandha Sarvangasana
1 minute, then either stay with Setu Bandha Sarvangasana 3 more times or set up for Urdhva Dhanurasana.

25. Urdhva Dhanurasana
5–10 breaths. Repeat 2–3 times. Either stay with Urdhva Dhanurasana or explore Viparita Dandasana.

26. Viparita Dandasana
5–10 breaths. If stable, explore the Eka Pada variation, holding each side for up to 5 breaths.

27. Apanasana
5 breaths.

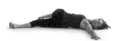

28. Supta Parivartanasana
5 breaths on each side.

29. Ananda Balasana
5 breaths.

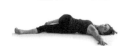

30. Supta Parivartanasana
10 breaths on each side.

31. Dandasana
1 minute.

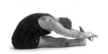

32. Paschimottanasana
2 minutes.

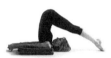

**33. Tiriang
Mukha Eka Pada
Paschimottanasana**
1 minute on each side.

34. Bharadvajrasana B
Hold each side for 1
minute.

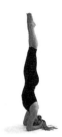

35. Salamba Sirsasana I
3–5 minutes. Rest in
Balasana.

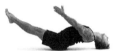

36. Balasana
5–10 breaths. Lie supine
(option: vinyasa and
float through).

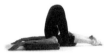

37. Halasana
5–10 breaths.

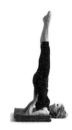

38. Salamba Sarvangasana
2–3 minutes.

39. Karnapidasana
5 breaths.

40. Uttana Padasana
5 breaths.

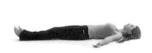

41. Savasana
5–10 minutes.

42. Padmasana or Sukhasana
Kapalabhati pranayama.

Sequence 16: Intermediate Level—Focus on Hip Opening

1. Padmasana or Sukhasana
3–5 minutes. Kapalabhati pranayama for 1 minute.

2. Classical Surya Namaskara
3 times, holding Anjaneyasana on each side on the last time.

3. Surya Namaskara A
3 times. In Adho Mukha Svanasana on the third time, hold Tail of the Dog for 1 minute on each side before doing the following pose on that side.

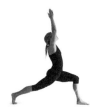

4. Ashta Chandrasana
Move dynamically in and out of the pose 5 times before holding for 5 breaths, then transition through Chaturanga, Urdhva Mukha Svanasana, Adho Mukha Svanasana.

5. Surya Namaskara B
3 times. On the third time, transition from Virabhadrasana I to Virabhadrasana II.

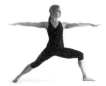

6. Virabhadrasana II
1 minute, then transition into Side Warrior for 5 breaths, and then to Utthita Parsvakonasana.

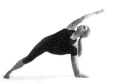

7. Utthita Parsvakonasana
Prepare in Virabhadrasana II. Hold each side for 2 minutes. Transition back to Virabhadrasana II and then vinyasa to Tadasana, or the following asana.

8. Eka Pada Koundinyasana A
From the wrapped variation of Utthita Parsvakonasana, transition through Eka Pada Koundinyasana A and then vinyasa to Tadasana, or add the following asana.

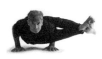

9. Astavakrasana
From Eka Pada Koundinyasana A transition to Astavakrasana, back to Eka Pada Koundinyasana A, then vinyasa to Tadasana.

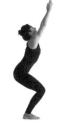

10. Utkatasana
Hold 5 breaths, maintaining pelvic neutrality in relation to the spine.

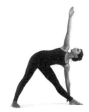

11. Utthita Trikonasana
Set up from Prasarita stance and hold 5 breaths.

12. Prasarita Padottanasana A
5 breaths. Cue using core muscles.

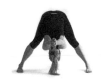

13. Prasarita Padottanasana C
5 breaths.

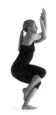

14. Garudasana
10 breaths on each side.

15. Parsvottanasana
10 breaths, then transition to the next asana.

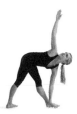

16. Parivrtta Trikonasana
5 breaths, release to Parsvottanasana, and switch sides.

Sequence 16: Intermediate Level—Focus on Hip Opening (continued)

17. Surya Namaskara A
Flow to Adho Mukha Svanasana.

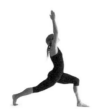

18. Ashta Chandrasana
5–10 breaths, then transition to the next asana.

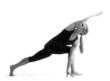

19. Parivrtta Ashta Chandrasana
5–10 breaths, do a vinyasa and switch sides, then vinyasa to Adho Mukha Svanasana.

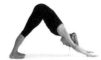

20. Adho Mukha Svanasana
5 breaths.

21. Malasana
5–10 breaths, then vinyasa to Adho Mukha Svanasana.

22. Eka Pada Raj Kapotasana
Explore on each side 2–3 minutes, bicycling out the legs in Adho Mukha Svanasana after each side.

23. Urdhva Dhanurasana
5–10 breaths. Repeat 3–4 times.

24. Ardha Matsyendrasana
10 breaths on each side.

25. Gomukhasana
10 breaths on each side.

26. Agnistambhasana
2 minutes on each side. Keep the feet strongly flexed (dorsiflexion).

27. Dandasana
Hold 5 breaths. Root the sit bones down and extend tall.

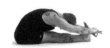

28. Paschimottanasana
1 minute. Move dynamically to slowly release.

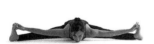

29. Upavista Konasana
2 minutes. Keep the legs awake.

30. Baddha Konasana
2 minutes. Breath through the heart, sternum lifted, spacious heart.

31. Swastikasana
2 minutes on each side. Explore letting go with each exhale.

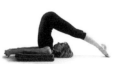

32. Halasana
5 breaths. Feed the legs to extend the spine.

Sequence 16: Intermediate Level—Focus on Hip Opening (continued)

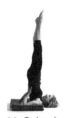

33. Salamba Sarvangasana
3–5 minutes. Play with leg variations.

34. Urdhva Padmasana
5 breaths. Use mula bandha to extend the spine.

35. Pindasana
5 breaths. Stronger inhales, slower exhales.

36. Matsyasana
5 breaths. Pull on the feet to leverage the heart center to the sky.

37. Uttana Padasana
5 breaths. Feed the legs. Be sensitive to the neck.

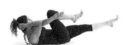

38. Savasana
5–10 minutes.

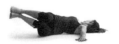

39. Padmasana
Sit in meditation.

Sequence 17: Intermediate Level—Focus on Twisting

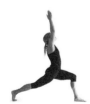

1. Sukhasana
3–5 minutes. Set intention, begin ujjayi pranayama, then lie supine.

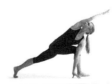

2. Yogic Bicycles
1–2 minutes, the rest in Apanasana 5 breaths.

3. Jathara Parivartanasana
5–10 cycles moving side to side, rest in Supta Baddha Konasana for 5 breaths, come to standing.

4. Surya Namaskara A
3 times. Transition to the next asana from Adho Mukha Svanasana.

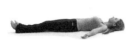

5. Ashta Chandrasana
Move in an out dynamically 5 times on the first side, then hold 5 breaths before transitioning to the next asana.

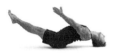

6. Parivrtta Ashta Chandrasana
5–10 breaths. Flow through a vinyasa and repeat 5–6 times on the other side.

7. Surya Namaskara B
3 times. Transition to the next asana from Utkatasana.

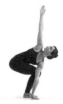

8. Parivrtta Utkatasana
5 breaths on each side. Transition to Tadasana, then to Prasarita stance.

9. Virabhadrasana II
10 breaths on the first side, then transition to the next asana.

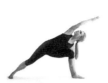

10. Utthita Parsvakonasana
10 breaths, come back to Virabhadrasana II, and repeat asanas 9 and 10 on the other side.

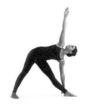

11. Utthita Trikonasana
10 breaths on the first side, then transition to the next asana.

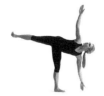

12. Ardha Chandrasana
10 breaths, come back to Utthita Trikonasana, and repeat asanas 11 and 12 on the other side.

13. Prasarita Padottanasana C
5 breaths.

14. Parsvottanasana
5 breaths on each side.

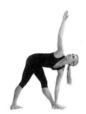

15. Parivrtta Trikonasana
10–15 breaths on the first side, then transition to the next asana.

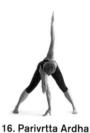

16. Parivrtta Ardha Chandrasana
10 breaths, release back to Parivrtta Trikonasana, switch sides and repeat asanas 15 and 16. Step to Tadasana.

17. Surya Namaskara A
1 breath.

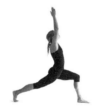

18. Ashta Chandrasana
5 breaths on the first side, then transition to the next asana.

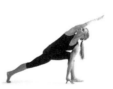

19. Parivrtta Ashta Chandrasana
10–15 breaths on the first side. Vinyasa to the other side of asanas 18 and 19. Do a vinyasa and transition to the other side or to the following asana.

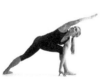

20. Parivrtta Parsvakonasana
Explore as a more challenging alternative to Parivrtta Ashta Chandrasana.

21. Balasana
Rest 5–10 breaths.

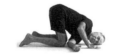

22. Urdhva Mukha Pasasana
2–3 minutes on each side.

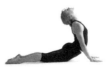

23. Bhujangasana
3 times, 5 breaths each time.

24. Ustrasana
3 times, 5–10 breaths each time.

Sequence 17: Intermediate Level—Focus on Twisting (continued)

25. Bharadvajrasana B
10 breaths on each side.

26. Swastikasana
1–2 minutes on each side.

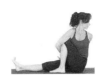

27. Marichyasana C
10 breaths on each side.

28. Dandasana
1 minute.

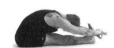

29. Paschimottanasana
Explore dynamically, then hold 1–2 minutes.

30. Parivrtta Janu Sirsasana
1–2 minutes.

31. Baddha Konasana
1–2 minutes, then come to all fours.

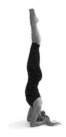

32. Salamba Sirsasana I
2–5 minutes, then rest in Balasana. As an alternative, do Viparita Karani.

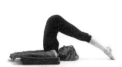

33. Halasana
5 breaths. As an alternative to this and the next 3 asanas, do Viparita Karani.

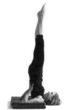

34. Salamba Sarvangasana
2–3 minutes. Play with leg variations.

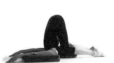

35. Karnapidasana
5 breaths.

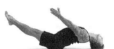

36. Uttana Padasana
5 breaths.

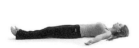

37. Savasana
5–10 minutes.

38. Sukhasana
Meditation, pranayama, complete the practice.

Sequence 18: Intermediate Level—Focus on Standing Balance

1. Virasana
3–5 minutes. Welcome, set intention, begin guiding.

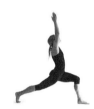

2. Adho Mukha Svanasana
Bicycle out the legs for 1 minute before coming to standing.

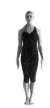

3. Tadasana
1 minute. Teach pada bandha, toots and extension, mula bandha.

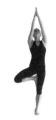

4. Vrksasana
1 minute on each side. Play with closing the eyes.

5. Surya Namaskara A
3 times. On the third time, transition from Tail of the Dog to Ashta Chandrasana.

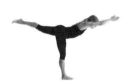

6. Ashta Chandrasana
5 breaths. Stay or transition to the next asana.

7. Virabhadrasana III Prep
10 breaths with the arms back by the sides, then release back to Ashta Chandrasana, vinyasa, and switch sides.

8. Surya Namaskara B
3 times. Move slowly and steadily.

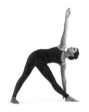

9. Utthita Trikonasana
10 breaths. Set up from Prasarita stance. Transition to the next asana before switching sides.

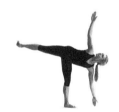

10. Ardha Chandrasana
10 breaths. Release to Utthita Trikonasana and switch sides on asanas 9 and 10. Hop to Tadasana.

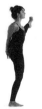

11. Surya Namaskara A
1 time, holding Adho Mukha Svanasana 1 breaths, then Tail of the Dog to Virabhadrasana I, then open to Virabhadrasana II.

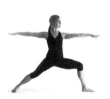

12. Virabhadrasana II
5 breaths.

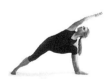

13. Utthita Parsvakonasana
5 breaths. If possible, take the wrapped variation. Either stay or transition to the next asana by first stepping the back foot next to the front foot.

14. Svarga Dvijasana
10 breaths. Stand tall with the wrapped leg bent at the knee. When tall and stable, explore straightening that leg, then release and reverse these steps to come back to Utthita Parsvakonasana and transition through a vinyasa (perhaps blend in Eka Pada Koundinyasana A). Switch sides on asanas 11–14.

Sequence 18: Intermediate Level—Focus on Standing Balance (continued)

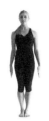

15. Tadasana
Revisit intention.

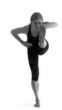

16. Utthita Hasta Padangusthasana
10 breaths on each side.

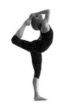

17. Natarajasana Prep
10 breaths on each side.

18. Garudasana
10 breaths on each side.

19. Parsvottanasana
5 breaths on the first side, then transition to the next asana.

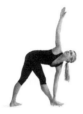

20. Parivrtta Trikonasana
5 breaths, then switch sides on asanas 19–20.

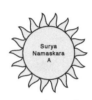

21. Surya Namaskara A
1 time, then Tail of the Dog in transition to the next asana.

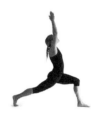

22. Ashta Chandrasana
5 breaths.

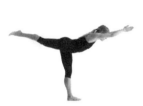

23. Virabhadrasana III
5 breaths. Keep the standing knee bent to take it easier on the knee, hip, and lower back, then stand tall, lifting the knee.

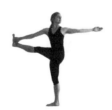

24. Parivrtta Hasta Padangusthasana
10 breaths. Encourage the twist with the hand to the knee or the foot, then release to the center, back to Virabhadrasana III, and to the next asana.

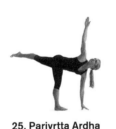

25. Parivrtta Ardha Chandrasana
5 breaths, then place both hands on the floor. Either step back and vinyasa to Adho Mukha Svanasana or do the next asana.

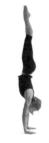

26. Adho Mukha Vrksasana
3 breaths in transition to Chaturanga Dandasana and vinyasa. Repeat asanas 22–26 on the other side.

27. Balasana
5 breaths. As an alternative, rest in Adho Mukha Svanasana or Adho Mukha Vrksasana, then lie prone.

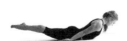

28. Salabhasana A
5 breaths. Repeat 3 times, resting between or vinyasa between.

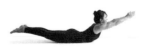

29. Salabhasana C
5 breaths, then rest or vinyasa.

30. Bhujangasana
5 breaths. Repeat 2–3 times.

Sequence 18: Intermediate Level—Focus on Standing Balance (continued)

31. Balasana
5 breaths.

**32. Ardha
Matsyendrasana**
5 breaths on each side.

33. Gomukhasana
10 breaths on each side.

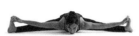
34. Upavista Konasana
2 minutes.

35. Dandasana
5 breaths.

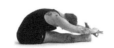
36. Paschimottanasana
2 minutes.

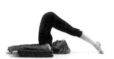
37. Halasana
5 breaths.

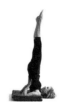
**38. Salamba
Sarvangasana**
2–5 minutes.

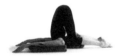
39. Karnapidasana
5 breaths.

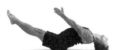
40. Uttana Padasana
5 breaths.

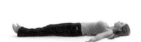
41. Savasana
5–10 minutes.

42. Sukhasana
Meditation.

Sequence 19: Intermediate Level—Focus on Arm Support I

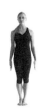

1. Tadasana
1–2 minutes. Welcome, set intention, begin guiding.

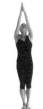

2. Urdhva Hastasana
1 minute, guiding students to maintain steady grounding, active legs, pelvic neutrality, and neutral extension of the spine.

3. Surya Namaskara A
3 times.

4. Surya Namaskara B
3 times. On the last time, hold Virabhadrasana I for 1 minute with the arms in Garudasana position, then stay in Adho Mukha Svanasana for 5 breaths.

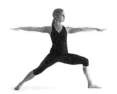

5. Virabhadrasana II
10 breaths on each side with the arms positioned as for Gomukhasana. Set up in Prasarita stance.

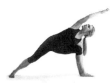

6. Utthita Parsvakonasana|
10 breaths on each side. Explore the wrapped variation and transition out through Eka Pada Koundinyasana and Astavakrasana.

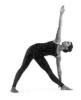

7. Utthita Trikonasana
10 breaths on each side.

8. Prasarita Padottanasana C
10 breaths.

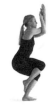

9. Garudasana
10 breaths on each side.

10. Surya Namaskara A
1 time, then float through to the next asana.

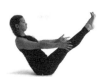

11. Navasana
5 breaths each of 5 times, then transition to the next asana.

12. Tolasana
1–5 breaths, then transition to the next asana.

13. Lolasana
1–5 breaths, then vinyasa.

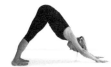

14. Adho Mukha Svanasana
10 breaths (or rest in Balasana).

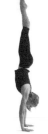

15. Adho Mukha Vrksasana
3 times for 5–10 breaths, then rest in Balasana. Do Wrist Therapy between each Handstand.

16. Wrist Therapy
1–2 minutes.

Sequence 19: Intermediate Level—Focus on Arm Support I (continued)

17. Virasana
1 minute with Garudasana arms, then 1 minute with Gomukhasana arms.

18. Shishulasana
5 breaths. Either keep exploring here or transition to the next asana.

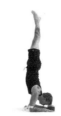

19. Pincha Mayurasana
3 times for 5–10 breaths, then rest in Balasana.

20. Balasana
10 breaths.

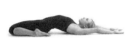

21. Supta Virasana
2 minutes. Prop the back if tightness prevents releasing the back to the floor.

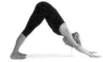

22. Adho Mukha Svanasana
10 breaths, bicycling out the legs, then lie prone.

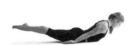

23. Salabhasana A
5 breaths. Repeat 3 times, resting between or vinyasa between.

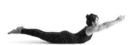

24. Salabhasana C
5 breaths, then rest or vinyasa.

25. Dhanurasana
3 times, 5–10 breaths each time, resting between or vinyasa between.

26. Bharadvajrasana A (or B)
10 breaths on each side.

27. Dandasana
5 breaths.

28. Gomukhasana
10 breaths on each side. Play with twisting rather than folding forward.

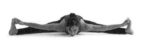

29. Upavista Konasana
1 minute.

30. Parivrtta Janu Sirsasana
10 breaths on each side.

31. Baddha Konasana
1 minute.

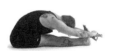

32. Paschimottanasana
2 minutes.

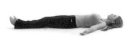

34. Savasana
5–10 minutes.

35. Sukhasana
Meditation.

Sequence 20: Intermediate Level—Focus on Arm Support II

1. Sukhasana
2–3 minutes. Welcome, set intention, begin guiding.

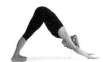

2. Adho Mukha Svanasana
2–3 minutes. Play with bicycling the legs and alternately resting in Balasana.

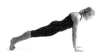

3. Phalakasana
10 breaths, using the belly and active legs for added support.

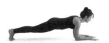

4. Shishula Phalakasana
10 breaths or optional kapalabhati pranayama.

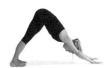

5. Adho Mukha Svanasana
5 breaths, then transition to Tadasana.

6. Surya Namaskara A
3 times.

7. Surya Namaskara B
3 times, then from Adho Mukha Svanasana leap from the feet around the arms to set up for the next asana.

8. Bhujapidasana
10 breaths, then vinyasa and transition to standing.

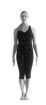

9. Tadasana
Wrist Therapy.

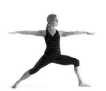

10. Virabhadrasana II
10 breaths on each side. Set up from Prasarita stance.

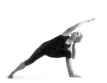

11. Utthita Parsvakonasana
10 breaths on each side. Offer wrapped variation and transition out through Eka Pada Koundinyasana A.

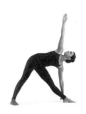

12. Utthita Trikonasana
10 breaths on each side.

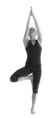

13. Vrksasana
10 breaths on each side, or do the following asana instead.

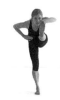

14. Utthita Hasta Padangusthasana
10 breaths on each side.

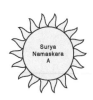

15. Surya Namaskara A
1 time. Transition to next asana from Adho Mukha Svanasana.

16. Vasisthasana
5–10 breaths on each side, then vinyasa.

17. Adho Mukha Svanasana
5 breaths, then float through to Dandasana.

18. Navasana
5 breaths, rest, repeat 4 times, then lie supine.

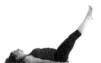

19. Leg Lifts
10–15 times.

20. Malasana
10 breaths.

21. Bhujapidasana
5 breaths. Either release and repeat or transition directly to the next asana.

22. Tittibhasana
5 breaths. Either release and repeat or transition directly to the next asana.

23. Bakasana
5 breaths. Either release and repeat or transition directly to the next asana.

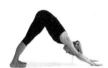

24. Adho Mukha Svanasana
5 breaths, or rest in Balasana, then hop forward.

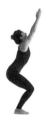

25. Utkatasana
5 breaths.

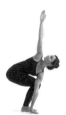

26. Parivrtta Utkatasana
5 breaths on each side, then vinyasa and float through to lying supine.

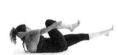

27. Yogic Bicycles
1–2 minutes.

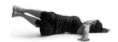

28. Jathara Parivartanasana
5 times each way, then transition to a simple squat.

29. Parsva Bakasana
5 breaths on each side, either transitioning on each side to the next asana or switching side and them repeating.

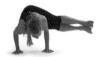

30. Dwi Pada Koundinyasana
5 breaths on each side, then vinyasa to Adho Mukha Svanasana.

31. Balasana
10 breaths.

32. Ardha Matsyendrasana
10 breaths on each side.

Sequence 20: Intermediate Level—Focus on Arm Support II (continued)

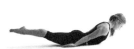

33. Salabhasana A
5 breaths. Repeat 3 times.
Optional vinyasa between
each time.

34. Dhanurasana
5 breaths. Repeat 3 times.
Optional vinyasa between
each time.

35. Balasana
5 breaths.

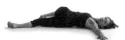

**36. Supta
Parivartanasana**
10 breaths on each side.

37. Ananda Balasana
5 breaths.

38. Dandasana
5 breaths.

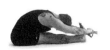

39. Paschimottanasana
1 minute.

40. Gomukhasana
10 breaths on each side.

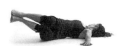

**41. Parivrtta Janu
Sirsasana**
10 breaths on each side.

42. Baddha Konasana
10 breaths.

**43. Supta Baddha
Konasana**
2 minutes.

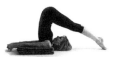

44. Halasana
5 breaths.

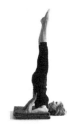

**45. Salamba
Sarvangasana**
3 minutes.

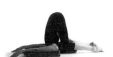

46. Karnapidasana
5 breaths.

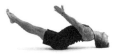

47. Uttana Padasana
5 breaths.

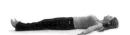

48. Savasana
5–10 minutes.

49. Sukhasana
Meditation.

Sequence 21: Intermediate Level—Focus on Forward Bends

1. Virasana
3–5 minutes. Welcome, set intention, begin guiding.

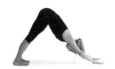

2. Adho Mukha Svanasana
2 minutes, bicycling out the legs.

3. Uttanasana
10 breaths.

4. Surya Namaskara A
3 times.

5. Surya Namaskara B
3 times.

6. Padangusthasana
5 breaths.

7. Pada Hastasana
5 breaths. Transition to Prasarita stance.

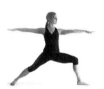

8. Virabhadrasana II
10 breaths on each side.

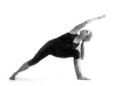

9. Utthita Parsvakonasana
10 breaths on each side.

10. Utthita Trikonasana
10 breaths on each side.

11. Prasarita Padottanasana A
5 breaths.

12. Prasarita Padottanasana B
5 breaths.

13. Prasarita Padottanasana C
5 breaths.

14. Prasarita Padottanasana D
5 breaths.

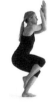

15. Garudasana
10 breaths on each side.

16. Parsvottanasana
5 breaths.

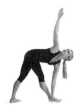

17. Parivrtta Trikonasana
5 breaths on each side,
then step to Tadasana.

18. Surya Namaskara A
1 time, hold Adho Mukha
Svanasana 5 breaths, float
through to sitting.

19. Dandasana
10 breaths. Emphasize rooting the sit bones as
the primary action of all
seated asanas.

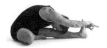

20. Janu Sirsasana A
10 breaths on each side.

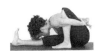

21. Marichyasana A
10 breaths on each side.

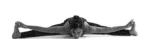

**22. Upavista
Konasana**
2 minutes.

**23. Parivrtta Janu
Sirsasana**
10 breaths on each side.

**24. Baddha
Konasana**
2 minutes.

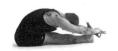

25. Paschimottanasana
2 minutes.

**26. Ardha
Matsyendrasana**
10 breaths on each side.

27. Swastikasana
1 minute on each side.

**28. Setu Bandha
Sarvangasana**
3 times, 5–10 breaths
each time. Repeat or do
the next asana.

**29. Urdhva
Dhanurasana**
3 times, 5–10 breaths
each time.

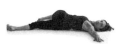

**30. Supta
Parivartanasana**
5 breaths on each side.
Transition to all fours and
Adho Mukha Svanasana.

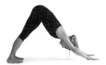

**31. Adho Mukha
Svanasana**
5 breaths.

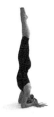

**32. Salamba
Sirsasana I**
2–5 minutes.

Sequence 21: Intermediate Level—Focus on Forward Bends (continued)

33. Balasana
5 breaths.

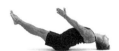

34. Uttana Padasana
5 breaths.

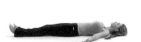

35. Savasana
5–10 minutes.

36. Sukhasana
Meditation.

Sequence 22: Intermediate Level—Focus on Inversions

1. Sukhasana
1–2 minutes. Welcome, set
intention, begin guiding.

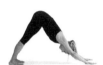

**2. Adho Mukha
Svanasana**
2–3 minutes, then rest
in Balasana.

3. Uttanasana
1 minute.

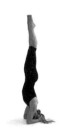

4. Salamba Sirsasana I
2–3 minutes, then rest in
Balasana.

5. Gomukhasana
10 breaths on each side,
then come to standing.

**6. Classical Surya
Namaskara**
2 times. Transition to Adho
Mukha Svanasana.

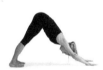

**7. Adho Mukha
Svanasana**
1 minute, then transition to
Tadasana.

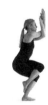

8. Garudasana
10 breaths on each side, then
a Sun Salutation to Adho
Mukha Svanasana.

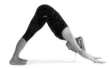

**9. Adho Mukha
Svanasana**
10 breaths, then float
through to the next asana.

10. Navasana
5 breaths. Repeat twice,
then vinyasa and release
to all fours.

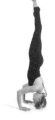

11. Salamba Sirsasana II
2 minutes, rest 5 breaths, 2
more minutes.

12. Balasana
5 breaths, then come
to Tadasana.

Sequence 22: Intermediate Level—Focus on Inversions (continued)

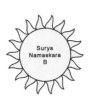

13. Surya Namaskara B
2 times, then come to
Adho Mukha Svanasana.

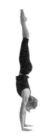

14. Adho Mukha Vrksasana
1–3 times, 5–10 breaths
each time.

15. Padangusthasana
5 breaths.

16. Pada Hastasana
5 breaths.

17. Malasana
10 breaths.

**18. Ardha
Matsyendrasana**
5 breaths on each side.

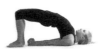

**19. Setu Bandha
Sarvangasana**
5–10 breaths. Repeat
twice or transition to the
next asana.

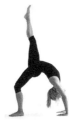

20. Urdhva Dhanurasana
5–10 breaths. Repeat twice.

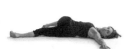

**21. Supta
Parivartanasana**
5 breaths on each side.

22. Ananda Balasana
10 breaths.

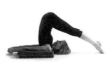

23. Halasana
5 breaths.

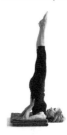

**24. Salamba
Sarvangasana**
2–3 minutes.

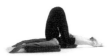

25. Karnapidasana
5 breaths.

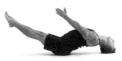

26. Uttana Padasana
5 breaths.

27. Dandasana
5 breaths.

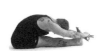

28. Paschimottanasana
10 breaths.

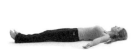

29. Savasana
5–10 minutes.

30. Sukhasana
Meditation.

Chapter Eight

Advanced-Level Classes

All great achievements require time.
—MAYA ANGELOU

In teaching yoga, we are very lucky when advanced students come to our classes. Rather than the acrobatically talented athlete with a flashy practice on display for all to admire or envy, the most seriously advanced yoga student is the one who shows up regularly in his or her practice with an attitude of beginner's mind. Practicing each day as though it is the first time, the advanced student appreciates that there is always something new to learn when doing yoga. Unattached to the outcome of the practice, he or she is fully present to the experience of doing yoga as a process through which to learn more about oneself while remaining open to changing in conscious ways that bring about greater freedom and happiness in life. Approached in this way, the yoga path is endless; there is no final asana or experience one attains and then says, "I'm done," or, "Now I'm a yoga master."

Given that there is nothing to master, but rather everything to endlessly explore, there is no such thing as a yoga master (despite an increasing number of self-anointed masters promoting their mastery in the burgeoning marketplace of yoga).[1] This sets the context for designing and teaching classes in which there is vast freedom to explore. Working with advanced students, we can anticipate that their ego is, largely, safely checked at the door. They are likely to step onto their yoga mat with refined somatic awareness born of years in the intensity of yogic self-exploration. They recognize the centrality of the breath in doing asana and know from experience how conscious pranayama opens and expands the horizons of awareness in the bodymind. Bringing this set of qualities to their practice, we are invited to craft sequences that further encourage them on their evolving path.

The advanced series in Ashtanga Vinyasa (there are four) is collectively called *sthira bhaga*, from *sthira*, meaning "steady," and *bhaga*, meaning "divine" or "serene." The idea is that advanced yoga practice is one of cultivating steadiness in the overall fruits of the practice, to be wholly in it. While in Ashtanga Vinyasa and other yoga systems we are given specific asana sequences as the path of advanced practice, doing advanced yoga is not necessarily about particular physical forms. Rather it is about how, in exploring more complex forms, we discover deeper and often unexamined or unconscious sources of tension, and in this discovery go further in releasing the emotional, mental, and physical sources of self-limitation invariably encountered on the path to greater serenity in our lives.

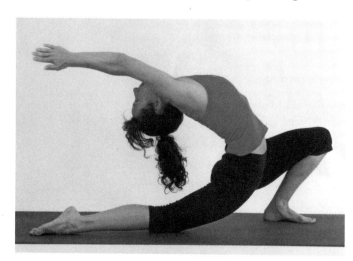

An advanced student in Anjaneyasana

Through years of consistent practice, we can come to a very subtle refinement of our awareness in doing yoga. What may have been a struggle some years before—starting with maintaining steady ujjayi pranayama throughout each practice—comes to feel more natural. We become more attuned to the nuances of the asanas, moving more slowly to move more deeply in the small self-adjustments that allow a sense of effortless ease even when the asanas are very

Designing Beginning, Intermediate, and Advanced Classes

complex. This more subtle practice renews the quality of beginner's mind that is ideally there for anyone doing yoga, allowing us to find and explore something new and transforming even in the simplest asanas. The truism that "the more we know, the more we know that we do not know" manifests with fascination in making even the most complex practice as simple as possible.

As we find greater ease in asanas and basic pranayama, we also discover that there are endless horizons yet to be explored in the world of pranayama. With the gross body strong and flexible, the nervous system fully turned on, the respiratory system tuned up, and the connection of breath to bodymind more refined, we can play with a variety of pranayamas that are the primary source for cultivating full energetic awakening. We come to sense that doing pranayama is like playing a musical instrument, with the slightest change in the pace, duration, texture, retention, or release of the breath bringing about the most subtle shifts in awareness.

We also come to recognize and respect our limitations, appreciating them as our teachers in a practice increasingly oriented around balance in our overall lives. In earlier years we might have obsessed over getting into some more complex asanas; now we tune in and find an inner invitation to go deeper, unconcerned with how our personal practice looks or compares with that of others. In every breath we slowly find more balance, clarity, and self-acceptance. The mind is becoming more familiar, more of a friend, quieter amid the syncopating rhythms of our lives. Here and now we come into doing advanced yoga.

In teaching advanced yoga classes, the world of asana and pranayama is wide open. Now you can look to the 840,000 asanas alluded to in the Hatha Yoga Pradipika as a way of suggesting that there is no end to asanas, and you can explore all pranayama techniques. You can also explore complex sequencing in which there is less limitation in how asanas are arranged across the arc of a class. Yet the body is still the body with all of its attendant systems and structures, which suggests the importance of staying attentive to the constituent elements of asanas and their sensible sequencing based on the same principles that apply in designing beginning and intermediate-level classes.

As always, teach what you know based on your experience and your ongoing study of the asanas. When you encounter students whose experience or ability surpasses your own, offer what insight you can while giving them the space to further develop their personal practice. Reminding yourself that it is not about how far one goes, but how one goes, encourage your advanced students to open to the challenge of keeping it all as simple as can be.

Creating and Teaching Advanced-Level Sequences

- Frequently review the sequencing sensibilities given to beginning and intermediate classes, including the risks, contraindications, and preparatory practices for any given asana.
- Teach the full range of pranayama practices.
- Teach *bhastrika* pranayama once students have established steadiness and ease with kapalabhati pranayama.
- Teach nadi shodhana pranayama with viloma pranayamas, kumbhakas, kapalabhati pranayama, all in conjunction with mula bandha, uddiyana bandha (only with retention of the exhalation), and jalandhara bandha.
- Begin asana practices with up to five consecutive Surya Namaskara (Sun Salutation) A and B sequences.
- Begin asana practices with three to five minutes Salamba Sirsasana I (Headstand), or one to two minutes in Adho Mukha Vrksasana (Handstand).
- Link multiple standing asanas together to develop warmth and build strength in the legs.
- Teach complex variations of standing asanas, including transitioning directly from internal to external rotation of the femurs (for example, transition from Utthita Parsvakonasana [Extended Side Angle Pose] to Parivrtta Parsvakonasana [Revolved Extended Side Angle Pose]). Still do not transition from internal to external rotation in standing balance asanas or vice versa.
- Fully integrate arm balances into transitions to Chaturanga Dandasana (Four-Limbed Staff Pose).
- Introduce "floating" practices for direct transition from Adho Mukha Svanasana (Downward-Facing Dog Pose) to arm balances such as Bakasana (Crane Pose) and Bhujapidasana (Shoulder-Squeezing Pose).

- Teach the back-bending arm balances of Vrschikasana (Scorpion Pose), variation I from Salamba Sirsasana, variation II from Pincha Mayurasana (Feathered Peacock Pose, or Forearm Balance), initially introducing them at the wall.

- Teach a variety of Sirsasana II–arm balance vinyasas, directly transitioning from Salamba Sirsasana (Tripod Headstand) to Bakasana and back up, Parsva Bakasana (Side Crane Pose), going back up between sides, and Dwi Pada and Eka Pada Koundinyasana B (Two-Leg and One-Leg Sage Koundinya's Pose), going back up between sides.

- Teach a variety of Sirsasana I vinyasas, transitioning in and out of Sirsasana I to explore Urdhva Dandasana (Upward Staff Pose), Parivrtta Sirsasana (Revolved Headstand), Parivrtta Eka Pada Sirsasana (Revolved One-leg Headstand), Eka Pada Sirsasana (One-leg Headstand), Parsva Eka Pada Sirsasana (One-leg Side Headstand), Urdhva Padma Sirsasana (Upward Lotus Headstand), Parivrtta Urdhva Padma Sirsasana (Revolved Upward Lotus Headstand), Prasarita Padottanasana Sirsasana (Spread-Leg Headstand), Baddha Kona Sirsasana (Bound Angle Headstand), Mukta Hasta Sirsasana (Free-Hand Headstand) and Baddha Hasta Sirsasana (Bound-Hand Headstand).

- Teach direct transition from Adho Mukha Vrksasana and Salamba Sirsasana to Chaturanga Dandasana.

- Use Laghu Vajrasana (Little Thunderbolt Pose) to develop the strength and understanding for transitioning directly from Ustrasana (Camel Pose) to Kapotasana (Pigeon Pose). Emphasize this as the preparatory practice for transitioning up and down between Tadasana (Mountain Pose) and Urdhva Dhanurasana (Upward-Facing Bow Pose).

- Introduce direct transition between Tadasana and Urdhva Dhanurasana at the wall. Teach going up and down while minimizing use of the wall and maintaining alignment of the feet and internal rotation of the legs.

- Introduce direct transition from Salamba Sirsasana I to Viparita Dandasana (Inverted Staff Pose).

- Introduce asymmetrical back bends, including eka pada (one-leg) and *eka hasta* (one-arm) variations of Urdhva Dhanurasana and Viparita Dandasana.
- Teach Bhekasana (Frog Pose) to students comfortable with both Virasana (Hero Pose) and Dhanurasana (Bow Pose).
- Teach Eka Pada Raj Kapotasana (One-Leg King Pigeon Pose). Encourage the use of props.
- Introduce Padangustha Dhanurasana (Big Toe Bow Pose) to students who are able to clasp their feet in Urdhva Dhanurasana. From there, explore the asymmetrical back bend of Gherandasana (Sage Gheranda's Pose).
- Introduce Natarajasana (King Dancer Pose).
- Teach more complex twists involving asymmetrical positioning of the legs, arms, and spine such as Bharadvajrasana II (Sage Bharadvaj's Pose).
- Offer sustained complex forward bend sequences, such as moving seamlessly from Dandasana (Staff Pose) to Paschimottanasana (West Stretching Pose) to Janu Sirsasana (Head to Knee Pose) to Baddha Konasana (Bound Angle Pose) to Upavista Konasana (Wide-Angle Forward Fold Pose) to Paschimottanasana to Tiriang Mukha Eka Pada Paschimottanasana (Three Limbs Facing One Foot West Stretching Pose), holding each asana for one to three minutes.
- Neutralize the spine and lower back with simple twists and Setu Bandha Sarvangasana (Bridge Pose) following deep sustained forward-bending sequences.
- Teach the full range of variations in Salamba Sarvangasana (Shoulder Stand), including back bends, forward bends, and twists with the legs in lotus position.
- Teach Niralamba Sarvangasana (Without Support Shoulder Stand) to students comfortable and fully vertical in Salamba Sarvangasana.
- Teach Baddha Pindasana (Bound Lotus Pose).
- Teach Tolasana (Scales Pose) with up to 108 kapalabhati cycles prior to Savasana (Corpse Pose).
- Allow at least five minutes for Savasana.

Advanced Class Sequences

Sequence 23: Advanced Level—Focus on Back Bends I

1. Surya Namaskara A
3 times.

2. Surya Namaskara B
3 times.

3. Padangusthasana
5 breaths.

4. Pada Hastasana
5 breaths.

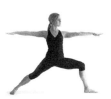

5. Virabhadrasana II
10 breaths on first side, then transition to the next asana.

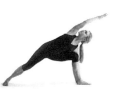

6. Utthita Parsvakonasana
10 breaths on first side, then transition to the next asana.

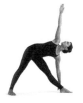

7. Utthita Trikonasana
10 breaths on first side, then transition to the next asana.

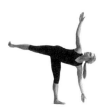

8. Ardha Chandrasana
10 breaths on first side, then switch sides on asanas 5–8.

9. Prasarita Padottanasana A
10 breaths. Transition to next asana from here, through Salamba Sirsasana II.

10. Urdhva Kukkutasana
10 breaths, then release to Salamba Sirsasana II and back to Prasarita Padottanasana A.

11. Parsvottanasana
5 breaths on first side, then transition to the next asana.

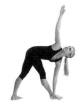

12. Parivrtta Trikonasana
5 breaths on first side, then transition to the next asana.

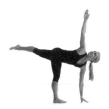

13. Parivrtta Ardha Chandrasana
10 breaths on first side, then switch sides on asanas 11–13.

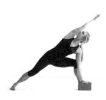

14. Surya Namaskara A
1 time.

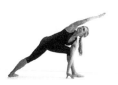

15. Parivrtta Parsvakonasana
10 breaths on each side, then vinyasa and lie supine.

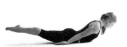

16. Salabhasana A, B, C
5 breaths in each asana, vinyasa between each asana.

Sequence 23: Advanced Level—Focus on Back Bends I (continued)

17. Dhanurasana
5 breaths, vinyasa, repeat, vinyasa.

18. Bhekasana
5 breaths, vinyasa, stand on the knees.

19. Ustrasana
5 breaths, then transition to the next asana.

20. Laghu Vajrasana
Drop back 5 times, hold 5 breaths, then transition to the next asana.

21. Kapotasana
10–15 breaths, then come back up to Ustrasana.

22. Balasana
10 breaths.

23. Ardha Matsyendrasana
5 breaths on each side.

24. Bharadvajrasana B
10 breaths on each side.

25. Dandasana
5 breaths.

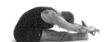

26. Paschimottanasana
10 breaths.

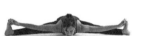

27. Upavista Konasana
10 breaths.

28. Kurmasana
5 breaths.

29. Baddha Konasana
10 breaths.

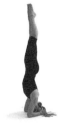

30. Salamba Sirsasana I
5 minutes.

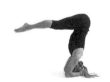

31. Urdhva Dandasana
5 breaths.

32. Balasana
5 breaths.

Sequence 23: Advanced Level—Focus on Back Bends I (continued)

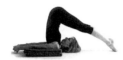

33. Halasana
5 breaths.

34. Urdhva Padmasana
5 breaths.

35. Pindasana
5 breaths.

36. Matsyasana
5 breaths.

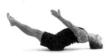

37. Uttana Padasana
5 breaths.

38. Padmasana
5 breaths.

39. Baddha Padmasana
5 breaths.

40. Tolasana
108 kapalabhati breaths,
then vinyasa and float
through.

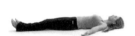

41. Savasana
5–10 minutes.

42. Padmasana
Meditation.

Sequence 24: Advanced Level—Focus on Back Bends II

1. Virasana
5 minutes. Welcome, set intention, begin guiding.

2. Surya Namaskara A
3 times.

3. Surya Namaskara B
3 times.

4. Dancing Warrior
5 times, then transition to Tadasana.

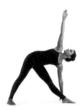

5. Utthita Trikonasana
5 breaths on first side, then the next asana.

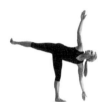

6. Ardha Chandrasana
5 breaths, then switch sides on asanas 5–6.

7. Prasarita Padottanasana C
10 breaths.

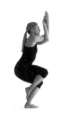

8. Garudasana
10 breaths on each side.

9. Parsvottanasana
5 breaths on each side.

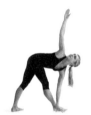

10. Parivrtta Trikonasana
5 breaths on each side.

11. Surya Namaskara A
1 time.

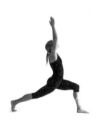

12. Ashta Chandrasana
5 breaths on first side, then transition to the next asana.

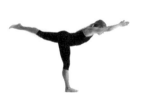

13. Virabhadrasana III
5 breaths on first side, then transition to the next asana.

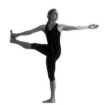

14. Parivrtta Hasta Padangusthasana
5 breaths on first side, then transition to the next asana.

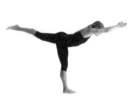

15. Virabhadrasana III
5 breaths on first side, then transition to the next asana.

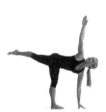

16. Parivrtta Ardha Chandrasana
5 breaths on first side, then transition to the next asana.

Sequence 24: Advanced Level—Focus on Back Bends II (continued)

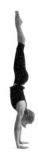

17. Adho Mukha Vrksasana
5 breaths, then vinyasa and switch sides on asanas 12–17.

18. Adho Mukha Svanasana
10 breaths.

19. Parivrtta Parsvakonasana
10 breaths on each side, then vinyasa to Adho Mukha Svanasana.

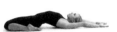

20. Supta Virasana
2 minutes.

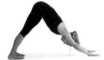

21. Adho Mukha Svanasana
5 breaths.

22. Shishulasana
10 breaths, press to Adho Mukha Svanasana, and float through to lying supine.

23. Urdhva Dhanurasana
5–10 breaths, repeat twice. Explore Eka Pada variation.

24. Viparita Dandasana
5–10 breaths, repeat twice. Explore Eka Pada variation. Come to Adho Mukha Svanasana.

25. Eka Pada Raj Kapotasana II
10 breaths on each side, then come to standing.

26. Natarajasana
10 breaths on each side, then repeat.

27. Ardha Matsyendrasana
5 breaths on each side.

28. Dandasana
5 breaths.

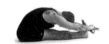

29. Paschimottanasana
10 breaths.

30. Ananda Balasana
5 breaths.

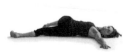

31. Supta Parivartanasana
5 breaths.

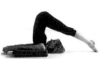

32. Halasana
5 breaths.

Sequence 24: Advanced Level—Focus on Back Bends II (continued)

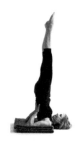

33. Salamba Sarvangasana
3 minutes.

34. Urdhva Padmasana
5 breaths.

35. Pindasana
5 breaths.

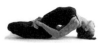

36. Matsyasana
5 breaths.

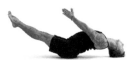

37. Uttana Padasana
5 breaths.

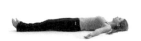

38. Savasana
5–10 minutes.

39. Padmasana
Meditation.

Sequence 25: Advanced Level—Focus on Hip Opening

1. Padmasana
5 minutes. Welcome, set intention, begin guiding.

2. Dandasana
5 breaths. Vinyasa to Adho Mukha Svanasana.

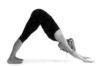

3. Adho Mukha Svanasana
2 minutes.

4. Surya Namaskara A
5 times.

5. Surya Namaskara B
5 times.

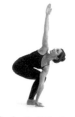

6. Parivrtta Utkatasana
10 breaths on each side.

7. Uttanasana
5 breaths, then come to standing in Prasarita stance.

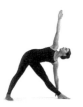

8. Utthita Trikonasana
10 breaths on first side, then transition to the next asana.

9. Ardha Chandrasana
10 breaths on first side, then transition to the next asana.

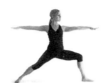

10. Virabhadrasana II
10 breaths on first side, then transition to the next asana.

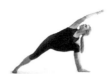

11. Utthita Parsvakonasana
10 breaths on first side, then transition to the next asana.

12. Eka Pada Koundinyasana A
5 breaths on first side, then transition to the next asana.

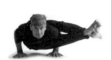

13. Astavakrasana
5 breaths on first side, then vinyasa and switch sides on asanas 8–13 and come to Tadasana.

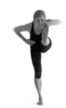

14. Utthita Hasta Padangusthasana
10 breaths on each side.

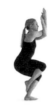

15. Garudasana
10 breaths on each side.

16. Prasarita Padottanasana A, B, C, D
5 breaths in each asana (B, C, and D are shown in Appendix B).

17. Parsvottanasana
5 breaths on first side, then transition to the next asana.

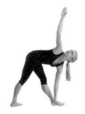

18. Parivrtta Trikonasana
5 breaths on first side, then transition to the next asana.

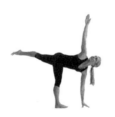

19. Parivrtta Ardha Chandrasana
5 breaths on first side, then transition to the next asana.

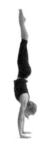

20. Adho Mukha Vrksasana
5 breaths, then vinyasa and repeat asanas 17–20 on the other side, then come to Adho Mukha Svanasana.

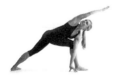

21. Parivrtta Parsvakonasana
10 breaths on first side, then transition to the next asana.

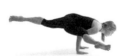

22. Eka Pada Koundin-yasana B
5 breaths on first side, then vinyasa and switch sides on asanas 21–22.

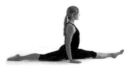

23. Hanumanasana
2 minutes on each side.

24. Eka Pada Raj Kapotasana II
10 breaths on each side.

25. Natarajasana
10 breaths on each side.

26. Ardha Matsyendrasana
5 breaths on each side.

27. Gomukhasana
5 breaths on each side.

28. Agnistambhasana
10 breaths on each side.

29. Eka Pada Sirsasana
10 breaths on the first side, then transition to the next asana.

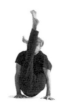

30. Chakorasana
5 breaths on first side, then vinyasa and switch sides on asanas 29–30.

31. Dandasana
5 breaths.

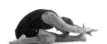

32. Tiriang Mukha Eka Pada Paschimottanasana
5 breaths on first side, then transition to the next asana.

33. Krounchasana
5 breaths on first side, then vinyasa and switch sides on asanas 32–33.

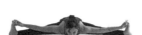

34. Upavista Konasana
10 breaths.

35. Kurmasana
5 breaths.

36. Baddha Konasana
10 breaths.

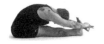

37. Paschimottanasana
10 breaths.

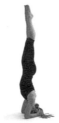

38. Sirsasana I
5 minutes with Lotus vinyasas (twist, forward bend, back bend).

39. Balasana
5 breaths.

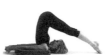

40. Halasana
5 breaths.

Sequence 25: Advanced Level—Focus on Hip Opening (continued)

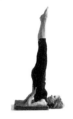

41. Salamba Sarvangasana
5 breaths.

42. Urdhva Padmasana
5 breaths.

43. Pindasana
5 breaths.

44. Matsyasana
5 breaths.

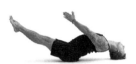

45. Uttana Padasana
5 breaths.

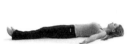

46. Savasana
5–10 minutes.

47. Padmasana
Meditation.

Sequence 26: Advanced Level—Focus on Twisting

1. Virasana
5 minutes. Welcome, set intention, begin guiding.

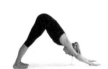

2. Adho Mukha Svanasana
10 breaths.

3. Surya Namaskara A
5 times.

4. Surya Namaskara B
5 times. Transition to the next asana from the last Utkatasana.

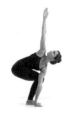

5. Parivrtta Utkatasana
10 breaths on each side. Explore Pasasana as an alternative.

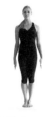

6. Tadasana
5 breaths, renewing intention.

7. Parsvottanasana
5 breaths on first side, then transition to the next asana.

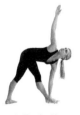

8. Parivrtta Trikonasana
5 breaths on first side, then transition to the next asana.

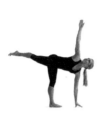

9. Parivrtta Ardha Chandrasana
5 breaths on first side, then transition to the next asana.

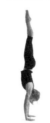

10. Adho Mukha Vrksasana
5 breaths, then vinyasa to Adho Mukha Svanasana and repeat asanas 7–10 on the other side.

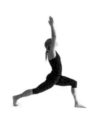

11. Ashta Chandrasana
5 breaths on first side, then transition to the next asana.

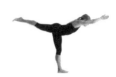

12. Virabhadrasana III
5 breaths on first side, then transition to the next asana.

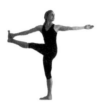

13. Parivrtta Hasta Padangusthasana
1 minute, then transition through Warrior III to Ashta Chandrasana, then vinyasa to Adho Mukha Svanasana.

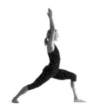

14. Virabhadrasana I
5 breaths on first side, then transition to the next asana.

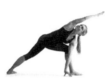

15. Parivrtta Parsvakonasana
5 breaths, then vinyasa to Adho Mukha Svanasana, repeat asanas 11–15 on the other side, and float through to sitting.

16. Dandasana
5 breaths.

17. Navasana
5 breaths, then lower to Ardha Navasana for 30 seconds of kapalabhati pranayama. 5 times, and then lie supine.

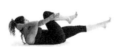

18. Yogic Bicycles
2 minutes.

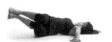

19. Jathara Parivartanasana
Chakorasana transition to a vinyasa, or pick up and float back.

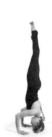

20. Salamba Sirsasana II
5 breaths, then transition to the first side of the next asana.

21. Parsva Bakasana
5 breaths, then transition to the first side of the next asana.

22. Dwi Pada Koundinyasana
5 breaths, then transition to the first side of the next asana.

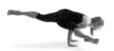

23. Eka Pada Koundinyasana B
5 breaths, then transition back up to Salamba Sirsasana II and switch sides on asanas 20–23, then release.

24. Balasana
5 breaths.

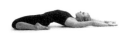

25. Supta Virasana
2 minutes, then transition to Adho Mukha Svanasana and hold for 1 minute before floating through to lying down supine.

26. Urdhva Dhanurasana
5–10 breaths; repeat 3 times. Explore Eka Pada variation.

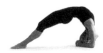

27. Viparita Dandasana
5–10 breaths; repeat 3 times. Explore Eka Pada variation.

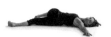

28. Supta Parivartanasana
5 breaths on each side.

29. Swastikasana
10 breaths on each side.

30. Ardha Matsyendrasana
10 breaths on each side.

31. Marichyasana C
10 breaths on each side.

32. Bharadvajrasana B
10 breaths on each side.

33. Dandasana
5 breaths.

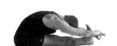

34. Paschimottanasana
10 breaths.

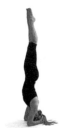

35. Sirsasana I
5 minutes.

36. Balasana
5 breaths.

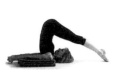

37. Halasana
5 breaths.

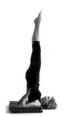

38. Salamba Sarvangasana
3minutes.

39. Urdhva Padmasana
5 breaths.

40. Pindasana
5 breaths.

Sequence 26: Advanced Level—Focus on Twisting (continued)

41. Matsyasana
5 breaths.

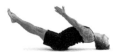

42. Uttana Padasana
5 breaths.

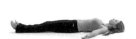

43. Savasana
5–10 minutes.

44. Padmasana
Meditation.

Sequence 27: Advanced Level—Focus on Standing Balance

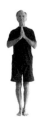

1. Samasthihi
2 minutes. Welcome, set intention, begin guiding.

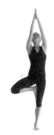

2. Vrksasana
1 minute on each side. Try with eyes closed.

3. Surya Namaskara A
5 times.

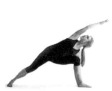

4. Surya Namaskara B
5 times.

5. Padangusthasana
5 breaths.

6. Pada Hastasana
5 breaths.

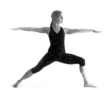

7. Virabhadrasana II
5 breaths on first side, then transition to the next asana.

8. Utthita Parsvakonasana
5 breaths on first side, then transition to the next asana.

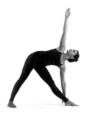

9. Utthita Trikonasana
5 breaths on first side, then transition to the next asana.

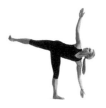

10. Ardha Chandrasana
2 minutes, release to Virabhadrasana II, repeat asanas 7–10 on the other side.

11. Gomukhasana
10 breaths on each side.

12. Parsvottanasana
5 breaths on first side, then transition to the next asana.

Sequence 27: Advanced Level—Focus on Standing Balance (continued)

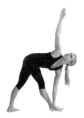

13. Parivrtta Trikonasana
5 breaths on first side, then transition to the next asana.

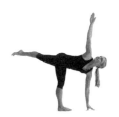

14. Parivrtta Ardha Chandrasana
1 minute, release to Parivrtta Trikonasana, repeat asanas 12–14 on the other side, and step to the front of the mat.

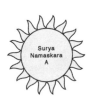

15. Surya Namaskara A
1 time, then 5 breaths in Adho Mukha Svanasana.

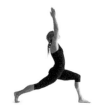

16. Ashta Chandrasana
5 breaths on first side, then transition to the next asana.

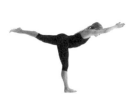

17. Virabhadrasana III
10 breaths on first side, then transition to the next asana.

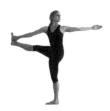

18. Parivrtta Hasta Padangusthasana
5 breaths on first side, then transition to the next asana.

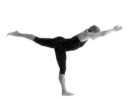

19. Virabhadrasana III
5 breaths on first side, then transition to the next asana.

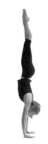

20. Adho Mukha Vrksasana
5 breaths, then vinyasa and switch sides on asanas 16–20, then come to Tadasana.

21. Ardha Baddha Padmottanasana
10 breaths on each side, then vinyasa and release to the knees.

22. Virasana
5 breaths.

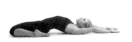

23. Supta Virasana
10 breaths.

24. Ustrasana
5 breaths; repeat twice and transition to the next asana from there.

25. Laghu Vajrasana
Drop back 5 times, hold 5 breaths, then transition to the next asana.

26. Kapotasana
5–10 breaths, then transition back to Ustrasana, vinyasa, and float through to lying supine.

27. Urdhva Dhanurasana
5 breaths. Repeat once or twice.

28. Apanasana
5 breaths.

Sequence 27: Advanced Level—Focus on Standing Balance (continued)

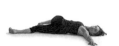

29. Supta Parivartanasana
5 breaths on each side.

30. Dandasana
5 breaths.

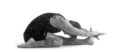

31. Tiriang Mukha Eka Pada Paschimottanasana
10 breaths on each side.

32. Bharadvajrasana B
10 breaths on each side.

33. Agnistambhasana
10 breaths on each side.

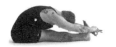

34. Paschimottanasana
2 minutes.

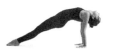

35. Pursvottanasana
5 breaths; Chakorasana or vinyasa transition to all fours.

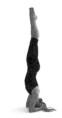

36. Sirsasana I
5 minutes.

37. Balasana
5 breaths.

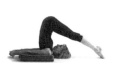

38. Halasana
5 breaths.

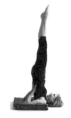

39. Salamba Sarvangasana
3–5 minutes.

40. Urdhva Padmasana
5 breaths.

41. Pindasana
5 breaths.

42. Matsyasana
5 breaths.

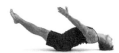

43. Uttana Padasana
5 breaths.

44. Savasana
5–10 breaths.

45. Padmasana
Meditation.

Sequence 28: Advanced Level—Focus on Arm Support I

1. Virasana
5 minutes. Welcome, set intention, begin guiding.

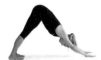

2. Adho Mukha Svanasana
10 breaths.

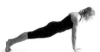

3. Phalakasana
10 breaths.

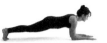

4. Shishula Phalakasana
27 kapalabhati pranayama breaths.

5. Shishulasana
10 breaths.

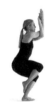

6. Virasana
1 minute with Garudasana arm position (reverse arms after 30 seconds).

7. Adho Mukha Svanasana
5 breaths.

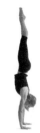

8. Adho Mukha Vrksasana
Explore coming up 3 times and holding for 1 minute. Scorpion option.

9. Uttanasana
5 breaths.

10. Pada Hastasana
10 breaths, then come to Tadasana.

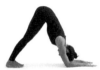

11. Garudasana
5 breaths on each side.

12. Surya Namaskara B
3 times, then transition from Adho Mukha Svanasana to the next asana.

13. Shishulasana
10 breaths.

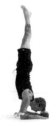

14. Pincha Mayurasana
Explore coming up 3 times and holding for 1 minute. Scorpion option.

15. Balasana
5 breaths.

16. Adho Mukha Svanasana
5 breaths.

17. Vasisthasana
10 breaths on each side.

18. Virasana
10 breaths with
Gomukhasana arms
(switch arm position
after 5 breaths).

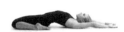

19. Supta Virasana
2 minutes.

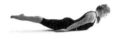

20. Salabhasana A, B, C
5 breaths in each asana, vinyasa between (B and C are
shown in Appendix B).

21. Ustrasana
10 breaths, vinyasa,
repeat twice.

22. Bhekasana
10 breaths, vinyasa, repeat
twice.

23. Balasana
5 breaths.

**24. Ardha
Matsyendrasana**
5 breaths.

25. Dandasana
5 breaths.

26. Navasana
5 breaths, then transition to
the next asana.

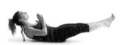

27. Ardha Navasana
30 seconds of kapalabhati
pranayama, then repeat asanas 26–27 four times.

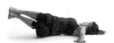

**28. Jathara
Parivartanasana**
10 times each direction.

29. Ananda Balasana
10 breaths.

30. Dandasana
5 breaths.

31. Gomukhasana
10 breaths on each side.

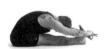

32. Paschimottanasana
10 breaths.

Sequence 28: Advanced Level—Focus on Arm Support I (continued)

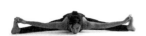

33. Upavista Konasana
10 breaths.

34. Parivrtta Janu Sirsasana
10 breaths on each side.

35. Baddha Konasana
10 breaths.

36. Supta Baddha Konasana
5 breaths.

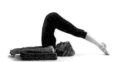

37. Halasana
5 breaths.

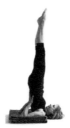

38. Salamba Sarvangasana
2–3 minutes.

39. Urdhva Padmasana
5 breaths.

40. Pindasana
5 breaths.

41. Matsyasana
5 breaths.

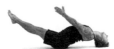

42. Uttana Padasana
5 breaths.

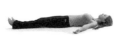

43. Savasana
5–10 minutes.

44. Padmasana

Sequence 29: Advanced Level—Focus on Arm Support II

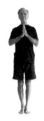

1. Samasthihi
1–2 minutes. Welcome, set intention, begin guiding.

2. Surya Namaskara A
3 cycles.

3. Surya Namaskara B
3 cycles. Transition to the next asana from the last Utkatasana.

4. Parivrtta Utkatasana
5 breaths on the first side, then transition to the next asana.

5. Parsva Bakasana
5 breaths on the first side, then transition to the next asana.

6. Dwi Pada Koundinyasana
5 breaths on the first side, then transition to the next asana.

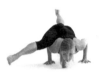

7. Eka Pada Koundinyasana B
5 breaths on the first side, then float back, vinyasa, and switch sides on asanas 4–7, then 5 breaths in Adho Mukha Svanasana.

8. Dancing Warrior
3 times, holding each standing asana 5 breaths, then transition to Tadasana.

9. Prasarita Padottanasana A
5 breaths, then transition to the next asana.

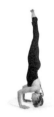

10. Salamba Sirsasana II
5 breaths, then transition to the next asana.

11. Bakasana
5 breaths, then move back into Salamba Sirsasana II and transition to the next asana.

12. Urdhva Kukkutasana
5 breaths, then transition back up into Salamba Sirsasana II and release to Prasarita Padottanasana A.

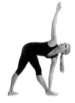

13. Parsvottanasana
5 breaths on each side.

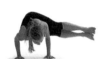

14. Parivrtta Trikonasana
5 breaths on each side, then step to Tadasana.

15. Surya Namaskara B
1 time, then transition to the next asana from Adho Mukha Svanasana.

16. Bhujapidasana
5 breaths, then transition to the next asana.

Sequence 29: Advanced Level—Focus on Arm Support II (continued)

17. Tittibhasana
5 breaths, then transition to the next asana.

18. Bakasana
5 breaths, then vinyasa and float through into the next asana or to Dandasana for easier preparation.

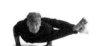

19. Astavakrasana
10 breaths on the first side, vinyasa, switch sides, then come to Tadasana.

20. Galavasana
5 breaths on the first side, vinyasa, then the other side.

21. Uttana Prasithasana
5 breaths on the first side, vinyasa, then the other side.

22. Virasana
Wrist therapy.

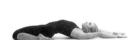

23. Supta Virasana
2 minutes.

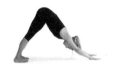

24. Adho Mukha Svanasana
10 breaths.

25. Eka Pada Raj Kapotasana II
5–10 breaths on each side. Repeat once or twice.

26. Ardha Matsyendrasana
10 breaths on each side.

27. Bharadvajrasana B
10 breaths on each side.

28. Dandasana
5 breaths.

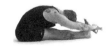

29. Paschimottanasana
2 minutes.

30. Gomukhasana
10 breaths on each side.

31. Parivrtta Janu Sirsasana
10 breaths on each side.

32. Baddha Konasana
2 minutes.

Sequence 29: Advanced Level—Focus on Arm Support II (continued)

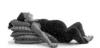

33. Supta Baddha Konasana
2 minutes.

34. Viparita Karani
5 minutes.

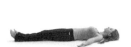

35. Savasana
5–10 minutes.

36. Padmasana
Meditation.

Sequence 30: Advanced Level—Focus on Forward Bends

1. Virasana
5 minutes. Welcome, set intention, begin guiding.

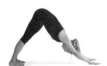

2. Adho Mukha Svanasana
2 minutes.

3. Uttanasana
2 minutes.

4. Malasana
10 breaths.

5. Navasana
5 breaths, then 5 breaths in the next asana. Repeat 4 times.

6. Tolasana
5 breaths each for 5 times, then transition to the next asana.

7. Lolasana
5 breaths, then vinyasa to Adho Mukha Svanasana.

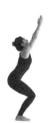

8. Utkatasana
5 breaths.

9. Malasana
5 breaths.

10. Bakasana
5 breaths, then vinyasa.

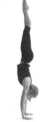

11. Adho Mukha Vrksasana
5 breaths.

12. Padangusthasana
5 breaths.

Designing Beginning, Intermediate, and Advanced Classes

13. Pada Hastasana
5 breaths.

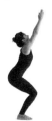

14. Surya Namaskara A
3 times.

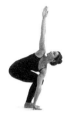

15. Utkatasana
5 breaths.

16. Parivrtta Utkatasana
5 breaths on the first side, then transition to the next asana.

17. Parsva Bakasana
5 breaths on the first side, then transition to the next asana

18. Dwi Pada Koundinyasana
5 breaths, float back to Chaturanga, Urdhva Mukha Svanasana, Adho Mukha Svanasana, then repeat asanas 15–17 on the other side, then Adho Mukha Svanasana.

19. Dancing Warrior
3 times, then come to Tadasana.

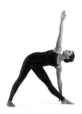

20. Utthita Trikonasana
10 breaths on each side. Set up from Prasarita stance.

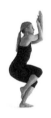

21. Garudasana
10 breaths on each side.

22. Prasarita Padottanasana A, B, C, D
5 breaths in each asana (B, C, and D are shown in Appendix B).

23. Parsvottanasana
10 breaths on each side.

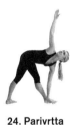

24. Parivrtta Trikonasana
10 breaths on each side, then transition to Tadasana.

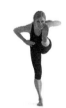

25. Utthita Hasta Padangusthasana
10 breaths on each side.

26. Ardha Baddha Padmottanasana
5 breaths, float to Chaturanga, keeping the Lotus leg in position, continuing through a vinyasa, and repeat on the other side.

27. Surya Namaskara A
1 time to Adho Mukha Svanasana.

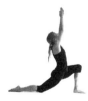

28. Anjaneyasana
2 minutes, alternative straightening and bending the front knee, and the gradually sliding the front heel forward.

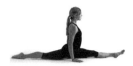

29. Hanumanasana
2 minutes. Explore forward bending and back bending. Repeat asanas 28–29 on the other side.

30. Ardha Matsyendrasana
10 breaths on each side.

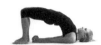

31. Setu Bandha Sarvangasana
10 breaths, pressing the hamstrings into the sitting bones.

32. Urdhva Dhanurasana
5–10 breaths. Repeat 2–4 times.

33. Bharadvajrasana B
5–10 breaths.

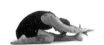

34. Tiriang Mukha Eka Pada Paschimottanasana
5–10 breaths.

35. Krounchasana
10 breaths, then vinyasa and switch sides, repeating asanas 33–35.

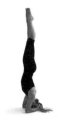

36. Salamba Sirsasana I
5 minutes. Transition directly to the next asana.

37. Salamba Sirsasana II
5 breaths, then fold the legs into Lotus.

38. Urdhva Kukkutasana
10 breaths, then transition to the next asana.

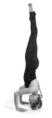

39. Salamba Sirsasana II
Release to Chaturanga, vinyasa, and float through to lying supine.

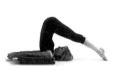

40. Halasana
10 breaths.

41. Niralamba Sarvangasana
2 minutes.

42. Urdhva Padmasana
5 breaths.

43. Pindasana
5 breaths.

44. Matsyasana
5 breaths.

Sequence 30: Advanced Level—Focus on Forward Bends (continued)

45. Uttana Padasana
5 breaths.

46. Savasana
5–10 minutes.

47. Padmasana
Meditation.

Sequence 31: Advanced Level—Focus on Inversions

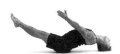

1. Virasana
5 minutes. Welcome, set
intention, begin guiding.

**2. Adho Mukha
Svanasana**
1 minute.

3. Uttanasana
1 minute.

**4. Adho Mukha
Svanasana**
2 minutes.

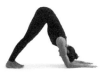

5. Shishulasana
2 minutes.

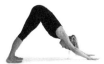

**6. Adho Mukha
Svanasana**
3 minutes.

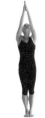

7. Urdhva Hastasana
1 minute.

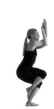

8. Garudasana
10 breaths on each side.

9. Surya Namaskara A
From Adho Mukha Svana-
sana, release the forearms
to the floor.

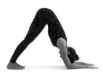

10. Shishulasana
5 breaths.

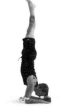

11. Pincha Mayurasana
1 minute, float to
Chaturanga, vinyasa, and
repeat 1–2 times.

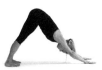

**12. Adho Mukha
Svanasana**
5 breaths.

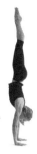

13. Adho Mukha Vrksasana
1 minute, float to Chaturanga, vinyasa, and repeat 1–2 times. On the last time, release the legs overhead into Urdhva Dhanurasana.

14. Urdhva Dhanurasana
5 breaths, release, rest, and repeat 2–3 times. Explore Eka Pada variation.

15. Viparita Dandasana
5 breaths, release, rest, and repeat 2–3 times. Explore Eka Pada variation. On the last time, spring into Pincha Mayurasana and hold for 5 breaths before resting in Balasana for 5 breaths.

16. Ardha Matsyendrasana
5 breaths on each side.

17. Bharadvajrasana B
5 breaths on each side.

18. Parighasana
5 breaths on each side.

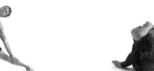

19. Gomukhasana
5 breaths on each side.

20. Dandasana
5 breaths.

21. Akarna Dhanurasana
5 breaths on each side.

22. Eka Pada Sirsasana
5 breaths on each side, vinyasa, and float through to Dandasana.

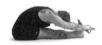

23. Paschimottanasana
2 minutes.

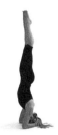

24. Salamba Sirsasana I
5 minutes.

25. Balasana
5 breaths.

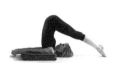

26. Halasana
5 breaths.

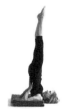

27. Salamba Sarvangasana
5 minutes.

28. Urdhva Padmasana
5 breaths.

Sequence 31: Advanced Level—Focus on Inversions (continued)

29. Pindasana
5 breaths.

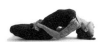

30. Matsyasana
5 breaths.

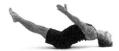

31. Uttana Padasana
5 breaths.

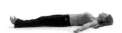

32. Savasana
5–10 minutes.

33. Padmasana
Meditation.

Part Three

Sequencing Across
the Life Cycle

Chapter Nine

Yoga Sequencing for Kids

You are worried about seeing him spend his early years in doing nothing. What! Is it nothing to be happy? Nothing to skip, play, and run around all day long? Never in his life will he be so busy again.
—JEAN-JACQUES ROUSSEAU, *ÉMILE,* 1762

In past generations, children tended to be much more physically active than today, whether playing with friends, active in organized sports or recreational programs, or working. Today, more and more children have a sedentary life that, coupled with poor eating habits, has more than tripled the obesity rate among children ages six to seventeen from five percent in 1976 to twenty percent in 2009.[1] Children are also under increasing pressure to perform academically in keeping with narrowly defined national and state standards of educational accomplishment, a trend that has combined with more limited spending on education to justify the reduction of physical education, the arts, and other activities in which children get exercise as well as a mental break that, if given, would enhance learning. With rising expectations on children to perform, they are increasingly experiencing stress and related emotional and psychological disorders. Close to ten percent of youth ages twelve to seventeen had a major depressive episode (MDE) in 2009, with a rate higher (thirteen percent) among female youth.[2] A significant percentage of children also have serious difficulties with emotions, concentration, or getting along with other people.[3]

Despite these trends, many children are very healthy. Kids who get regular exercise have stronger muscles and bones, leaner body mass, are less likely to develop type-2 diabetes, and are likelier to feel better about themselves, have strong social relationships, and have a better outlook on life. They also tend to sleep better and are better at handling stressful situations, whether preparing for a test at school or dealing with a disappointing event. By getting more exercise these children have greater endurance, strength, and flexibility than their more sedentary peers. When combined with a healthy diet, children who exercise regularly are on the path of a healthier and happier life.

Most children who do yoga came to it by mimicking their parents or by having parents who introduced them to yoga. Children can certainly benefit from doing yoga on a regular basis just as much as adults, developing or maintaining flexibility, strength, coordination, and balance in their physical bodies while reducing stress and gaining a more positive outlook on life. However, the yoga that parents do may not be appropriate for kids.

It is important to take children's stage of development into consideration when crafting sequences for kids yoga classes. Children's bodies are still growing. Their bones are softer and their ligaments more elastic. Asanas that give healthy stress to the bones of an adult can overstress a child's bones. Movement that involves maximum range of motion in an adult joint can overstretch a child's ligaments, leading to long-term instability in the joint. While it may seem that kids can run and play forever, adult yoga classes—typically an hour to an hour and a half—can cause fatigue in a child. And while many adults enjoy doing yoga in a highly heated room, a child doing that practice in the same room is considerably more prone to heat exhaustion.

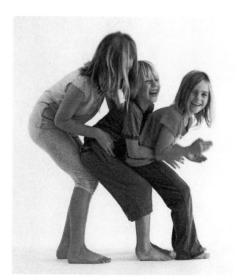
Kids playing yoga

Many simple and popular yoga asanas are contraindicated in the broader literature on children's physical fitness. For example, in the California Department of Education's (2009, 292–97) Physical Education Framework for California Public Schools, several positions that mimic or are identical to basic yoga asanas are listed as contraindicated for all children in kindergarten through twelfth grade, including: Utkatasana (Chair Pose), Uttanasana (Standing Forward Bend Pose), Halasana (Plow Pose), Salamba Sarvangasana (Shoulder Stand), Utthita Trikonasana (Extended Triangle Pose), the arm position of Virabhadrasana II (Warrior II Pose), and Baddha Konasana (Bound Angle Pose, often called Butterfly Pose). In several instances the recommended alternative appears riskier than the contraindicated position: a high lunge with the knee projected beyond the foot is the alternative to Baddha Konasana, while a slumped expression of Marichyasana A (Sage Marichi's Pose) is given as the alternative to Uttanasana. On strength training, the biomechanics of which are similar to some repetitive actions in yoga such as Plank-Chaturanga, the American Association of Pediatrician's position is that "children and adolescents should avoid the practice of weight lifting, power lifting, and bodybuilding, as well as the repetitive use of maximal amounts of weight in strength training programs, until they have reached Tanner stage 5 level of developmental maturity."[4] At the other end of the caution continuum, we find many professional fitness organizations and yoga styles that advocate positions and practices that are widely considered risky for children, including bodybuilding with resistance weights, doing yoga in an extremely hot room, and stretching to one's greatest ability.

Here we take a middle path, respecting the insights provided by leading sources of research and education on children's physical fitness, mental health, and overall well-being while suggesting practices that fall outside that research, including the ways that asanas are linked together in coherent sequences, as well as meditation practices.

In teaching yoga to children it is best to divide them into age groups. Here we will focus on three age groups associated with school grade levels: elementary school, middle school, and high school. While infants and toddlers often find abundant joy playing around with their parents while their parents are attempting to do yoga, often doing their best to mimic their parents, it is best to let them simply play; this is a beautiful expression of a child's fascination with movement, energy, and interaction. Enjoy watching and playing—and try to leave it at that until your toddler gets closer to school age.

In Sequencing Yoga for Elementary School–Age Children ...

- Appreciate that most children are inherently active (unless led into a sedentary lifestyle) and that with yoga you are giving children an opportunity to direct their physical activity in specific ways to help them to develop keener awareness of being in their bodies.

- Appreciate that young children are inherently creative and that they will spontaneously express their creativity with the asanas.

- Play with offering yoga as a form of play rather than as a disciplined practice so that children feel a sense of freedom in their physical exploration.

- Limit the practice to twenty-five to forty-five minutes, depending on fitness.

- Offer natural breathing exercises to highlight the four natural phases of the breath (inhale, pause, exhale, pause).

- Teach ujjayi pranayama.

- Guide children in feeling the movements and overall sensations in their bodies that happen with the fluctuations of the breath.

- Create a variety of different ways to explore yoga, tapping into and further encouraging children to develop their yogic intelligence though thinking, listening, speaking, interacting, and demonstrating.

- Sprinkle classes with mythology,[5] storytelling, music, and games to more fully engage each child.

- Maximize the use of natural names for asanas such as tree, frog, cat, cobra, butterfly, and so on, and encourage imaginative and expressive ways of bringing the asanas more to life by "acting" these parts.

- Offer partner play to encourage trust and communication skills.

- Take a few minutes at the beginning of each class to check in with how the children in your class are doing. Get creative in making the check-in session fun.

- Guide kids in exploring the different qualities of awareness that happen with their eyes open versus closed.

- Keep the asanas simple. Be aware that as flexible as young kids are, they can easily overstretch.

- Teach standing asanas one at a time, with a brief rest between each asana.

- Keep the room temperature moderate and comfortable. There is absolutely no benefit to children in doing yoga in a room heated above seventy-five degrees Fahrenheit.
- Offer natural warming of the body through dynamic movement, including Classical Surya Namaskara.
- Do not teach young children Sirsasana (Headstand).
- Craft sequences of asanas that develop the three elements of children's fitness: strength, flexibility, and endurance.
- Appreciate that different children are different from one another and can benefit from sequences that address their uniqueness.
- In working with hyperactive children, help to channel their energy by offering sequences that involve movement. Standing and balancing asanas are an excellent way for these children direct their more impulsive energy in healthy ways.
- Use creative visualization in Savasana (Corpse Pose) to encourage relaxation. Read a short story during their Savasana.
- Listen; children will teach you how to guide them.

Sequence 32: Yoga for Elementary School–Age Children

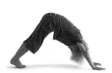

1. Lotus
Sitting in a circle in a simple cross-legged position, eyes closed, ask the kids to check in with how they're feeling and share about their intention.

2. Peace Breath
Take 5 deep breaths, then each child hums his or her name with the exhale.

3. Twisting Lotus
Simple twist, holding 5 breaths, then switching sides.

4. Cat/Cow
5 times.

5. Dog
A few breaths here.

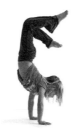

6. Donkey Kick
Play with kicking the legs up high for a minute.

7. Frog
A few breaths here to rest, then stand up.

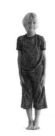

8. Mountain
Feel the feet and legs awakening, rounding, and growing taller.

Sequence 32: Yoga for Elementary School-Age Children (continued)

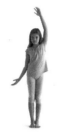

9. Half Moon
5 breaths on each side.

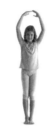

10. Full Moon
5 breaths.

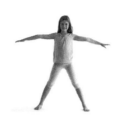

11. Star
Press the feet, stretch the arms, 5 breaths

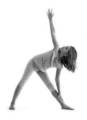

12. Triangle
5 breaths on each side.

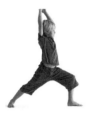

13. Bold Warrior
5 breaths on each side.

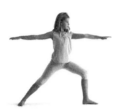

14. Brave Warrior
5 breaths on each side.

15. Reading Break
Stories with ideas for asanas, then do one of them.

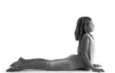

16. Snake
Stay up for 5 breaths.

17. Swan
Stay for 5 breaths, then rest or do the next asana.

18. Owl
Take 5 breaths on each side.

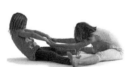

19. Seesaw
With a partner, go back and forth several times.

20. Butterfly
5 more breaths.

**21. Wings of
the Butterfly**
5 breaths on each side!

23. Lotus
Sitting in a circle, thank one another for the practice with "Namaste."

In Sequencing Yoga for Middle School–Age Children ...

- Review all of the guidelines for teaching younger children; they all apply to guiding children in the middle school years.
- Limit the practice to thirty to forty-five minutes, depending on fitness.
- Offer gradually more vigorous sequences of standing asanas.
- Gradually build up to doing three standing asanas linked together in a sequence.
- Offer variations so that children can self-select more or less vigorous activity; the needs and interests of the child should take precedence over doing a certain sequence.
- Introduce resistance practices, including holding Phalakasana (Plank Pose) and Adho Mukha Svanasana (Downward-Facing Dog Pose) for up to a minute each and lowering slowly from Plank to Chaturanga.
- Introduce Surya Namaskara A and B one asana at a time and give alternatives that make the asanas and transitions accessible to every child.
- Offer guided meditation up to five minutes.

Sequence 33: Yoga for Middle School–Age Children

1. Lotus
Sitting in a circle in a simple cross-legged position, eyes closed, checking in.

2. Peace Breath
Take 5 deep breaths, then each kid hums his or her name with the exhale.

3. Twisting Lotus
Simple twist, holding 5 breaths, then switching sides.

4. Cat/Cow
Moving with the breath, 5–10 times.

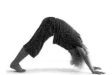

5. Dog
A few breaths here.

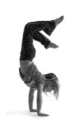

6. Donkey Kick
Play with it for a minute.

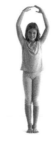

11. Full Moon
5 breaths.

12. Classical Surya Namaskara
1 time, rest in Child's Pose, then come up to standing.

Sequence 33: Yoga for Middle School-Age Children (continued)

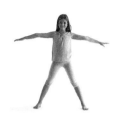

13. Star
Press the feet, stretch the arms, 5 breaths.

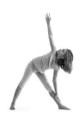

14. Triangle
5 breaths on each side.

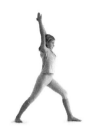

15. Bold Warrior
5 breaths on each side.

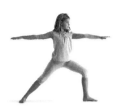

16. Brave Warrior
5 breaths on each side.

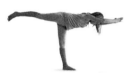

17. Warrior in My Power
5 breaths on each side with a partner to hold hands and share support.

18. Reading Break
Stories with ideas for poses, then do one of them.

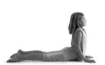

19. Snake
Stay up for 5 breaths.

20. Bridge
Stay up for 5–10 breaths, then rest or do the next pose.

21. Wheel
Stay up for 5–10 breaths, then rest or do the next pose.

22. Swan
Stay for 5 breaths, then rest or do the next pose.

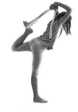

23. Dancer
Play on each side for a minute or so.

24. Owl
Take 5 breaths on each side.

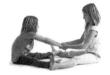

25. Seesaw
With a partner, go back and forth several times.

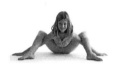

26. Turtle
Just 5 breaths!

27. Butterfly
5 more breaths.

28. Wings of the Butterfly
5 breaths on each side!

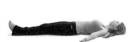

29. Savasana
Rest!

30. Lotus
Sitting in a circle, thank one another for the practice with "Namaste."

In Sequencing Yoga for High School-Age Youth …

- Review all of the guidelines for teaching younger children; most apply to guiding high school age youth.
- Limit the practice to forty-five to sixty minutes, depending on fitness.
- Gradually build up to doing three standing asanas linked together in a sequence.
- Explore viloma, vritti, and nadi shodhana pranayamas.
- Introduce arm balances, starting with Bakasana (Crane Pose) and Adho Mukha Vrksasana (Handstand) Prep at a wall.
- Offer creative flowing sequences such as Dancing Warrior.
- Invite physically adept and motivated youth to attend regular adult yoga classes.

Sequence 34: Yoga for High School-Age Youth

1. Sukhasana
Eyes closed, tune in, explore ujjayi breath, set intention.

2. Parivrtta Sukhasana
5 breaths on each side.

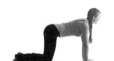

3. Bidalasana
Move through the spine and pelvis 5 times, then press to Adho Mukha Svanasana.

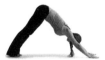

4. Adho Mukha Svanasana
10 breaths, getting aligned, rooting, extending.

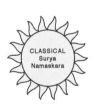

5. Classical Surya Namaskara
3 times, then come back to Adho Mukha Svanasana.

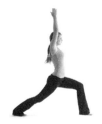

6. Ashta Chandrasana
Stay 5 breaths on the first side, then do the next asana.

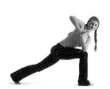

7. Parivrtta Ashta Chandrasana
5 breaths, then vinyasa to Adho Mukha Svanasana and then to standing in Tadasana.

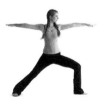

8. Virabhadrasana II
Set up from Prasarita stance, hold the first side 5 breaths, then transition to the next asana.

Sequence 34: Yoga for High School-Age Youth (continued)

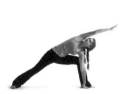

9. Utthita Parsvakonasana
5 breaths, then switch sides for asanas 8–9.

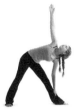

10. Utthita Trikonasana
10 breaths.

11. Prasarita Padottanasana C
5 breaths.

12. Parsvottanasana
5 breaths on the first side, then transition to the next asana.

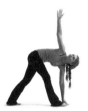

13. Parivrtta Trikonasana
5 breaths, then switch sides for asanas 12–13.

14. Surya Namaskara A
Flow to Adho Mukha Svanasana.

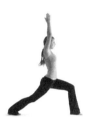

15. Ashta Chandrasana
Hold 5 breaths on the first side, then transition to the next asana.

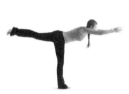

16. Virabhadrasana III
5 breaths on the first side, then transition back to Ashta Chandrasana and to the next asana.

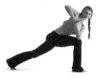

17. Parivrtta Ashta Chandrasana
5 breaths, come back to Ashta Chandrasana, then vinyasa to Adho Mukha Svanasana and switch sides for asanas 15–17.

18. Balasana
Rest for 1 minute.

19. Ustrasana
5 breaths, then either rest and repeat once or transition to the next asana.

20. Laghu Vajrasana
5 breaths, then come back to Ustrasana 1 breath, then lie supine.

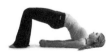

21. Setu Bandha Sarvangasana
1–3 times, holding for 5–10 breaths. After the first time, consider transitioning to Urdhva Dhanurasana.

22. Urdhva Dhanurasana
1–2 times, holding for 5–10 breaths.

23. Bharadvajrasana A
5 breaths on each side.

24. Ardha Matsyendrasana
5 breaths on each side.

Sequence 34: Yoga for High School-Age Youth (continued)

25. Swastikasana
2 minutes on each side.

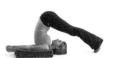

26. Parivrtta Janu Sirsasana
10 breaths on each side.

27. Baddha Konasana
10 breaths.

28. Dandasana
5 breaths.

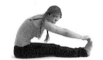

29. Paschimottanasana
1 minute.

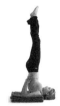

30. Halasana
5 breaths.

31. Salamba Sarvangasana
2–3 minutes.

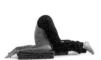

32. Karnapidasana
5 breaths.

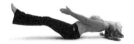

33. Uttana Padasana
5 breaths.

34. Savasana
5 minutes.

35. Sukhasana
Sit in meditation, set intention, namaste.

Chapter Ten

Sequencing for Special Conditions of Women

I am not afraid. I was born to do this.

—JOAN OF ARC

The conditions of men and women change considerably across the broad span of one's life. Most of the changes are similar when considering the broad scope of human physical, emotional, and mental development from early childhood to the latest moments of life. Yet along the way there are several factors that bring us to give the conditions of women in yoga special consideration in crafting yoga sequences. While there is no question that the onset of puberty is very significant in boys, the changes in boys pale in comparison with the hormonal and larger physical and physiological changes experienced by girls with menarche (the onset of menstruation) and the cyclical recurrence of menstruation until menopause. While sharing in the experience of pregnancy and childbirth can be very significant to men, this experience pales even more in contrast to the experience of being pregnant, giving birth, breast-feeding, and healing in the postpartum period. And while men often have a variety of emotional and physical challenges in midlife, the hormonal changes that occur with menopause can greatly amplify the sense of dramatic change that signifies moving into a new phase of life.

Until the late twentieth century most writings on yoga practice did not differentiate between men and women primarily because yoga was largely the province of men (and mostly men of the upper castes in India's hierarchical social system). Indeed, across the broad span of yoga history, women were largely excluded from yoga, reflecting the "oppressive social and cultural context out of which the yoga tradition arose" in India, particularly during the Brahmanic period in which women, as Janice Gates (2006, 7–16) reminds us, were defined as "impure" and thus pronounced by male yoga gurus as being ill-fit for the spiritually enlightening practices of yoga.[1] It is only much later that, with the development of yoga in the West, we begin to find specific guidance that addresses the special needs and conditions of women in yoga, albeit still often adhering to age-old patriarchal and sexist assumptions about women.

Even when not sexist, we find that many of the yoga practice prescriptions for women—often given by women—are based less on science than anecdotal assumption, superstition, or unfounded supposition that is repeatedly passed from teacher to student. For example, in the leading book on yoga for women, *Yoga: A Gem for Women* (1995), Geeta Iyengar reiterates her father's admonition against doing yoga during menstruation, as follows: "During the monthly period (48–72 hours) complete rest is advisable. Asanas should not be practiced.... Normal practice may be resumed from the fourth or fifth day." She goes on to say that a few forward bends may be done during menstruation to reduce tension. More recently, in *The Women's Book of Yoga: Asana and Pranayama for All Phases of the Menstrual Cycle* (2007), Bobby Clennell allows certain practices during the menstrual cycle while following the teachings on B. K. S. Iyengar, Geeta Iyengar, and other leading teachers in making this questionable assertion regarding the relationship between inversion and menstruation:

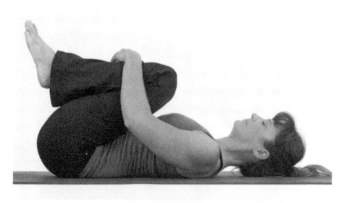

Yoga can help relieve menstrual discomfort.

> If the body is turned upside down, this process [of menstrual discharge] is disturbed and may force the menstrual flow back up into the menstrual cavity and up through the fallopian tubes, causing the uterus to perform an adapted function instead of its normal function.... Since the menstrual process is one of discharge, it is a commonsense precaution to avoid these poses. Do not practice any inversions until the menstrual flow has completely stopped.

This is now a "commonsense" notion in the yoga community if only because it has been repeated mutatis mutandis, ad nauseam for the past two generations. Yet menstrual discharge is no more affected by one's relationship to gravity than the passage of food or water through the body. Try swallowing a mouthful of water when in Adho Mukha Svanasana (Downward-Facing Dog Pose) or Sirsasana (Headstand); does the water stay in your mouth, flood your sinuses, or move through your throat and into your stomach? As the NASA Medical Division has confirmed through studies of women in zero-gravity environments, medical science in general has established that menstrual egress is caused by intrauterine and intravaginal pressure along with the peristaltic action of muscles, which are not measurably influenced by gravity.[2] This is also why four-legged females have no problem with healthy menstrual flow despite not having a vertical orientation to gravity, and why a menstruating woman will flow just as normally whether sleeping on her belly or back despite her uterus and vagina being turned in opposite relation to gravity.[3]

We use this as one example of misinformation becoming urban yoga myth and then parading as fact in informing yoga sequences for women and others. Whether, how, or to what degree this and other fallacies are rooted in patriarchal or sexist assumptions would make for an interesting study that is far beyond the scope and purpose of this book. Rather, for our purposes, it points to the value of always asking "why" or "why not" when told that something must not be done or must be done only in a certain way or at a certain time. Whether the various admonitions about women in yoga (indeed, about everyone in yoga) are valid deserves to be studied, discussed, and ultimately considered through one's personal yoga experience. It is with these sensibilities—evidence combined with shared understanding and experience—that women (and men) ideally make decisions for what to do or not do in their personal yoga practice throughout the larger cycle of life. In advising students on the question of menstruation and inversion, longtime yoga teacher Barbara Benagh (2003) says that since "no studies or research make a compelling argument to avoid inversions during menstruation, and since menstruation affects each woman differently and can vary from cycle to cycle, I am of the opinion that each woman is responsible for her own decision."

Practicing Yoga During Menstruation

Just as each student comes to the practice in a unique way, women experience their menstrual cycle in different ways. For some women, menstruation is simple and easy, while for others it can be painful and distressing. As discussed above, most of the literature on yoga for women advises a highly modified practice emphasizing basic restorative poses, no inversions, or no practice at all. Yet many active yoga students maintain their regular practice while menstruating—including doing inversions—across the span of decades with no signs of ill effects. This suggests that the best guide to practice when menstruating is each student's personal experience and intuition. The basic question to ask is, "How do I feel?" It is entirely possible that cramps, bloating, fatigue, or other discomfort will be present, indicating a relaxing practice that helps to reduce pressure in the uterus and abdomen, as described in the following sequence.

Sequence 35: Yoga for Easing Menstrual Discomfort

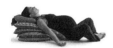

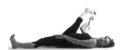

1. Supta Baddha Konasana
Prop the back and head onto a set of bolsters or folded blankets and allow the thighs and arms to release toward the floor. Stay for 5–10 minutes.

2. Apanasana
Gently draw the knees toward the chest and move them around in increasingly large circles for 1–2 minutes.

3. Ananda Balasana
Clasp the feet to drawn the knees toward the floor, slightly and gently rocking from side to side for 1 minute.

4. Supta Padangusthasana B
Extend one leg out to the side, resting it on a bolster. Stay for 1 minute, switch sides, and then repeat.

Sequence 35: Yoga for Easing Menstrual Discomfort (continued)

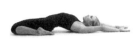

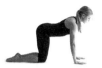

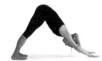

5. Supta Virasana
Propped as for Supta Baddha Konasana, place strap around the thighs to keep them from splaying out and to reduce pressure in the lower back. Stay for 2–5 minutes.

6. Bidalasana
Hold for 1 minute, alternately extending the legs back to release tension through the knees.

7. Adho Mukha Svanasana
Hold for 1 minute before resting in Balasana for 5 breaths. Repeat 2–4 times.

8. Setu Bandha Sarvangasana
Keep the tailbone tucked to maintain ease in the lower back while focusing the back bend more up the spine and into the heart center. Repeat once or twice.

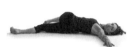

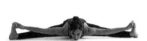

9. Supta Parivartanasana
Press the upper hip away from the shoulder while pressing the lower leg back to reduce pressure in the lower back and sacroiliac joints. Hold for 1 minute, switch sides, and repeat 2 times.

10. Gomukhasana
Hold for 1–3 minutes on each side.

11. Upavista Konasana
Hold for 2–5 minutes. Consider placing a stack of bolsters under the torso and head.

12. Paschimottanasana
Hold for 1–3 minutes. Consider placing a stack of bolsters under the torso and head.

13. Viparita Karani
Elevate the pelvis on bolsters, release the arms overhead onto the floor, and stay for 5–10 minutes.

Practicing Yoga During and After Pregnancy

Which yoga asana sequences are beneficial or possibly risky during pregnancy and in the early postpartum period (and during extended periods of lactation)? Which asanas are indicated and contraindicated during each trimester? How do these prescriptions vary depending on the unique woman and specific conditions such as age, number of previous pregnancies, and other factors?

These and other questions pertaining to working with pregnant students did not appear in the yoga literature until the late twentieth century. Looking more broadly to the general question of exercise and pregnancy, we find very different views in the modern historical literature, starting with Alexander Hamilton's 1781 "Treatise on Midwifery," which encouraged moderate exercise avoiding "agitation of the body from violent or improper exercise, as jolting in a carriage riding on horseback, dancing and whatever disturbs the body or mind" (Mittelmark et al. 1991). Nineteenth-century scientific examination of exercise and birth outcomes all have similar findings showing an association between robust activity and lower birth weight, leading to legislation in several countries (but not the United States) prohibiting employment of women in the weeks preceding and following delivery.

By the early twentieth century we find a growing list of arbitrary restrictions on activity, derived more from cultural and social biases than scientific study. A 1935 issue of *Modern Motherhood* says to "bathe, swim, golf, and dance, but no excessive walking, horseback riding, or tennis," while noting that some expectant mothers experience no ill effects from such activities. Yet also in the 1930s, British writer and maternal advocate Kathleen Vaughan advocated

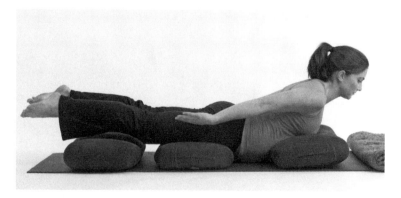

Pregnant students can use props to safely practice prone asanas.

improving joint flexibility through squats to widen the pelvic outlet as well as Baddha Konasana–like positions and pelvic floor exercises to prevent tears of the perineum. Still, during the 1940s and 1950s, most of the literature suggested very moderate activity and no sports, giving way in the 1950s to Vaughan's criticism of the sedentary life of English women in *Exercises before Childbirth* (1951), which presents both physical and psychological benefits of regular group exercise during pregnancy.

In the 1970s and early 1980s, we find the emphasis shifting to control over the body and a sense of well-being, but the advice typically ignores basic physiological changes such as aortal compression syndrome, laxity of joints and ligaments, exaggerated lumbar lordosis, and abdominal compression issues. We also start to find the unexamined assumption that some minor dietary error or failure to engage in some specific regimen of prenatal exercises could damage the unborn child or mother, motivating many pregnant women to quickly immerse themselves in exercise programs, often predisposing them (and their babies) to injury. In the past twenty years we have come to much greater insight into the relationship between exercise and pregnancy, including clear evidence that normal daily activities in no way compromise the mother or baby unless there's some significant pathological condition. The emergent conventional wisdom offers several suggestions regarding exercise during pregnancy: it should be regular, not intermittent, and not competitive; if vigorous, it should not be in intense heat or humidity or with high fever; ballistic and jarring movements as well as deep flexion and extension of joints should be avoided; and if starting from a sedentary lifestyle, begin with very simple exercises.

These insights come largely through the lens of a Western medical and scientific model, which still mostly assumes the separation of body and mind. Taken to the extreme, this perspective considers thoughts and feeling largely irrelevant to physical welfare, addressing physical anomalies and problems with purely physical therapy, drugs, or surgery. Yet we find considerable evidence that emotion is a highly significant factor in pregnancy and delivery; holding onto a secret fear, having commitment issues and other emotional complexes can have a direct effect on the physiology of the body.[4] An increasing number of hospitals and birthing centers recognize that discharging emotions eases the way in labor, and so they offer a more peaceful environment and even encourage conscious breathing and meditation practices to ease labor and delivery.

All pregnant students can benefit from bringing greater awareness and support to the structure, muscles, and organs of their pelvis. This ideally begins well before pregnancy with a more focused practice of mula bandha as a tool for toning and refining one's awareness of the lower pelvic muscles and organs. Mula bandha helps to develop a stronger and more flexible set of perineal muscles, more awareness of the lower pelvic organs and their surrounding support structure, greater ease in the delivery process, and a reduction in several physical risks that often naturally occur during pregnancy, labor, and delivery, including perineal tears (or reduced indication of episiotomy), urinary incontinence, and vaginal prolapse. Building on the basic mula bandha practice, women can develop more subtle awareness and control of all of the superficial muscles of the perineal floor and higher up into the layers of deep pelvic muscles that surround and give support to the bladder, vagina, and rectum, as well as the ability to differentiate and differentially engage or release muscles acting on the pelvis from above and below.[5] With this awareness, women can participate in their birthing process in a safer and more conscious fashion.

We can usefully divide pregnant students into two general categories: (1) those with sedentary lifestyles, poor physical health, or high-risk pregnancy, and (2) those with active lifestyles, good overall health, and minimal pregnancy risks. Women in the first category should be encouraged to attend yoga classes designed specifically for pregnant students, typically referred to as prenatal yoga. Women in the second category should be encouraged to explore practicing in regular yoga classes with teachers who are prepared to give them informed guidance on when and how to modify their practice. Women in the second category and already regularly practicing yoga should be encouraged to do a maintenance practice along with the modifications discussed below; pregnancy is not the time to begin a vigorous yoga practice, nor the time to attempt new or more complex asanas.[6] Below we offer separate sequences for these two relatively distinct groups of pregnant women in each trimester of pregnancy.

Yoga Sequences by Stage of Pregnancy

General Guidelines and Sequences for the First Trimester

- During the early period of pregnancy up to around the thirteenth week, pregnant students should take it easy as they adjust to changing hormones and energy during an often intense and delicate period of transformation. This is a time for getting more grounded, slowing down a bit, focusing more inside, and creating a favorable environment for the ovum to grow into a healthy fetus.

- Stay with ujjayi pranayama. Do not do kapalabhati pranayama or other breathing techniques that involve pumping action in the belly.

- Do not jolt the body by jumping into asanas (if the student has a well-developed floating practice, she might feel comfortable staying with it).

- Minimize twisting (to minimize pulling on the broad ligament that attaches to the uterus); when twisting, focus the movement in the upper thoracic spine.

- Do basic pelvic awareness exercises.

- The fetus is very small and the uterus well protected inside the pelvis, so students can lie on their belly (until they are "showing").

- Develop more pelvic awareness by doing Bridge Rolls (undulating the pelvis and spine slowly in and out of Setu Bandhasana [Supported Bridge Pose]), Supta Baddha Konasana (Reclined Bound Angle Pose), Swastikasana, Vajrasana (Thunderbolt Pose), Virasana (Hero Pose), Upavista Konasana (Wide-Angle Forward Fold Pose), Gomukhasana (Cow Face Pose), Ananda Balasana (Happy Baby Pose), and Eka Pada Raj Kapotasana Prep (One-Leg King Pigeon Pose Prep). Become very familiar with Malasana (Garland Pose).

- Do a variety of shoulder strengtheners and openers (see the discussion on shoulders above).

- Explore Utthita Trikonasana (Extended Triangle Pose), Virabhadrasana II (Warrior II Pose), and Utthita Parsvakonasana (Extended Side Angle Pose) as hip openers that stimulate circulation in the legs and contribute to strong feet and legs, creating a more stable foundation for the off-kilter weight distribution soon to come.

- While still in the first trimester, begin to explore asanas and props that are used in the second and third trimesters.

Sequence 36: Yoga in the First Trimester of Pregnancy—New to Yoga

1. Sukhasana
1–2 minutes. Welcome, set intention, begin guiding.

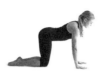

2. Bidalasana
2 minutes, moving through the spine and pelvis with Cat and Dog Tilts.

3. Virasana
Introduce mula bandha.

4. Bidalasana
5 breaths.

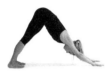

5. Adho Mukha Svanasana
10 breaths. Explain basic alignment and energetic actions.

6. Classical Surya Namaskara
3 times.

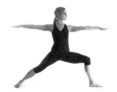

7. Virabhadrasana II
5 breaths on each side. Set up from Prasarita stance.

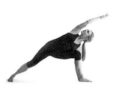

8. Utthita Parsvakonasana
5 breaths on each side.

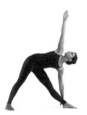

9. Utthita Trikonasana
5 breaths on each side, then step to Tadasana.

10. Malasana
1–2 minutes. Use props to make it accessible.

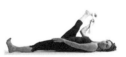

11. Supta Padangusthasana B
5 breaths on each side.

12. Apanasana
5 breaths.

13. Ananda Balasana
10 breaths.

14. Setu Bandha Sarvangasana
5 breaths. Repeat once or twice.

15. Bharadvajrasana A
5 breaths on each side; a 60% twist focused up the spine.

16. Gomukhasana
5 breaths on each side.

Sequence 36: Yoga in the First Trimester of Pregnancy—New to Yoga (continued)

17. Dandasana
5 breaths.

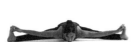

18. Upavista Konasana
2 minutes.

19. Baddha Konasana
2 minutes.

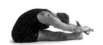

20. Paschimottanasana
2 minutes.

21. Viparita Karani
5 minutes.

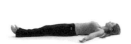

22. Savasana
5–10 minutes.

23. Sukhasana
Meditation.

Sequence 37: Yoga in the First Trimester of Pregnancy—Healthy and Experienced Yogini

1. Sukhasana
3–5 minutes. Welcome, set intention, begin guiding.

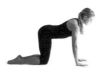

2. Bidalasana
5 rounds of Cat and Dog Tilts.

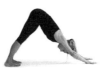

3. Adho Mukha Svanasana
10 breaths.

4. Classical Surya Namaskara
2 times.

5. Malasana
Hold for 1 minute while repeatedly engaging and releasing mula bandha.

6. Surya Namaskara A
2 times.

7. Malasana
Hold for 1 minute while repeatedly engaging and releasing mula bandha.

8. Surya Namaskara B
2 times.

Sequence 37: Yoga in the First Trimester of Pregnancy—Healthy and Experienced Yogini (continued)

9. Balasana
Rest for 1 minute, then come to Tadasana.

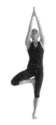

10. Vrksasana
10 breaths on each side.

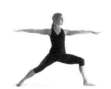

11. Virabhadrasana II
5 breaths on each side. Set up from Prasarita stance.

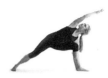

12. Utthita Parsvakonasana
5 breaths on each side.

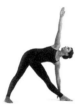

13. Utthita Trikonasana
5 breaths on each side.

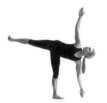

14. Ardha Chandrasana
5 breaths on each side.

15. Garudasana
5 breaths on each side.

16. Prasarita Padottanasana A
10 breaths.

17. Prasarita Padottanasana C
10 breaths.

18. Malasana
2 minutes.

19. Dandasana
5 breaths.

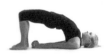

20. Setu Bandha Sarvangasana
5 breaths.
Repeat 3–4 times.

21. Apanasana
10 breaths. Move the knees around in circles.

22. Bharadvajrasana A
5 breaths on each side.

23. Gomukhasana
5 breaths on each side.

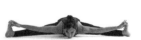

24. Upavista Konasana
10 breaths.

25. Baddha Konasana
10 breaths.

26. Dandasana
5 breaths.

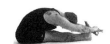

27. Paschimottanasana
2 minutes.

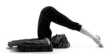

28. Halasana
5 breaths.

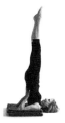

29. Salamba Sarvangasana
2–3 minutes.

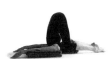

30. Karnapidasana
5 breaths.

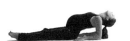

31. Uttana Padasana Prep
5 breaths.

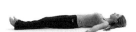

32. Savasana
5–10 minutes.

33. Sukhasana
5 minutes of guided heart-to-belly meditation.

General Guidelines and Sequences for the Second Trimester

- With the placenta fully functional, hormone levels balance out and the pregnancy is generally well established. This is the perfect time to focus on cultivating strength and stamina, to refine awareness of the pelvis and spine, and to build more internal support for the inevitable challenge to balance and ease that will happen as the baby grows.

- The size of the belly varies greatly in the second trimester; different women show at different points in time. As a woman's pregnancy start to show, the pelvis no longer protects the uterus, so it is time to start adapting asanas accordingly.

- Toward the middle of the second trimester, students should tune in more to any sense of numbness while lying on their back as the increasing weight of the baby may place pressure on the vena cava, restricting the flow of blood back to the mother's heart.

- Avoid jarring movements, intense abdominal work such as Yogic Bicycles and Navasana (Boat Pose), and kapalabhati pranayama. It is important to avoid pressure on the abdomen and to develop a supple belly; female athletes with tight abdominal muscles are at highest risk of perineal tears and urinary incontinence arising from downward pressure.

- Use pelvic neutrality exercises in Tadasana (Mountain Pose) and Urdhva Hastasana (Upward Hands Pose) to cultivate alignment of the spine, and stay with the Bridge Roll practice.

- Practice Surya Namaskara (Sun Salutations) with the feet apart in Tadasana, step back to Phalakasana (Plank Pose), and use folded blankets to support the ribs and hips when lying prone in preparation for either Salabhasana (Locust Pose) or Urdhva Mukha Svanasana (Upward-Facing Dog Pose). Integrate squats into the salutations.

- Practice standing asanas to develop or maintain leg strength and open the hips and pelvis (modify and use a wall or chair for support as needed): Vrksasana (Tree Pose), Garudasana (Eagle Pose), Anjaneyasana (Low Lunge Pose), Ashta Chandrasana (Crescent Pose), Virabhadrasana I and II, Utthita Trikonasana, Parsvottanasana (Intense Extended Side Stretch Pose), Utthita Parsvakonasana.

- Explore a variety of seated hip openers and forward folds: Baddha Konasana; Upavista Konasana; Parivrtta Janu Sirsasana (Revolved Head to Knee Pose); Bharadvajrasana (Sage Bharadvaj's Pose); Eka Pada Raj Kapotasana Prep; Gomukhasana; Dandasana (Staff Pose); Paschimottanasana (West Stretching Pose), with legs apart; Marichyasana A (Sage Marichi's Pose); and Janu Sirsasana (Head to Knee Pose). Release pressure in the sacroiliac joint with the knees wide apart in Supta Parivartanasana (Reclined Revolved Pose).

- For relaxation, explore Viparita Karani (Active Reversal Pose) with legs straight up the wall, apart, and with the feet together and knees apart; elevate the feet in Baddha Konasana; raise the hips and legs onto a long bolster in Savasana.

- From around the twenty-fifth week of pregnancy, become more aware of any numbness or tingling sensations when lying on your back as this may be an indication of the baby pressing down on the vena cava, the "vein of life" that returns blood to the heart from the lower extremities. Increasingly prop up your back, shoulders, and head when on your back, eventually propped to about forty-five degrees when close to term.

Sequence 38: Yoga in the Second Trimester of Pregnancy—New to Yoga

1. Sukhasana
1–2 minutes. Welcome, set intention, begin guiding.

2. Parivrtta Sukhasana
Hold each side for 10 breaths, focusing on creating the twist from the mid-thoracic spine upward, keeping the belly soft and spacious.

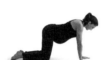

3. Bidalasana
5 times of Cat and Dog movements.

4. Virasana
Hold for 2 minutes, alternately engaging and releasing mula bandha.

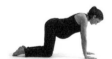

5. Bidalasana
Stretch one leg back at a time, pressing back through the heel to release tension in the knees.

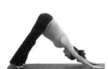

6. Adho Mukha Svanasana
1 minute.

7. Classical Surya Namaskara
3 times, pausing for several breaths in Tadasana between each time.

CLASSICAL Surya Namaskara

8. Balasana
1 minute.

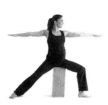

9. Virabhadrasana II
Set up from Prasarita
stance and hold each side
5–10 breaths.

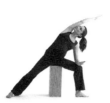

**10. Utthita
Parsvakonasana**
5–10 breaths on
each side.

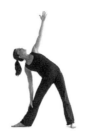

11. Utthita Trikonasana
5–10 breaths on each side.
Practice at a wall for
added support.

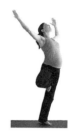

12. Vrksasana
Encourage use of a wall for
added support. Hold each
side for 1 minute.

**13. Prasarita
Padottanasana C**
1 minute.

14. Malasana
2 minutes.

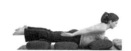

15. Salabhasana A
Place props under the hips,
legs, chest, and forehead
to ensure the belly is free.
Lift and release 5 times
before holding for 5 breaths.
Repeat 3 times.

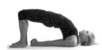

**16. Setu Bandha
Sarvangasana**
Keep the tailbone tucked to
bring the arch up the spine
and minimize pressure in the
belly. Hold for 5 breaths and
repeat once or twice.

17. Ananda Balasana
1 minute, gently rocking side
to side on the sacrum.

18. Bharadvajrasana A
5–10 breaths on each side,
focusing the twist in the
upper thoracic area.

19. Dandasana
1 minute, concentrating on
rooting the sit bones to fully
extend the legs and spine.

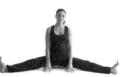

20. Upavista Konasana
2 minutes.

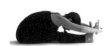

21. Paschimottanasana
2 minutes.

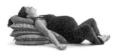

**22. Supta Baddha
Konasana**
Do deep heart-centered
breathing practice
for 3–5 minutes.

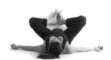

23. Viparita Karani
5–10 minutes with a bolster
under the sacrum. Alternate
leg positions (basic form,
wide apart, knees apart,
with feet together).

24. Sukhasana
5 minutes of guided heart-to-
belly meditation.

Sequence 39: Yoga in the Second Trimester of Pregnancy—Healthy and Experienced Yogini

1. Sukhasana
3–5 minutes. Welcome, set intention, begin guiding.

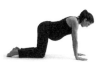

2. Bidalasana
5 times of Cat and Dog stretches.

3. Classical Surya Namaskara
2 times.

4. Malasana
Hold 1 minute while repeatedly engaging and releasing mula bandha.

5. Surya Namaskara B
3 times.

6. Malasana
2 minutes while repeatedly engaging and releasing mula bandha.

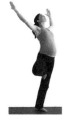

7. Vrksasana
1 minute on each side.

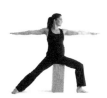

8. Virabhadrasana II
5–10 breaths on each side. Set up from Prasarita stance.

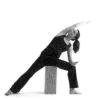

9. Utthita Parsvakonasana
5–10 breaths on each side.

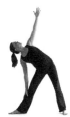

10. Utthita Trikonasana
5–10 breaths on each side.

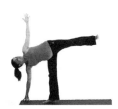

11. Ardha Chandrasana
5 breaths on each side. Practice next to a wall if uncertain of balance.

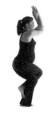

12. Garudasana
1 minute on each side.

13. Prasarita Padottanasana A
5 breaths.

14. Prasarita Padottanasana C
5 breaths.

15. Malasana
1 minute while repeatedly engaging and releasing mula bandha.

16. Uttanasana
5 breaths. Step back to Adho Mukha Svanasana.

Sequence 39: Yoga in the Second Trimester of Pregnancy—Healthy and Experienced Yogini (continued)

17. Adho Mukha Svanasana
1 minute.

18. Balasana
1 minute.

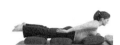

19. Salabhasana A
Place props under the hips, legs, chest, and forehead to ensure the belly is free. Lift and release 5 times before holding for 5 breaths. Repeat 3 times.

20. Ustrasana
5–10 breaths.
Repeat once or twice.

21. Balasana
5–10 breaths.

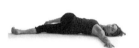

22. Supta Parivartanasana
1 minute on each side.

23. Ananda Balasana
1 minute.

24. Dandasana
1 minute, cultivating mula bandha.

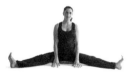

25. Upavista Konasana
1–2 minutes.

26. Baddha Konasana
1–2 minutes.

27. Parivrtta Janu Sirsasana
5–10 breaths on each side.

28. Paschimottanasana
Hold for 1 minute, separating the legs wider to accommodate the belly.

29. Balasana
5 breaths.

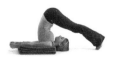

30. Halasana
5 breaths.

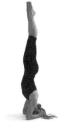

31. Salamba Sarvangasana
2–3 minutes. Explore leg variations.

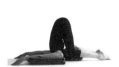

32. Karnapidasana
5 breaths.

**Sequence 39: Yoga in the Second Trimester of Pregnancy—
Healthy and Experienced Yogini (continued)**

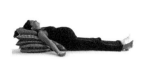

34. Savasana
5–10 minutes.

35. Sukhasana
5 minutes of guided heart-
to-belly meditation.

General Guidelines and Sequences for the Third Trimester

This is the time to refocus on cultivating energy, especially by resting amid the flow of asanas to allow the body to integrate the practice more fully. It is increasingly important to limit time lying supine as the weight of the baby puts greater pressure on the vena cava. Relaxin hormone levels are now sufficiently high to cause the softening of ligaments throughout the body (not just in the pelvis), potentially causing fallen arches (as the calcaneonavicular ligaments stretch), weakness in the knees, and instability in the sacroiliac and other joints throughout the body.

- Continue working on postural alignment to give support to the spine.
- Become increasingly familiar with using a chair to support a variety of standing and sitting asanas (including Virabhadrasana and Malasana).
- Become increasingly aware of any numbness or tingling sensation when lying on your back as this may be an indication of excessive pressure on the vena cava.
- After the thirty-fourth week, be aware that Adho Mukha Svanasana and other inversions can cause (or reverse!) breech presentation.

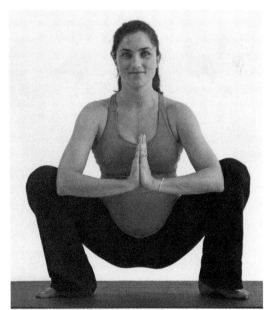

Malasana—the queen of prenatal asanas

- Begin doing birthing visualizations in squatting and other abducted hip-opening positions.
- Explore using a high bolster for long holds in Supta Baddha Konasana.
- Increasingly rest in Savasana, lying on the side of the body with props between the knees, under the head, and under the upper arm for easy comfort and relaxation.

Sequence 40: Yoga in the Third Trimester of Pregnancy—New to Yoga

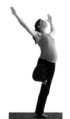

1. Supta Baddha Konasana
5–10 minutes. Prop the back at a 45-degree angle, and give ample support to the head and arms.

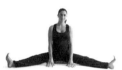

2. Upavista Konasana
5 minutes. Prop the chest and forehead.

3. Marichyasana A Variation
2 minutes on each side. Sit tall and use one hand to pull on the lifted knee, the other hand to pull on the opposite knee, and relieve pressure on the pubic symphysis.

4. Parivrtta Janu Sirsasana
5–10 breaths on each side, then repeat.

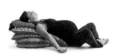

5. Bidalasana
10 times of Cat and Dog tilts, then rest in Balasana with the knees wide apart.

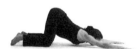

6. Anahatasana
10 breaths.

7. Malasana
1–2 minutes. Use a wall for added support.

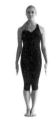

8. Tadasana
5 breaths.

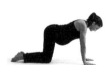

9. Vrksasana
1 minute on each side, the repeat. Use a wall for added support.

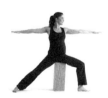

10. Virabhadrasana II
1–2 minutes. Place a chair under the sitting bone of the bent leg.

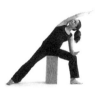

11. Utthita Parsvakonasana
5–10 breaths on each side.

12. Dandasana
1 minute.

Sequence 40: Yoga in the Third Trimester of Pregnancy—New to Yoga (continued)

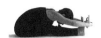

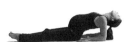

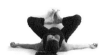

13. Paschimottanasana
2–3 minutes.

14. Uttana Padasana Prep
1 minute.

15. Viparita Karani
5–10 minutes.

16. Sukhasana
5 minutes of guided heart-to-belly meditation.

Sequence 41: Yoga in the Third Trimester of Pregnancy—Healthy and Experienced Yogini

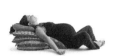

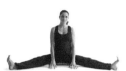

1. Supta Baddha Konasana
5–10 minutes. Prop the back at a 45-degree angle.

2. Upavista Konasana
5 minutes. Prop the chest and forehead.

3. Marichyasana A Variation
2 minutes on each side. Sit tall and use one arm to press out on the lifted knee, the other hand to pull on the opposite foot (use a strap to keep the spine extended).

4. Parivrtta Janu Sirsasana
5–10 breaths on each side.

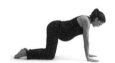

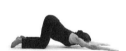

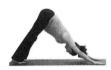

5. Bidalasana
10 times of Cat and Dog tilts, then rest in Balasana.

6. Anahatasana
10 breaths.

7. Adho Mukha Svanasana
1 minute. Discontinue this inverted asana starting at 33 weeks.

8. Uttanasana
2 minutes.

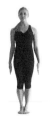

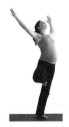

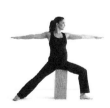

9. Malasana
2–3 minutes. Use a wall for added support.

10. Tadasana
5 breaths.

11. Vrksasana
1 minute on each side. Use a wall for added support.

12. Virabhadrasana II
5–10 breaths on each side.

Sequence 41: Yoga in the Third Trimester of Pregnancy—
Healthy and Experienced Yogini (continued)

13. Utthita Parsvakonasana
5–10 breaths on each side.

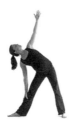

14. Utthita Trikonasana
5–10 breaths on each side.

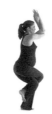

15. Garudasana
2 minutes on each side.

16. Prasarita Padottanasana C
1 minute. Slowly roll up to standing to minimize light-headedness.

17. Dandasana
1 minute.

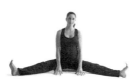

18. Upavista Konasana
1–2 minutes.

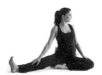

19. Parivrtta Janu Sirsasana
2 minutes on each side.

20. Baddha Konasana
2 minutes.

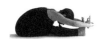

21. Paschimottanasana
2–3 minutes.

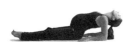

22. Uttana Padasana Prep
1 minute.

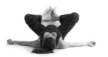

23. Viparita Karani Variation
5–10 minutes.

24. Sukhasana
5 minutes of guided heart-to-belly meditation.

Sequence 42: Yoga in the Third Trimester of Pregnancy—During Labor

1. Standing Pelvic Rocking
Stand with the feet mat width apart about 2 feet from a wall, extend the hands up the wall, and move the hips side to side in a circular motion to encourage labor and reduce discomfort.

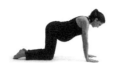

2. Bidalasana
Sway the hips from side to side while arching the spine like a cat during contractions.

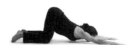

3. Anahatasana
Explore Anahatasana if the labor is moving fast and too intensely.

4. Balasana
Modify by positioning the knees wide apart, keeping the torso relatively upright, placing the hands on the floor, and leaning slightly forward.

5. Malasana
Sit on a bolster and recline slightly back against an exercise ball. Have a partner sitting behind to lift the shoulders and help relieve pressure in the pelvis.

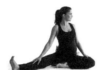

6. Parivrtta Janu Sirsasana
Keeping the bent knee lifted, press it outward while pulling on the opposite foot or leg to reduce pressure in the pubic symphysis.

7. Anjaneyasana
With a wide lateral yet short stance, shift the hips forward and back, first on one side and then the other to reduce pressure at the pubic symphysis.

General Guidelines and Sequences for Postpartum Reintegration

It is important for new mothers to slowly increase energy, redevelop muscle strength, and cultivate more endurance after giving birth. There should be no abdominal pressure from core work or kapalabhati pranayama for at least six weeks (longer if there was an episiotomy or perineal tear, allowing complete healing before starting pelvic floor exercises); gradually move back into toning the abdominal core. There are heightened levels of relaxin hormone until around two months postpartum or postlactation if breast-feeding, so encourage students to stay with an eighty percent practice when doing deep stretches (especially forward folds and back bends).

Sequence 43: Yoga for Postpartum Reintegration

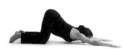

1. Anahatasana
1 minute, moving the joined knees in circles.

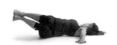

2. Jathara Parivartanasana
Keep the knees bent and move them slowly and slightly side to side to gently stretch and strengthen the abdominal muscles.

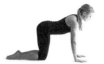

3. Bidalasana
Rotate the pelvis forward and back while undulating up along the spine 2–3 minutes.

4. Urdhva Mukha Pasasana
1–2 minutes on each side.

5. Balasana
5 breaths.

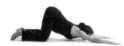

6. Anahatasana
Breathe deeply while stretching the shoulders and chest.

7. Salabhasana A
Moving in and out with the flow of the breath for 5 cycles of breath, then release and rest.

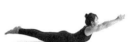

8. Salabhasana C
5–10 breaths.

9. Adho Mukha Svanasana
5 breaths, then rest in Balasana.

10. Prasarita Padottanasana C
1 minute.

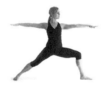

11. Virabhadrasana II
5 breaths on each side. Use a shorter than usual stance, and don't lunge so deeply.

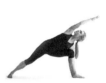

12. Utthita Parsvakonasana
5 breaths. Keep a shorter than usual stance, and still don't lunge so deeply.

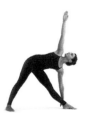

13. Utthita Trikonasana
5 breaths on each side, sensitive to over-stretching in the groins and lower pelvis.

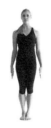

14. Tadasana
Refocus on clear intention.

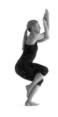

15. Garudasana
5–10 breaths on each side.

17. Balasana
1 minute.

17. Balasana
1 minute.

18. Gomukhasana
1–2 minutes on each side.

19. Apanasana
5 breaths.

20. Pelvic Tilts
10 times.

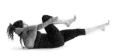

21. Yogic Bicycles
1 minute.

22. Dandasana
5 breaths.

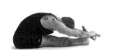

23. Paschimottanasana
2 minutes.

24. Viparita Karani
5 minutes.

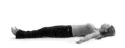

25. Savasana
5 minutes.

26. Sukhasana
Heart-centered calming
meditation.

Yoga Sequences for Menopause

Just as menarche and pregnancy signal potentially profound life changes, the transition to menopause is a powerful cause for pause and reflection in a woman's life. Contrary to popular misconception, menopause is not a disease but rather a natural transition that every fertile woman experiences in her life cycle, normally between the ages of forty-five and fifty-five, with symptoms lasting for five or more years after her last period.[7] The ovaries are gradually reducing their production of estrogen and progesterone, which causes changes in a woman's entire reproductive system. The vagina gradually shortens, its walls become thinner and less elastic, lubricating secretions become watery, and the labia atrophy. Menstruation becomes irregular for a period of up to three years before ending completely.

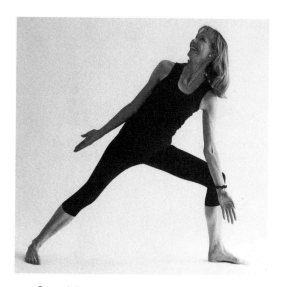

Gracefully sequencing through life with yoga

Along the way, common symptoms include hot flashes, night sweats, insomnia, flushed skin, an irregular heartbeat, mood swings, headaches, forgetfulness, diminished libido, urinary incontinence, and aches and pains in the joints. Many women describe feeling misunderstood or unappreciated by their partner, children, and friends, exacerbating feelings of loneliness, anxiety, depression, and other emotional and mental imbalances. Many women with severe symptoms turn to hormone therapy, which is contraindicated for some women, while many others take other prescription drugs to alleviate specific symptoms such as depression and hot flashes. One of the long-term effects of decreased estrogen levels may be bone loss and eventual osteopenia or osteoporosis, which can lead to several further health challenges.

The surest path to reducing or eliminating some of the symptoms of menopause is to maintain one's overall health, starting with not smoking, maintaining regular exercise, and maintaining a nutritious diet. There are also many alternative health practices such as acupuncture and yoga that have proven helpful in making the symptoms of menopause more tolerable. Here we focus on yoga asana sequences that can help maintain overall comfort and health by reducing the effects of hot flashes, osteoporosis, and emotional fluctuations.[8]

Sequence 44: Yoga for Symptoms of Hot Flashes

1. Viparita Karani
Place a bolster under the sacrum and stay 5–10 minutes. Play with alternating leg position to reduce tension in the legs.

2. Apanasana
1 minute.

3. Ananda Balasana
1 minute, and then come onto all fours.

4. Adho Mukha Svanasana
1–2 minutes. If too intense, do Anahatasana.

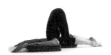

5. Balasana
1 minute.

6. Uttanasana
2 minutes.

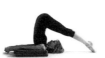

7. Halasana
3–5 minutes with the shoulders and back propped on blankets and the legs resting on a chair.

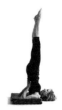

8. Salamba Sarvangasana
3–5 minutes.

9. Karnapidasana
5–10 breaths.

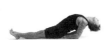

10. Uttana Padasana Prep
Stay in the prep position with the legs on the floor.

11. Viparita Karani
Rest for 5 minutes with bolster and alternative positions as in the first pose in this sequence.

Sequence 45: Yoga for Bone Health—Preventing Osteoporosis

1. Sukhasana
3–5 minutes. Welcome, set intention, begin guiding.

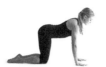

2. Bidalasana
Alternately extend the opposite arm and leg and hold for 5 breaths on each side. Alternatively, extend the lifted arm and leg out and back to center 5 times.

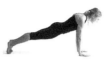

3. Phalakasana
5–10 breaths.

4. Balasana
5 breaths.

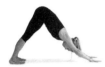

5. Adho Mukha Svanasana
10 breaths. Explain basic alignment and energetic actions.

6. Ardha Uttanasana
5 breaths.

7. Uttanasana
5 breaths.

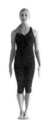

8. Tadasana
10 breaths.

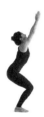

9. Utkatasana
5 breaths. Press to standing and repeat twice.

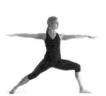

10. Virabhadrasana II
5–10 breaths on each side. Set up from Prasarita stance.

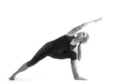

11. Utthita Parsvakonasana
5–10 breaths on each side.

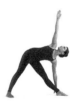

12. Utthita Trikonasana
5–10 breaths on each side.

13. Prasarita Padottanasana A
1 minute, come up slowly, and step to Tadasana.

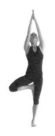

14. Vrksasana
Hold each side 1 minute.

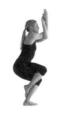

15. Garudasana
1 minute on each side. Step back into Adho Mukha Svanasana.

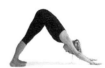

16. Adho Mukha Svanasana
1–2 minutes. Stronger students can come to a wall and explore Handstand for up to 1 minute, rest, and repeat.

Sequence 45: Yoga for Bone Health—Preventing Osteoporosis (continued)

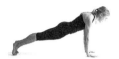

17. Phalakasana
5 breaths, the release
to the floor and rest.

18. Salabhasana A
5 breaths each for 3 times.

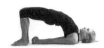

**19. Setu Bandha
Sarvangasana**
5 breaths each for 2–3
times. Either rest in Apanasana, Supta Baddha
Konasana, or do the
following asana.

**20. Urdhva
Dhanurasana**
5 breaths each for
1–3 times.

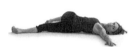

**21. Supta
Parivartanasana**
5 breaths on each side.

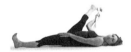

**22. Supta
Padangusthasana B**
10 breaths on each side.

23. Ananda Balasana
5 breaths.

24. Apanasana
5 breaths.

25. Dandasana
5 breaths.

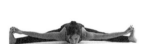

26. Upavista Konasana
10 breaths.

27. Baddha Konasana
10 breaths.

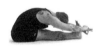

28. Paschimottanasana
2 minutes.

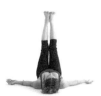

29. Viparita Karani
5 minutes.

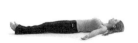

30. Savasana
5–10 minutes.

31. Sukhasana
Meditation.

Sequence 46: Yoga for Reducing Mood Swings

1. Sukhasana
Set intention, explore ujjayi pranayama, aum.

2. Supta Baddha Konasana
5–10 minutes, propped comfortably.

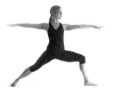

3. Swastikasana
2–3 minutes on each side.

4. Bidalasana
5 times of Cat and Dog stretches.

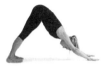

5. Adho Mukha Svanasana
1–2 minutes.

6. Balasana
5–10 breaths.

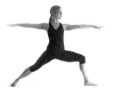

7. Virabhadrasana II
5–10 breaths on each side.

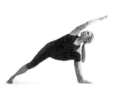

8. Utthita Parsvakonasana
5–10 breaths on each side.

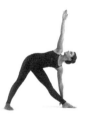

9. Utthita Trikonasana
5–10 breaths on each side.

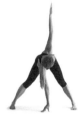

10. Parivrtta Ardha Prasarita
5–10 breaths on each side.

11. Malasana
1 minute, then come to Tadasana.

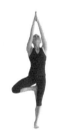

12. Vrksasana
1 minute on each side.

13. Surya Namaskara A
1 minute, then lie prone.

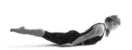

14. Salabhasana A
3 times for 1, 3, then 5 breaths.

15. Dhanurasana
5–10 breaths; repeat 2–3 times.

16. Balasana
5–10 breaths.

Sequence 46: Yoga for Reducing Mood Swings (continued)

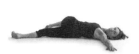

17. Supta Parivartanasana
5 breaths on each side. Repeat twice.

18. Dandasana
1 minute.

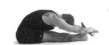

19. Paschimottanasana
1–2 minutes.

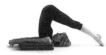

20. Halasana
5 breaths, or do Viparita Karani until Savasana.

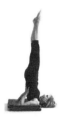

21. Salamba Sarvangasana
2–3 minutes.

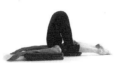

22. Karnapidasana
5 breaths.

23. Uttana Padasana
5 breaths.

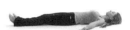

24. Savasana
5–10 minutes.

25. Sukhasana
Do nadi shodhana pranayama for 5 minutes, then settle into heart-centered meditation.

Chapter Eleven

Yoga Sequencing for Seniors

I could not, at any age, be content to take my place by
the fireside and simply look on. Life was meant to be
lived. Curiosity must be kept alive. One must never,
for whatever reason, turn his back on life.
—ELEANOR ROOSEVELT

Many portrayals of yoga in the media convey the impression that yoga is
primarily for young people. Yet as recently as 2005, *Yoga Journal*'s "Yoga in
America" survey revealed nearly twenty percent of the 15.8 million Americans
who practice yoga regularly are fifty-five or older. With life expectancy
continuing to climb—from forty-eight in 1900 to seventy-eight in 2000—
and fertility gradually diminishing, the senior age demographic is projected
to become proportionally greater in the coming years. Today, seniors age
sixty-five and older are already the fastest growing age group in the United
States. We can therefore anticipate more and more seniors doing yoga, and
with them we can anticipate more challenges in ensuring that yoga sequences
are designed appropriately for their needs.

In teaching an aging population, it is important to give careful consideration to the unique conditions of each individual student while letting go of the assumption that sequences that make sense for a twenty-five-year-old make just as much sense for the "uniquely vulnerable group" of yoga students in their sixties or older.[1] For instance, some seniors come to yoga for the first time and find themselves in an Ashtanga Vinyasa class described as helping with balance, strength, and flexibility. While this style of yoga might be appropriate for a very small percentage of exceptionally athletic, fit, and energetic seniors already experienced with yoga, it is important to appreciate that Ashtanga (and it's many branded variations, such as Power Yoga) was designed for youthful students (starting with young Brahman-caste boys at the Mysore Palace in the 1920s). It may be true that anyone can safely explore any sequence as long as they adhere to the yogic precepts of steadiness and ease; "explore" might mean a student sees what is being asked of them and possesses the confidence, clarity, and wisdom to say, "no thanks."[2] But in the reality of actual classes, students tend to push toward what they see others doing or what the teacher is suggesting; if the teacher is narrowly committed to a certain style rather than adapting yoga sequences to the needs of the real people in an actual class, many students—seniors included—will often push too hard or too far and get injured. Many others will simply disappear from yoga, convinced from the first experience that it just does not work for them.

Fortunately, wisdom does tend to come with age, as long as one continues learning. This is the conclusion made by Gene D. Cohen, MD (2006) in research on the aging brain in which he makes other insightful findings: the brain evolves throughout life in response to experience and learning; new brain cells form throughout life; the brain's emotional circuitry becomes more balanced with age; and the brain's two hemispheres are used more equally by older adults.[3] These findings point to the mental health value of yoga for seniors as they learn not merely asanas but rather a feeling for what is happening at a more subtle level of awareness within and between the asanas. Keeping the mind active while feeling their way into asanas that make sense given the reality of their condition, seniors further

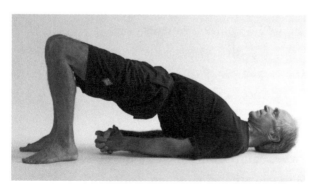

A healthy yogi enhancing his life

Sequencing Across the Life Cycle

stimulate both physical and mental vitality even as the forces of aging present new challenges and opportunities.

As with children, pregnant women, or indeed anyone interested in doing yoga, factors such as age may or may not be what is most significant. As with anyone anywhere in the life cycle, it is important first to assess their condition and intention before prescribing or suggesting a style of yoga or a particular yoga sequence. There are, to be sure, many active, fit, healthy seniors capable of doing a variety of practices. Yet taken as a whole, we can reasonable say that seniors tend to face a number of challenges that are altogether less common among their younger yoga peers. As we age, the body tends to become less mobile and weaker. There is an increased likelihood of having or developing arthritis, osteopenia, and osteoporosis, which contraindicates many asanas in which there is pressure in the joints while indicating the value of certain other asanas and actions that can help release joint pressure and restore strength to bones. There is also an increased fear of falling, even among seniors who have never experienced a serious fall, which often leads to less social and physical activity.[4] Heart disease, cancer, Alzheimer's disease, dementia, and vision and hearing loss are all increasingly common the older one gets.

Clearly, these conditions indicate the importance of adaptive and therapeutic yoga sequences for seniors. Perhaps the greatest insights into yoga for seniors have been developed through the research projects conducted through the Therapeutic Yoga for Seniors Program at Duke University Medicine as well as through research articles published in the *International Journal of Yoga Therapy*. Here we draw from those resources as well as direct experience in working with a diverse population of seniors in various yoga settings (yoga studios, hospitals, hospices, prisons, community centers, and privately).

Creating and Teaching Yoga Sequences for Seniors

- Appreciate that many healthy, physically fit seniors are best served in regular yoga classes in which age is not a distinction.
- Create a safe environment in which seniors are invited to feel whole.
- Welcome seniors—as with any student—as they are and provide appropriate yoga sequences based on their actual assessed conditions.
- Emphasize steadiness and ease in exploring asanas and pranayamas over attainment of poses or performance in breathing practices.

- Make ample use of props, including chairs, to help create adaptive accommodations.
- Teach the Joel Kramer method of "playing the edge" as a way to feel one's way into appropriate positioning.[5]
- Emphasize dynamic movement in connection with conscious ujjayi pranayama to stimulate the circulatory and respiratory systems.
- Provide ample time for rest and integration during practices over thirty minutes.
- Encourage seniors to do yoga five days per week for thirty to forty-five minutes per session, shortening or lengthening sessions based on ability.
- Include moderate strength and resistance activities to build or maintain muscle strength and to help maintain bone density.
- Include asanas and energetic actions within them that require and develop balance, including pada bandha as a technique for stabilizing the feet and ankles, as well as a variety of standing asanas.
- Include meditation and creative visualization practices that emphasize a sense of wholeness, body-mind integration, and self-acceptance.
- Offer end-of-life meditations as appropriate.[6]
- Create space for playfulness, encouraging seniors to spontaneously explore movement and to give mutual support to other seniors through safe partner yoga exercises.

Yoga Sequences for Seniors

Sequence 47: Yoga for Seniors with Arthritis

1. Classical Surya Namaskara
3–5 times to warm the body.

2. Balasana
1 minute. Place a blanket under the hips to reduce pressure in the knees and lower back.

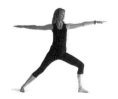

3. Virabhadrasana II
5 breaths on each side. Set up from Prasarita stance.

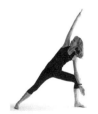

4. Utthita Parsvakonasana
5 breaths on each side.

Sequence 47: Yoga for Seniors with Arthritis (continued)

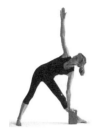

5. Utthita Trikonasana
5 breaths on each side.

6. Prasarita Padottanasana A Prep
1 minute.

7. Classical Surya Namaskara
After lunging on the second side, transition to Adho Mukha Svanasana and hold for 5 breaths.

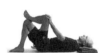

8. Balasana
5–10 breaths, then come back to Adho Mukha Svanasana.

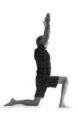

9. Ashta Chandrasana Prep
1 minute, then transition to the next pose before switching sides.

10. Salabhasana A
Move in and out 5 times before holding for 5 breaths, then release and roll onto the back.

11. Setu Bandha Sarvangasana
5–10 breaths, then repeat once or twice.

12. Thread the Needle Prep
2 minutes on each side.

13. Ardha Matsyendrasana
5–10 breaths on each side.

14. Dandasana
1 minute.

15. Janu Sirsasana
Hold each side 1 minute. Consider placing a block under the bent knee.

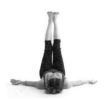

16. Viparita Karani
5 minutes with a folded blanket under the pelvis.

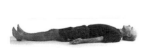

17. Savasana
5–10 minutes.

18. Sukhasana
Meditation.

Sequence 48: Yoga for Seniors with Osteoporosis

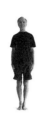

1. Tadasana
1–2 minutes. Set intention, welcome, begin guiding.

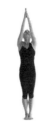

2. Urdhva Hastasana
10 breaths.

3. Ardha Uttanasana
10 breaths. Keep the spine fully extended (bent knees will help).

4. Phalakasana
10 breaths.

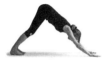

5. Adho Mukha Svanasana
10 breaths. Keep the spine fully extended (bent knees will help).

6. Balasana
5–10 breaths. Position the knees wide apart to help keep the spine from rounding into flexion.

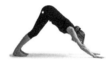

7. Adho Mukha Svanasana
5 breaths, then walk forward.

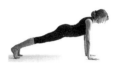

8. Ardha Uttanasana
10 breaths. Keep the spine fully extended.

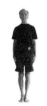

9. Tadasana
5 breaths. Step to Prasarita stance.

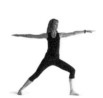

10. Virabhadrasana II
10 breaths on each side.

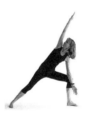

11. Utthita Parsvakonasana
10 breaths on each side.

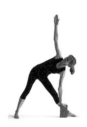

12. Utthita Trikonasana
10 breaths on each side.

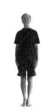

13. Tadasana
5 breaths.

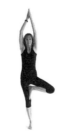

14. Vrksasana
Hold each side 10–15 breaths.

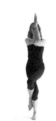

15. Garudasana
Hold each side 10–15 breaths. Contraindicated with hip replacement.

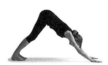

16. Adho Mukha Svanasana
1–2 minutes. Stronger students come to a wall and come into Handstand for up to 1 minute, rest, and repeat.

Sequence 48: Yoga for Seniors with Osteoporosis (continued)

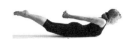

17. Salabhasana A
5 breaths each for 3 times.

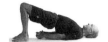

18. Setu Bandha Sarvangasana
5 breaths each for 3 times.

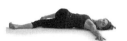

19. Supta Parivartanasana
5 breaths on each side.

20. Thread the Needle Prep
2 minutes on each side.

21. Dandasana
5 breaths.

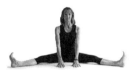

22. Upavista Konasana
10 breaths; keep the spine fully extended.

23. Baddha Konasana
10 breaths; keep the spine fully extended.

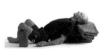

24. Supta Baddha Konasana
2 minutes, fully propped.

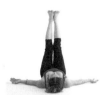

25. Viparita Karani
5 minutes. Prop the sacrum to reduce pressure along the spine.

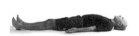

26. Savasana
5–10 minutes.

27. Sukhasana
Meditation.

Sequence 49: Yoga for Seniors with Difficulty Balancing

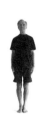

1. Tadasana
1–2 minutes. Welcome, set intention, begin guiding.

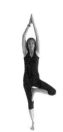

2. Vrksasana
10 breaths on each side. Use a wall for added support.

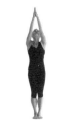

3. Tadasana
5 breaths.

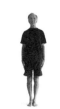

4. Urdhva Hastasana
5 breaths.

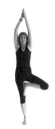

5. Vrksasana
10 breaths on each side. Use a wall for added support.

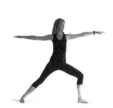

6. Virabhadrasana II
5 breaths on each side. Set up from Prasarita stance.

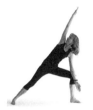

7. Utthita Parsvakonasana
5 breaths on each side.

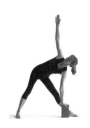

8. Utthita Trikonasana
5 breaths on each side.

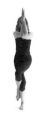

9. Garudasana
5 breaths on each side. Contraindicated with hip replacement.

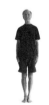

10. Tadasana
5 breaths.

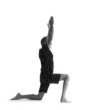

11. Ashta Chandrasana Prep
5 breaths on each side.

12. Salabhasana A
5 breaths each for 3 times, then hold 5 breaths with hands clasped.

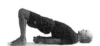

13. Setu Bandha Sarvangasana
5 breaths each for 3 times.

14. Apanasana
5 breaths.

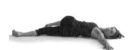

15. Supta Parivartanasana
5 breaths on each side.

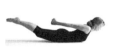

16. Dandasana
5 breaths.

Sequence 49: Yoga for Seniors with Difficulty Balancing (continued)

17. Janu Sirsasana
5 breaths on each side.

18. Baddha Konasana
10 breaths.

19. Ardha Matsyendrasana
5 breaths on each side.

20. Paschimottanasana
10 breaths.

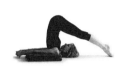

21. Halasana
5 breaths. Viparita Karani as an alternative.

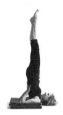

22. Salamba Sarvangasana
2–3 minutes. Stay in Viparita Karani as an alternative.

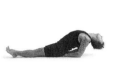

23. Uttana Padasana Prep
5 breaths.

24. Savasana
5–10 minutes.

25. Sukhasana
Meditation.

Sequence 50: Yoga for Seniors with Heart Disease

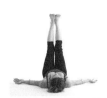

1. Viparita Karani
5 minutes. Focus on light ujjayi breathing.

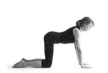

2. Bidalasana
5 times of Cat and Dog tilts, then rest in Balasana.

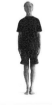

3. Tadasana
1 minute, exploring roots and extension.

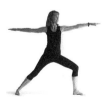

4. Virabhadrasana II
5–10 breaths on each side.

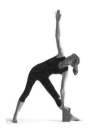

5. Utthita Trikonasana
5–10 breaths on each side.

6. Prasarita Padottanasana A Prep
Hold 1 minute.

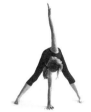

7. Parivrtta Prasarita Padottanasana
5 breaths on each side.

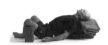

8. Supta Baddha Konasana
1 minute, breathing deeply and relaxing.

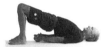

9. Setu Bandha Sarvangasana
1 minute, repeating 2–4 times.

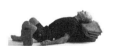

10. Supta Baddha Konasana
5 minutes.

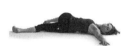

11. Supta Parivartanasana
5–10 breaths on each side.

12. Dandasana
1 minute.

13. Ardha Matsyendrasana
5–10 breaths on each side.

14. Paschimottanasana
2–3 minutes.

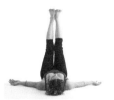

15. Viparita Karani
5–10 minutes.

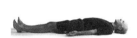

16. Savasana
5–10 minutes.

17. Sukhasana
Nadi shodhana pranayama 5 minutes, then 5 minutes of heart-centered meditation.

Part Four

Sequencing for
More Radiant Health
and Well-Being

Chapter Twelve

Cultivating Emotional
and Mental Health

This happiness consisted of nothing else but the
harmony of the few things around me with my own
existence, a feeling of contentment and well-being
that needed no changes and no intensification.
—HERMAN HESSE

We live in a world in which stress and anxiety are increasingly commonplace. According to the Stress in America Study by the American Psychological Association (2010), forty-two percent of American adults reported an increase in stress over the previous year, with a total of seventy-five percent of adults experiencing moderate to high stress levels. The top three stress responses are trouble sleeping (forty-seven percent), irritability or anger (forty-five percent), and fatigue (forty-three percent). Even kids—twenty-four percent of teens and fourteen percent of younger children—are reporting stress, with forty-five percent of kids overall reporting trouble sleeping and thirty-six percent reporting stress-related headaches. And while the proximate causes are not

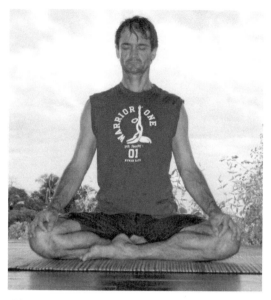
Yoga creates an opening to clarity and inner peace.

surprising—money, work, family responsibilities, relationship issues, and personal health concerns top the adult list—the means of managing it are disturbingly stressful themselves, even if not entirely surprising: thirty-five percent surf the internet, twenty-six percent eat, and thirteen percent smoke tobacco in order to reduce stress. Many of these and other short-term solutions are ultimately sources of further stress and anxiety.

Not surprisingly, the pharmaceutical industry sees a market opportunity in this, selling over $10 billion in antipsychotic and antidepressant prescription drugs to Americans in 2010 alone, nearly twice the amount of money spent by nearly twenty million Americans on yoga in the same year (DeNoon 2011). While prescription drugs are vitally necessary for some people experiencing symptoms of emotional or mental imbalance, many others might find a more wholesome and sustainable solution through such bodymind awareness practices as offered by yoga. Indeed, the American Psychological Association study finds that seven percent of Americans do turn to yoga to reduce stress. The question is: are they getting a stress-reducing yoga practice?

Before addressing this question, it is important to consider the other side of the emotional and mental health coin: depression. While anxiety and depression are often closely associated, many people are depressed or "feeling down" yet not anxious (or vice versa). Meanwhile, it is important to note that feeling sad or down, usually thought of negatively, can be subtly beneficial in helping a person cope with certain circumstances. The perceived sadness attracts social support, can help calm a person suffering from other ailments, and can have a "sadder but wiser" effect as the person comes to see the world more realistically.[1] Yet surely with chronic depression we want to be able to find a healthy way to steadier emotions and a deeper sense of contentment in life.

In the traditional yogic perspective, the tendencies toward anxiety and depression are symptomatic of an underlying energetic imbalance reflecting either a rajasic or tamasic state: rajasic when restless or anxious, tamasic when lethargic or depressed. Each of these conditions can be given a very general yogic prescription:

- If rajasic, offer students a slower asana practice that includes long holds in forward bends, a long Savasana, calming forms of pranayama such as nadi shodhana (simply breathing consciously is calming), and meditation practices in which the eyes are closed and students explore the slowing rhythms of thought.
- If tamasic, offer students a more vigorous, flowing style of asanas that includes a sustained series of stimulating back bends and twists and invigorating forms of pranayama such as kapalabhati along with meditation practices in which the eyes remain open with clear *dristi* and the quality of mindfulness is oriented toward being fully awake.

These alternative prescriptions can be given in the context of regular classes in which you offer modifications and variations that address the relative emotional or energetic imbalances of students. You can also offer entire class sequences designed to address these conditions. Here we offer four such sequences, two for reducing stress and two for relieving depression.

Sequence 51: Simple Relaxation Class for Beginning-Intermediate Students

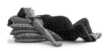

1. Supta Baddha Konasana
10 minutes. Prop the back and head on bolsters. Place blocks under the knees to reduce pressure in the knees and inner thighs.

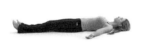

2. Savasana (modified)
5–10 minutes. Place a rolled blanket across under the shoulder blades and knees.

3. Swastikasana
5 minutes on each side.

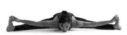

4. Upavista Konasana
5 minutes. Place bolsters under the chest and forehead to make this effortless.

5. Balasana
2 minutes. Keep the knees wide apart.

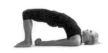

6. Setu Bandha Sarvangasana (modified)
5–10 minutes. Place block under the sacrum.

7. Viparita Karani
10 minutes. Place a strap around the legs and a sandbag on the feet.

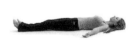

8. Savasana
5 minutes.

9. Sukhasana
Nadi shodhana pranayama for 2 minutes, then sit in meditation.

Sequence 52: Relax Deeply Class for Intermediate–Advanced Students

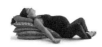

1. Supta Baddha Konasana
10 minutes. Prop the back
and head on bolsters.
Place blocks under the
knees to reduce pressure in
the knees and inner thighs.

2. Swastikasana
Stay on each side
5 minutes.

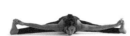

3. Upavista Konasana
Place bolsters under
the chest and forehead to
make this effortless.
Stay 10 minutes.

**4. Setu Bandha
Sarvangasana**
Place block under the
sacrum. Stay 5 minutes.
Now place a bolster under the
shoulders, legs extended,
and stay 5 minutes.

5. Swastikasana
2 minutes on each side.

6. Gomukhasana
3–5 minutes on each side.

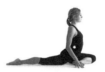

**7. Eka Pada Raj
Kapotasana I**
3–5 minutes on each side.

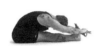

8. Paschimottanasana
5 minutes. Place bolsters
under the chest and forehead
to make this effortless.

9. Bharadvajrasana A
10–15 breaths
on each side.

10. Viparita Karani
10 minutes. Place a strap
around the legs and a sandbag on the feet.

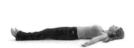

11. Savasana
5 minutes.

12. Sukhasana
Nadi shodhana pranayama
for 5 minutes, then sit in
meditation.

Sequence 53: Mildly Stimulating Class for Beginning-Intermediate Students

1. Classical Surya Namaskara
2 times.

2. Surya Namaskara A
3 times.

3. Surya Namaskara B
2 times.

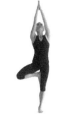

4. Vrksasana
1 minute on each side, then repeat on both sides.

5. Surya Namaskara A
1 time, then from Adho Mukha Svanasana transition to the next asana.

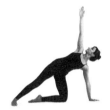

6. Vasisthasana Prep
5–10 breaths on each side, then transition to Adho Mukha Svanasana and to Tadasana.

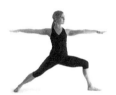

7. Virabhadrasana II
5 breaths on each side.

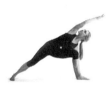

8. Utthita Parsvakonasana
5 breaths on each side.

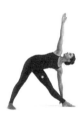

9. Utthita Trikonasana
5 breaths on each side.

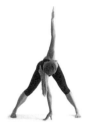

10. Parivrtta Ardha Prasarita
10 breaths on each side, then step to Tadasana.

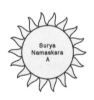

11. Surya Namaskara A
1 time, then from Adho Mukha Svanasana, release to Balasana.

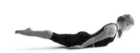

12. Salabhasana A
Raise and lower with the breath 5 times, hold for 5 breaths with the fingers interlaced behind the back, then rest for 5–10 breaths.

13. Dhanurasana
5 breaths, then repeat 1–3 times.

14. Balasana
5 breaths.

15. Bharadvajrasana A
5 breaths on each side.

16. Dandasana
5 breaths.

Sequence 53: Mildly Stimulating Class for Beginning-Intermediate Students (continued)

17. Parivrtta Janu Sirsasana
10 breaths on each side.

18. Baddha Konasana
10 breaths.

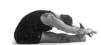

19. Paschimottanasana
5 breaths, then transition to the next asana.

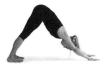

20. Adho Mukha Svanasana
1 minute.

21. Balasana
5 breaths.

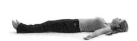

22. Savasana
5 minutes.

23. Sukhasana
Sit in meditation 5–15 minutes.

Sequence 54: Mildly Stimulating Class for Intermediate-Advanced Students

1. Surya Namaskara A
5 times.

2. Surya Namaskara B
5 times.

3. Navasana
Hold for 5 breaths, then transition to the next asana.

4. Tolasana
3–5 breaths, then repeat asanas 3–4 before transitioning to the next asana.

5. Lolasana
1–5 breaths, then transition to Chaturanga Dandasana.

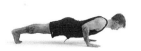

6. Chaturanga Dandasana
1–5 breaths, then press into the next asana.

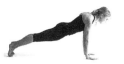

7. Phalakasana
5 breaths.

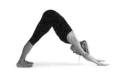

8. Adho Mukha Svanasana
5–10 breaths, or rest in Balasana.

Sequence 54: Mildly Stimulating Class for Intermediate–Advanced Students (continued)

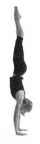

9. Adho Mukha Vrksasana
Hold up to 1 minute, rest, and repeat 2 times.

10. Pada Hastasana
1 minute.

11. Shishulasana
5 breaths or rest in Balasana.

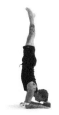

12. Pincha Mayurasana
1 minute, rest, and repeat 2 times.

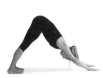

13. Balasana
Rest 1 minute, transition to Adho Mukha Svanasana, Tadasana, and a wide Prasarita stance.

14. Virabhadrasana II
Hold the first side 10 breaths.

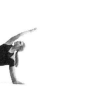

15. Utthita Parsvakonasana
Hold the first side 10 breaths.

16. Svarga Dvijasana
Hold the first side 5–10 breaths, then release back into Utthita Parsvakonasana and switch sides. After the second side, transition to Eka Pada Koundinyasana A or directly to Chaturanga Dandasana.

17. Adho Mukha Svanasana
5 breaths, then jump forward into Ardha Uttanasana.

18. Uttanasana
5 breaths.

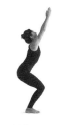

19. Utkatasana
5 breaths.

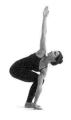

20. Parivrtta Utkatasana
5 breaths on each side, then press into Tadasana.

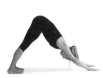

21. Surya Namaskara A
Hold Adho Mukha Svanasana 1 breath.

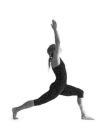

22. Ashta Chandrasana
Hold first side 5 breaths.

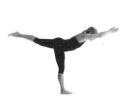

23. Virabhadrasana III
Hold first side 5 breaths.

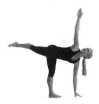

24. Parivrtta Ardha Chandrasana
1 minute, come back to Virabhadrasana III, then to Ashta Chandrasana, and do a vinyasa in transition to the other side.

25. Balasana
1 minute.

26. Ustrasana
5–10 breaths,
repeat 1–2 times.

27. Laghu Vajrasana
Drop back 1–5 times, holding the final dropped-back
position 5 breaths, then
either come up and rest or
do the next asana.

28. Kapotasana
5–10 breaths.

**29. Ardha
Matsyendrasana**
5–10 breaths on each side.

30. Dandasana
5 breaths.

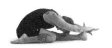

**31. Tiriang Mukha Eka
Pada Paschimottanasana**
1–2 minutes on each side.

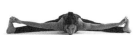

32. Upavista Konasana
10 breaths.

33. Gomukhasana
5–10 breaths on each
side, then pick up and do
a vinyasa to Adho Mukha
Svanasana.

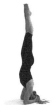

34. Salamba Sirsasana I
1–5 minutes. Explore twisting through the torso, holding each side 5 breaths.

35. Urdhva Dandasana
5 breaths, raise the legs
back to Sirsasana, then rest.

36. Balasana
5 breaths, then do a
vinyasa and float through
to lying supine.

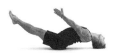

37. Uttana Padasana
5–10 breaths.

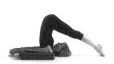

38. Savasana
5 minutes.

39. Virasana
108 kapalabhati pranayama
breaths, then sit in
meditation.

Chapter Thirteen

Chakra Sequences

I found I could say things with color and shapes
that I could not say any other way—things I had
no words for.
—GEORGIA O'KEEFFE

As with everything in the world of yoga, with chakras there are numerous contrasting and even conflicting views about what they are, how they work, their number, location, and even whether location is a relevant concept. Different chakra models found in historical, philosophical, and literary works have as few as five chakras or infinite chakras throughout the subtle body. In the traditional yogic literature the number varies from chakras at the intersection of every nadi to the identification of the major chakras, usually said to number between five and eight, that are located at the junctions of the major nadis as they spiral and rise along the spine and give us the major psycho-spiritual-energetic centers of the subtle body. The tantric model of chakras, which we will use here in looking at chakra sequences, was developed around the eleventh century and described in the Sat-Cakra-Narupana. It

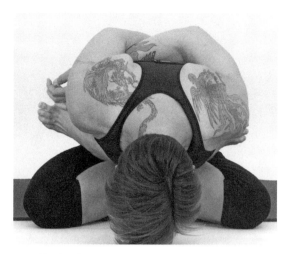

Turning inward, we can awaken to something deeper, clearer, and sweeter.

is the most widely accepted model, giving seven chakras described as emanations of divine consciousness (Avalon 1974, 318).

Just as the movement of prana is felt in the physical body and in our mental awareness despite being invisible, the chakras can be usefully visualized as psychic centers of energetic and spiritual experience, not physical locations that can be palpated, x-rayed, or detected with magnetic resonance imaging technology. "Concentration on physical organs or spots in the body as prescribed by many spiritual masters," says Harish Johari (1987, 15), "is misleading, for the chakras are not material." Yet the chakras may correlate with the major nerve plexuses of the physical body; some schools of thought associate chakras with particular sensations in the body.[1] More commonly they are correlated to psychological, emotional, and mental qualities. Lecturing in 1932, Carl Jung emphasized that "they symbolize highly complex psychic facts which at the present moment we could not possibly express except in images" (Shamdasani 1996, 61). Whether the relationships indicated by these symbols are useful is a question best answered in personal practice.

Chakras are said to be part of a much higher energy system than the physical body. Traditionally it is said that awakening of the chakras depends on opening a higher source of energy than the physical body can provide, that it takes a concentrated quality level of awareness (Frawley 1999). During normal consciousness, this energy is dormant. When awakened through conscious awareness, this energy rises through the core of one's being, creating ecstatic bliss. For this to happen there must be balance in each of the seven chakras, each of which symbolizes certain aspects of one's physical, psychological, and spiritual condition.

The chakra model offers an approach to integration in the entire being, unifying the physical, emotional, and spiritual. This model provides a useful approach to sequencing asanas while exploring deeper qualities of self-awareness that embody a more multidimensional self-understanding. Whether applied as the model for a complete class or to stimulate specific areas of energetic balance or self-awareness, a chakra model class has a variety of creative possibilities for sequencing asana and pranayama practices. Here we will look at separate sequences for cultivating balance in each chakra as well as a complete integrated chakra class.

Muladhara Chakra

The muladhara chakra (from *mul,* "base," and *adhara,* "support") symbolizes our present psychic condition, bound as we are in normal consciousness to the physical body and intertwined in the web of earthly forces. The base chakra, muladhara is associated with the earth element and the grounding aspects of life, including the basics of food, shelter, and livelihood. Finger (2005, 39) and others locate this chakra at the base of the pelvis. It is out of balance when we lack grounding or are so rigidly grounded as to lack mobility or resilience in navigating the evolving path of our life. If constantly feeling out of control, insecure, irresponsible, or caught up in matters of money, it is suggested that the muladhara chakra is out of balance. In the yoga practice, we cultivate muladhara chakra balance by establishing a sense of grounding, particularly through the feet, legs, and pelvis, as well as a sense of moving into stillness through grounded forward bends that evoke a feeling of surrendering to the earth. Amid these grounding actions and sensations, one can deepen their sense of physical, emotional, and mental stability through visualization practices that help embody these qualities of awareness.

Sequence 55: Muladhara Chakra Class

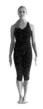

1. Tadasana
3 minutes. Teach pada bandha, mula bandha, pelvic neutrality, neutral spinal extension, and heart-centered ujjayi pranayama. Set intention.

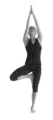

2. Vrksasana
Explore all the qualities taught in Tadasana amid the challenge of standing on one leg. Emphasize mula bandha.

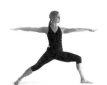

3. Virabhadrasana II
From Prasarita stance, move in and out 5 times, then hold 2 minutes before switching sides.

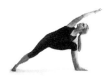

4. Utthita Parsvakonasana
2 minutes on each side.

Sequence 55: Muladhara Chakra Class (continued)

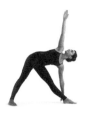

5. Utthita Trikonasana
1 minute on each side.

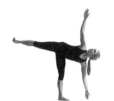

6. Ardha Chandrasana
1 minute on each side.

7. Prasarita Padottanasana A, B, C, D
5 breaths in each asana (B, C, and D are shown in Appendix B).

8. Garudasana
15 breaths on each side.

9. Parsvottanasana
5 breaths on each side.

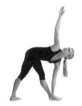

10. Parivrtta Trikonasana
5 breaths on the first side, then either switch sides or transition to the next asana.

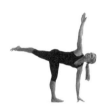

11. Parivrtta Ardha Chandrasana
5 breaths, then release to Parivrtta Trikonasana and switch sides.

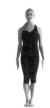

12. Tadasana
5 breaths. Focus on pada bandha, mula bandha, roots and extension.

13. Surya Namaskara A
1 time, then 5 breaths in Adho Mukha Svanasana.

14. Ashta Chandrasana
10 breaths on the first side, then transition into the next asana.

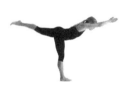

15. Virabhadrasana III
5 breaths, then release back to Ashta Chandrasana.

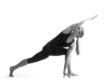

16. Parivrtta Ashta Chandrasana
10 breaths, then vinyasa and switch sides on asanas 14–16.

17. Balasana
5–10 breaths, then lie supine.

18. Dhanurasana
5 breaths. Repeat once or twice.

19. Ustrasana
5 breaths. Repeat once or twice.

20. Ardha Matsyendrasana
5 breaths on each side.

Sequence 55: Muladhara Chakra Class (continued)

21. Dandasana
5 breaths.

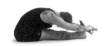

22. Paschimottanasana
10 breaths.

23. Apanasana
5 breaths.

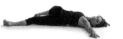

**24. Supta
Parivartanasana**
5 breaths on each side.

25. Ananda Balasana
5 breaths.

26. Viparita Karani
2–5 minutes.

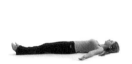

27. Savasana
5–10 minutes.

28. Sukhasana
Meditation.

Svadhisthana Chakra

The svadhisthana chakra (from *sva*, "self," and *adhisthana*, "dwelling place") symbolizes the core feelings we have around our likes and dislikes, reflecting what we gravitate toward or resist in our lives. Representing the water element, svadhisthana reflects the shifting tides of attraction and repulsion. It is often associated with the reproductive organs and the way these qualities are expressed in one's sex life. When the muladhara chakra is balanced, we more easily come to balance here as well, creatively expressing ourselves in the world of relationships in a way that helps to sustain our contentment. If we find ourselves being easily addicted (even to yoga), compulsive, lacking desire, or having difficulty sustaining relationships, this suggests that the svadhisthana chakra is imbalanced. We can cultivate svadhisthana balance by first recognizing the behavioral and emotional patterns that drive our lives around matters of sensuality, sexuality, creativity, and relationship. With this awareness, we can then explore these tendencies in our yoga practice, noticing where we flow more or less easily and comfortably. Fluid sequences such as Surya Namaskaras (Sun Salutations) stimulate circulation and a sense of creative expression, opening us to enjoy the simple flow and flavor of creative energy as the movement of delight. We can also suggest the fluid awareness evoked in the svadhisthana chakra by bringing more awareness to how to use the breath and energetic actions in all asanas in a way that balances the sharing of awakened energy throughout the entirety of our being, especially in the joints and other areas where we tend not to have much circulation.

Sequence 56: Svadhisthana Chakra Class

1. Sukhasana
2–3 minutes. Welcome, set intention, begin guiding.

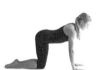

2. Bidalasana
10 cycles of Cat and Dog Tilts.

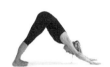

3. Adho Mukha Svanasana
10 breaths, bicycling the legs.

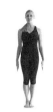

4. Tadasana
5 breaths.

5. Classical Surya Namaskara
3 times. Pause in the first Salabhasana B to alternately lift and release the right and left shoulders, swiveling through the spine, then continue, doing the complete Sun Salutation 3 times.

6. Balasana
5–10 breaths, or alternately rest in Adho Mukha Svanasana.

7. Dancing Warrior
5 times.

8. Balasana
5–10 breaths.

9. Utthita Trikonasana
10 breaths on each side.

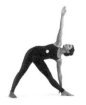

10. Ardha Chandrasana
10 breaths on each side.

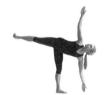

11. Prasarita Padottanasana A
2 minutes, or do the following arm balance exploration.

12. Salamba Sirsasana II
Inhaling, extend the legs overhead; exhaling, draw the knees to the shoulders for Bakasana, or fold the legs into lotus position for Urdhva Kukkutasana.

Sequence 56: Svadhisthana Chakra Class (continued)

13. Bakasana
5 breaths before placing the head on the floor and coming back up into Salamba Sirsasana II. As an alternative, do the following asana.

14. Urdhva Kukkutasana
5 breaths before placing the head on the floor and coming back up into Salamba Sirsasana II.

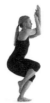

15. Garudasana
10 breaths on each side.

16. Parsvottanasana
5 breaths, then transition to the next asana on the same side.

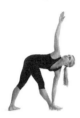

17. Parivrtta Trikonasana
Hold 5 breaths, then transition to the next asana on the same side.

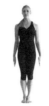

18. Parivrtta Ardha Chandrasana
5 breaths, release back to Parivrtta Trikonasana, then transition to the other side of Parsvottanasana, repeating asanas 16–18 on the other side.

19. Tadasana
5 breaths.

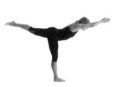

Surya Namaskara B

20. Surya Namaskara B
1 time, 5 breaths in Adho Mukha Svanasana. Newer students skip to asana 26 or 30.

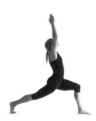

21. Ashta Chandrasana
5 breaths on the first side, then transition to the next asana.

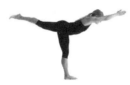

22. Virabhadrasana III
5 breaths on the first side, then transition to the next asana.

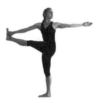

23. Parivrtta Hasta Padangusthasana
5 breaths on the first side, then transition to the next asana.

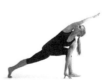

24. Virabhadrasana III
5 breaths on the first side, then transition to the next asana.

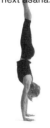

25. Adho Mukha Vrksasana
5 breaths, then vinyasa and switch sides on asanas 21–25.

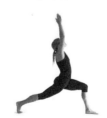

26. Ashta Chandrasana
5 breaths on the first side, then transition to the next asana.

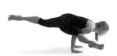

27. Parivrtta Ashta Chandrasana
5 breaths on the first side, then transition to the next asana.

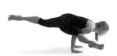

28. Eka Pada Koundinyasana B
Flow through this arm balance in transition to a vinyasa and switch sides on asanas 26–28.

Sequence 56: Svadhisthana Chakra Class (continued)

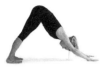

29. Adho Mukha Svanasana
5 breaths.

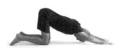

30. Anahatasana
10 breaths.

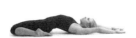

31. Supta Virasana
2 minutes.

32. Ustrasana
5 breaths. Repeat 1–2 times.

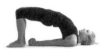

33. Setu Bandha Sarvangasana
5 breaths.
Repeat 1–2 times.

34. Urdhva Dhanurasana
5 breaths.
Repeat 1–2 times.

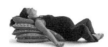

35. Supta Baddha Konasana
10 breaths.

36. Apanasana
5 breaths.

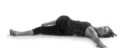

37. Supta Parivartanasana
5 breaths on each side.

38. Swastikasana
15 breaths on each side.

39. Ardha Matsyendrasana
5 breaths on each side.

40. Dandasana
5 breaths.

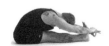

41. Paschimottanasana
3–5 minutes, then transition to the next asana, or skip to asana 49.

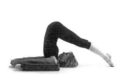

42. Halasana
5 breaths.

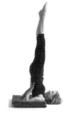

43. Salamba Sarvangasana
2–5 minutes.

44. Urdhva Padmasana
5 breaths.

45. Pindasana
5 breaths.

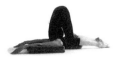

46. Karnapidasana
5 breaths.

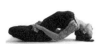

47. Matsyasana
5 breaths.

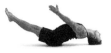

48. Uttana Padasana
5 breaths.

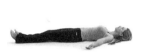

49. Savasana
5–10 minutes.

50. Sukhasana
Meditation.

Manipura Chakra

The manipura chakra (from *mani,* "gems," and *pura,* "town"), or "city of jewels," symbolizes the qualities that affect how we manifest ourselves in the world. Representing the fire element, manipura is about how we stoke our inner fire and thereby glow in the world. Often associated with the abdominal core, when the fire of manifestation blazes out of control we tend to be domineering, insensitive to other's needs, arrogant, and have difficulty in developing harmonious relationships in life. When dim, we tend to fade from action, have difficulty making decisions, are prone to self-destructive behavior, and constantly question ourselves in ways that lead to giving up or being timid. With balance in the muladhara and svadhisthana chakras, we more easily find balance in manipura qualities. With this we have the courage to face difficult circumstances with a sense of openness, the intensity to stay with challenges, and a balance of confidence and humility that enables us to more instinctively establish respectful and comfortable relationships. Assertive without being aggressive, determined without being forceful, we can more easily come to emotional balance even when faced with complexity. Core awakening asana and pranayama sequences can help develop the strong yet supple center, stoking the inner fire of motivation and embodying a clearer, stronger, yet softer way of moving, being, and manifesting. Applied to more intense action, we can cultivate grounded levity through applied abdominal action in arm balance sequences, yet also a sense of greater radiance by moving more from our core in asana transitions. With twists we can both stimulate and dampen the fire, thereby cultivating and directing energy in a way that is in keeping with our intention in any given practice.

Sequence 57: Manipura Chakra Class

1. Virasana
Awaken mula bandha and ujj-ayi pranayama for 2 minutes, then do 3 one-minute rounds of Kapalabhati pranayama.

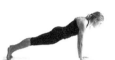

2. Phalakasana
2 minutes. Offer the option of having the knees on the floor.

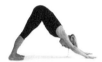

3. Adho Mukha Svanasana
1 minute, awakening the relationship between roots and extension.

4. Balasana
5–10 breaths.

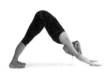

5. Adho Mukha Svanasana
1 minute, awakening a deeper connection of breath and awareness in the abdominal core. Teach "uddiyana bandha light."

6. Tadasana
Teach pada bandha and use it to access mula bandha.

7. Surya Namaskara A
3 times, emphasizing moving from the core.

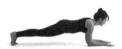

8. Shishula Phalakasana
If this pose is too intense, place the knees on the floor. Otherwise hold for 1 minute while doing kapalabhati pranayama.

9. Shishulasana
5 breaths, then press to Adho Mukha Svanasana (consider placing the knees on the floor first to reduce pressure in the shoulders).

10. Adho Mukha Svanasana
5 breaths. Consider resting in Balasana.

11. Dancing Warrior
3 times, holding each standing asana for 5–10 breaths.

12. Balasana
5–10 breaths.

Sequence 57: Manipura Chakra Class (continued)

13. Adho Mukha Svanasana
5 breaths, then float through to Dandasana.

14. Navasana
5 breaths, then transition to the next asana.

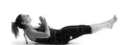

15. Ardha Navasana
30 seconds of kapalabhati pranayama, come back up into Paripurna Navasana for 1 breath, and transition to the next asana.

16. Tolasana
1–5 breaths, repeat asanas 16–18 one to four times, then transition to the next asana.

17. Lolasana
1–5 breaths, then vinyasa.

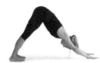

18. Adho Mukha Svanasana
5 breaths, then either rest in Balasana and skip to asana 24, or leap-frog the feet around the hands for the next asana.

19. Bhujapidasana
5 breaths, then transition to the next asana.

20. Tittibhasana
5 breaths, then transition to the next asana.

21. Bakasana
5 breaths, then vinyasa and float through to lying supine.

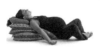

22. Supta Baddha Konasana
10 breaths.

23. Ananda Balasana
5 breaths.

24. Setu Bandha Sarvangasana
5 breaths. Repeat once or twice.

25. Urdhva Dhanurasana
5 breaths. Repeat once or twice.

26. Apanasana
5 breaths.

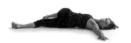

27. Supta Parivartanasana
5 breaths on each side.

28. Apanasana
5 breaths.

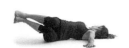

29. Jathara Parivartanasana
5 times each way.

30. Ananda Balasana
Laughing out loud!

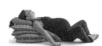

31. Supta Baddha Konasana
1–2 minutes.

32. Dandasana
5–10 breaths.

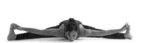

33. Upavista Konasana
2 minutes.

34. Parivrtta Janu Sirsasana
1–2 minutes on each side.

35. Ardha Matsyendrasana
5 breaths on each side.

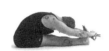

36. Paschimottanasana
1–2 minutes.

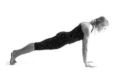

37. Parsvottanasana
5 breaths.

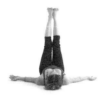

38. Viparita Karani
2–3 minutes.

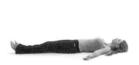

39. Savasana
5–10 minutes.

40. Sukhasana
Meditation.

Anahata Chakra

The anahata chakra (*anahata* means "unstruck sound") symbolizes awareness and manifestation of love. Representing the air element, anahata is about the heart of our feelings. Often associated with the heart or the spiritual heart center, here we tune in to the very pulse of life and expand it through the conscious cultivation of prana in breathing as though through our heart. With balance in the lower chakras, we can more easily come to balance in matters of emotional connection, thereby opening to the higher consciousness that naturally manifests when compassion, joy, and love are fully part of our life. Going beyond personal emotions to understand the love in all emotional fluctuations, becoming love itself, we begin to sense the greater possibilities for heightened awareness that creates a feeling of transcending the more mundane aspects of existence. While we can cultivate a heart-centered quality of awareness in all asana and pranayama practices, back bends accompanied by ujjayi pranayama most directly stimulate the opening and awakening of these qualities of being. Practicing viloma pranayama with antara kumbhaka (retention of the inhale) deepens this experience. We can also tap into a variety of heart-centered meditation practices to bring every cell of our being and consciousness more alive with compassion and love.

Sequence 58: Anahata Chakra Class

1. Sukhasana
5 minutes of heart-centered ujjayi pranayama, set intention, begin guiding.

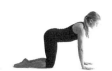

2. Bidalasana
5 cycles of Cat and Dog Tilts.

3. Balasana
5 breaths, then come to standing.

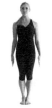

4. Tadasana
5 breaths.

5. Classical Surya Namaskara
3 times.

6. Surya Namaskara A
3 times. New students skip to asana 8.

7. Surya Namaskara B
3 times. New students skip to asana 8.

8. Balasana
10 breaths.

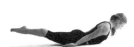

9. Salabhasana A
Lift a little and release, repeating 5 times with a higher lift each time, then hold 5 breaths.

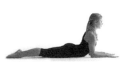

10. Niravalasana
10 breaths.

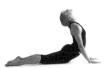

11. Bhujangasana
5 breaths; repeat once or twice. New students skip to asana 15.

12. Bhekasana
10 breaths, then vinyasa to Adho Mukha Svanasana.

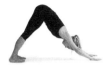

13. Adho Mukha Svanasana
10 breaths.

14. Ardha Matsyendrasana
5 breaths on each side.

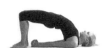

15. Setu Bandha Sarvangasana
5 breaths; repeat once or twice. New students skip to asana 18.

16. Urdhva Dhanurasana
5 breaths; repeat once or twice.

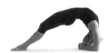

17. Viparita Dandasana
5 breaths; repeat once or twice.

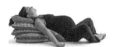

18. Supta Baddha Konasana
Propped to open heart.

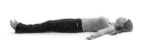

19. Savasana
1 minute. Yes, Savasana.

20. Swastikasana
1 minute on each side.

21. Dandasana
5 breaths.

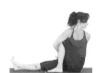

22. Marichyasana C
5 breaths on each side.

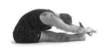

23. Paschimottanasana
2 minutes.

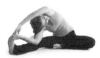

24. Parivrtta Janu Sirsasana
5 breaths on each side.

25. Baddha Konasana
10 breaths.

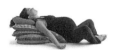

26. Supta Baddha Konasana
2–3 minutes. Prop the back and head.

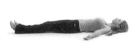

27. Savasana
5–10 minutes.

28. Sukhasana
Heart-centered meditation.

Vishuddha Chakra

The vishuddha chakra (*vishuddha* means "pure," "clear," or "virtuous") symbolizes purity and harmony in the entirety of one's being. Representing the element of ether or space that hosts the other four elements, when the lower chakras are balanced and the anahata chakra awakened, we find greater ease in every aspect of balance in our lives. Often associated with the throat, here we come to more closely sense the flow of prana and the expressions of voice. No longer feeling conflicted or pulled in opposing directions, filled with the light of compassion and love, we more easily find balance in the flow of breath, and with it, simpler energetic balance. With wisdom rising from our heart, we more easily know and share the truth as we experience it. Communication is clearer, expressing the stability, creativity, willfulness, and love emanating from the balanced quality of the muladhara, svadhisthana, manipura, and anahata chakras. In asana practice, we bring greater awareness to the vishuddha chakra with Uttana Padasana (Extended Leg Pose), Matsyasana (Fish Pose), Halasana (Plow Pose), Salamba Sarvangasana (Supported Shoulder Stand), and other asanas that draw awareness and release to the region of the throat and neck. Simhasana (Lion's Breath Pose), ujjayi pranayama, bahya kumbhaka (retention of the exhalation), and jalandhara bandha (throat lock) bring even greater awareness of vishuddha chakra energy and an opening to feeling the emergence of clearer consciousness.

Sequence 59: Vishuddha Chakra Class

1. Sukhasana
Ujjayi pranayama, set intention, chant "aum" 5 times.

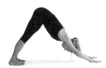

2. Adho Mukha Svanasana
1–3 minutes.

3. Balasana
5 breaths.

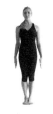

4. Tadasana
5 breaths.

Sequence 59: Vishuddha Chakra Class (continued)

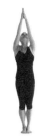

5. Urdhva Hastasana
1 minute.

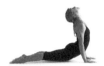

6. Classical Surya Namaskara
Do 5 times. In Ardha Uttanasana, emphasize space from the heart through the throat, then maintain it throughout the Sun Salutations.

7. Urdhva Mukha Svanasana
5 breaths, with strong audible Lion's Breath exhalations (out the mouth, gaze to the third eye, tongue to chin).

8. Balasana
5 breaths.

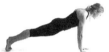

9. Phalakasana
5 breaths.

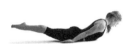

10. Salabhasana A
Move in and out 5 times before holding for 5 breaths, release, then come up 2 more times, holding for 5–10 breaths each time.

11. Dhanurasana
5 breaths, release, rest, and repeat.

12. Ustrasana
5 breaths, release, rest, and repeat, or do the following asana.

13. Laghu Vajrasana
Drop back 5 times, hold 5 breaths, come up, and either repeat or do the following asana.

14. Kapotasana
5 breaths.

15. Balasana
5–10 breaths.

16. Ardha Matsyendrasana
5 breaths on each side.

17. Bharadvajrasana A
5 breaths on each side. Either repeat or do the following asana.

18. Bharadvajrasana B
5 breaths on each side.

19. Dandasana
5 breaths

20. Paschimottanasana
Hold 1–2 minutes.

Sequence 59: Vishuddha Chakra Class (continued)

21. Pursvottanasana
5 breaths. Consider keeping the knees bent to take it easier.

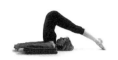

22. Halasana
5 breaths.

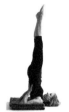

23. Salamba Sarvangasana
2 minutes.

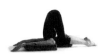

24. Karnapidasana
5 breaths.

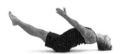

25. Uttana Padasana
5 breaths.

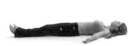

26. Savasana
5–10 minutes.

27. Sukhasana
Meditate for 5–25 minutes, focusing awareness in the throat while breathing through the heart and opening to clearer awareness.

Ajna Chakra

The ajna chakra (*ajna* means "command" or "authority") symbolizes the overarching intelligence and wisdom that brings all of the other chakras to life and balance. Representing the *mahat* ("great") element of pure awareness that envelops and animates the lower five chakras, here the conditions of our life come fully to consciousness. All that we have inherited and all that we manifest in the moment is brought into a sense of clarity and wholeness through the prism of the ajna chakra. As though "seeing" through our third eye, we witness our life and world as though transcending time and space, especially by opening through meditation to dimensions of consciousness that are otherwise obfuscated or blurred. Often associated with the mysterious pineal gland, which René Descartes referred to as the "seat of the soul,"[2] the ajna chakra reflects learning to live with the purest insight. In ajna chakra sequencing, the ajna chakra itself guides the practice, giving us an intuitive approach to practice as presently exemplified and encouraged in the teachings of Erich Schiffmann's Freedom-style yoga. Nadi shodhana pranayama (alternate nostril breathing) stimulates energetic balance in the ajna chakra and can be refined through suryabheda and chandrabheda (sun and moon piercing, respectively) pranayamas. These practices will contribute to simpler awakening of intuitive awareness in mediation, opening to more balanced awareness of one's being in the universe.

Sequence 60: Ajna Chakra Class

1. Sukhasana
Set intention, aum, 5 minutes of nadi shodhana pranayama.

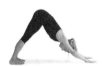

2. Adho Mukha Svanasana
Bicycle out the legs for 1 minute.

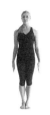

3. Tadasana
Cultivate pada bandha, roots and extension.

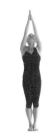

4. Urdhva Hastasana
1 minute.

5. Uttanasana
3 minutes.

6. Shishulasana
1–2 minutes, then rest in Balasana 5–10 breaths.

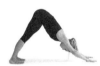

7. Adho Mukha Svanasana
1 minute, then release to all fours.

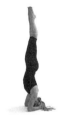

8. Salamba Sirsasana I
3–5 minutes, then rest in Balasana 5–10 breaths.

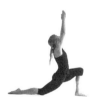

9. Anjaneyasana
1–2 minutes on each side.

10. Setu Bandha Sarvangasana
5–10 breaths.
Repeat 2–3 times, or do the following asana.

11. Urdhva Dhanurasana
5–10 breaths.
Repeat 1–2 times.

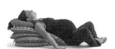

12. Supta Baddha Konasana
1 minute, then come up to sitting.

13. Bharadvajrasana A
5 breaths on each side.
Either repeat or do the
following asana.

14. Bharadvajrasana B
5 breaths on each side.

15. Dandasana
5 breaths.

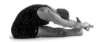

16. Paschimottanasana
1–2 minutes.

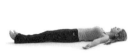

17. Savasana
5–10 minutes.

18. Sukhasana
Meditate for 5–55 minutes.

Sahasrara Chakra

The sahasrara chakra (*sahasrara* means "thousand petals") symbolizes the full manifestation of enlightened awareness. The number one thousand is given to signify the infinite; beyond the elements, it is said to be the seat of the soul, representing the abiding quality of consciousness that pervades the universe. Reflecting the overall condition of one's life, once one has brought balance and integration to the qualities of existence symbolized by the other chakras, one comes to a sense of integrated, blissful being, wholly at peace and at one in the world. Flowing along the path of asana, pranayama, and mediation, one is now in the fullest fruits of yoga practice.

Sequence 61: Sahasrara: An Integrated Chakra Class (Intermediate Level)

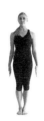

1. Tadasana
Set intention, aum, ujjayi pranayama, pada bandha, mula bandha.

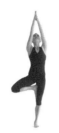

2. Vrksasana
1–2 minutes on each side.

3. Classical Surya Namaskara
3 times.

4. Dancing Warrior
3–5 times, flowing continuously.

5. Dandasana
1 minute, focused on roots and extension.

6. Navasana
5 times, holding 5 breaths each time. Do the following asana between each side.

7. Tolasana
5 breaths each time. On the final time, transition to the following asana.

8. Lolasana
5 breaths, then step or float back.

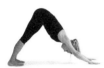

9. Adho Mukha Svanasana
1 minute.

10. Bakasana
5 breaths, applying the awakened core to create grounded levity.

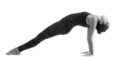

11. Pursvottanasana
5–10 breaths, then do a vinyasa and come to lying supine.

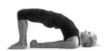

12. Setu Bandha Sarvangasana
5–10 breaths. Repeat 2–3 times, or do the following asana.

13. Urdhva Dhanurasana
5–10 breaths. Repeat 1–2 times.

14. Ustrasana
5–10 breaths. Repeat twice, or do Laghu Vajrasana and/or Kapotasana.

15. Balasana
5–10 breaths.

16. Ardha Matsyendrasana
5–10 breaths on each side.

17. Dandasana
5–10 breaths.

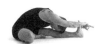

18. Janu Sirsasana
1 minute on each side.

19. Baddha Konasana
1–2 minutes.

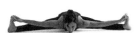

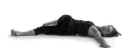

20. Upavista Konasana
1–2 minutes. Consider
Kurmasana as an alternative.

21. Gomukhasana
1 minute on each side.

22. Dandasana
1 minute.

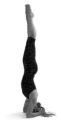

23. Salamba Sirsasana I
2–5 minutes, rest in Balasana, then lie supine; or, do
Viparita Karani at a wall.

**24. Supta
Parivartanasana**
5–10 breaths on each side.

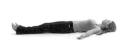

25. Savasana
5–10 minutes.

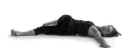

26. Sukhasana
Nadi shodhana pranayama,
heart-centered meditation,
crown-centered meditation.

Chapter Fourteen

Ayurvedic Yoga Sequencing

It's bizarre that the produce manager is
more important to my children's health than
the pediatrician.
—MERYL STREEP

As prana manifests in the physical body, it moves in different ways in different people, depending on all of life's circumstances. In yoga's sister science of ayurveda—"the science of life"—the manifestation of prana in the body is described by the energetic interplay of the universal elements: air, fire, water, earth, and ether. The various combinations of these elements give us several qualities, from hot to cold, dry to wet, light to heavy, hard to soft, as well as functional tendencies such as grounded or floating, spaciousness or constraint. According to ayurveda, how these elements interact creates patterns in three expressions of prana in the physical body called *doshas* (literally, "deviations"). The relative constitution of the balance of doshas is affected by diet and lifestyle, giving any individual a unique energetic fingerprint. While ayurvedic doctors give advice and treatments to help cultivate doshic balance, in yoga we can offer asana and pranayama practices designed to complement the larger lifestyle choices that affect this balance and thus overall health.

In ayurveda, the balance of doshas governs all physiological processes in the physical body. The three main doshas are *vata, pitta,* and *kapha,* which together make up the *tridoshas* ("three doshas"). One dosha tends to be dominant in any individual, giving him or her a specific doshic constitution. Sometimes two are equally present, or when all three are in balance, one's constitution is described as "tridoshic." Ayurveda provides a science of the body that is largely predicated on looking at individuals through the prism of their doshic constitution. It is in the combination of the basic elements that the doshas are determined:

- Vata, similar to *vayu,* arises from the combination of air and ether, creating the subtle energy of movement in the mind and body. It governs breathing, the flow of blood, muscle and tissue movement, even the movement of thoughts in the mind. In activating the nervous system, when vata is in good balance it is a source of creativity, enthusiasm, and flexibility. With excessive vata one becomes fearful, worrisome, and prone to insomnia.

- Pitta arises from fire (and some air, as fire requires air), creating the heat that governs digestion, absorption, metabolism, and transformation in the body and mind. Put differently, heat in the body is the product of metabolic activity, thus placing this process under pitta. In balance, pitta is a source of intelligence and understanding, helping us discriminate between right and wrong. Excessive pitta lends to anger and hatred.

- Kapha, formed from earth and water, creates the body's physical structure—bones, muscles, tendons—and cements the body together. Kapha supplies the body with water, lubricating the joints, moisturizing the skin, reinforcing the body's resistances, helping to heal wounds and give biological strength. Associated with emotions, kapha is expressed as love, compassion, and calmness. Out of balance, it creates lethargy, attachment, and envy.

To learn one's doshic constitution, it is best to get a comprehensive doshic analysis from an ayurvedic doctor. There are also hundreds of free online doshic typing tests that can provide an initial, very rough approximation of one's doshic constitution and imbalances. Based on this understanding, one can then undertake a variety of practices to promote better health, including specific diets, cleansing practices, and yoga sequences. Here we offer basic sequences for each dosha.

Yoga Sequences for Dosha Balancing

Vata types—filled with air, tending toward being dry and cold, flexible when young but typically stiff and prone to arthritis later in life—benefit from exploring poses more gradually and steadily, moving very slowly through their Surya Namaskaras (Sun Salutations), focusing more on grounding in standing and balancing poses, and lingering longer than most in deep asanas. Nadi shodhana (alternate nostril breathing), emphasizing the right nostril in the morning for energy and warmth and the left at night to promote calm and sleep, should be done in a gentle and grounding way.

Sequence 62: Vata Balancing Class

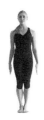

1. Tadasana
2–3 minutes. Focus on balancing the breath, awakening pada bandha, and cultivating a firm grounding through the feet and legs.

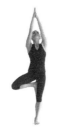

2. Vrksasana
1–2 minutes on each side.

3. Classical Surya Namaskara
5 times. Move slowly yet steadily, pausing in each asana for one complete breath cycle. Keep the gaze slightly toward the earth.

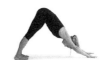

4. Adho Mukha Svanasana
1–2 minutes. Focus on grounding evenly through the hands and feet while staying present in the breath.

5. Balasana
Rest 5 breaths.

6. Surya Namaskara B
3 times. Move slowly yet steadily, pausing in each asana for 1 complete breath cycle.

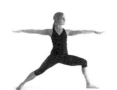

7. Virabhadrasana II
10 breaths on each side, moving dynamically in and out of the lunge.

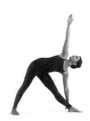

8. Utthita Trikonasana
5 breaths, then transition to the next asana.

Ayurvedic Yoga Sequencing

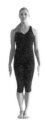

9. Utthita Parsvakonasana
5 breaths, then switch sides on asanas 8–9.

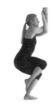

10. Garudasana
1 minute on each side.

11. Prasarita Padottanasana B
5–10 breaths.

12. Parsvottanasana
1 minute on each side, focusing on strong roots.

13. Tadasana
1 minute, renewing intention and strong roots.

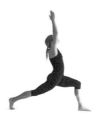

14. Surya Namaskara A
2 times. Move slowly, stretching the breath, then hold Adho Mukha Svanasana.

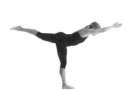

15. Ashta Chandrasana
5 breaths on the first side, moving dynamically in and out of the lunge.

16. Virabhadrasana III
5–10 breaths on the first side, then release to Ashta Chandrasana, vinyasa, and switch sides on asanas 15–16.

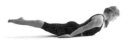

17. Salabhasana A
5 breaths, then vinyasa.

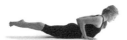

18. Salabhasana B
5 breaths, then vinyasa.

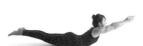

19. Salabhasana C
5 breaths, then vinyasa.

20. Ustrasana
3 times, 5 breaths each time, optional vinyasa between each time.

Sequence 62: Vata Balancing Class (continued)

21. Balasana
5 breaths.

22. Bharadvajrasana A
5 breaths on each side.

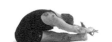

23. Paschimottanasana
1 minute.

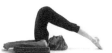

24. Halasana
5 breaths.

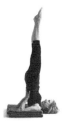

**25. Salamba
Sarvangasana**
2–3 minutes.

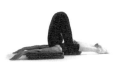

26. Karnapidasana
5 breaths.

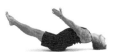

27. Uttana Padasana
5 breaths.

28. Savasana
5–10 minutes, wrapped in a
blanket to stay warm.

29. Sukhasana
Meditation.

Pittas tend to push hard and gravitate toward hot, vigorous practices. In cultivating balance, pittas benefit from letting go of their competitive tendencies, tapping into asana as a cooling, nurturing, and relaxing practice. Rather than moving quickly into the next pose, the pitta student benefits from a longer pause, especially after strong sequences, being mindful of relaxing and letting go of tension. Rather than going for the hot and sweaty practice, pittas are better advised to go slow and learn to relax deeply by moving more slowly and consciously in their practice. Cooling pranayamas such as *sitali* can help with further balancing, allowing them to come away from the practice with a calmer, clearer mind and a lighter, more relaxed body.

Sequence 63: Pitta Balancing Class

1. Sukhasana
2–3 minutes. Set intention. 2 minutes of nadi shodhana pranayama, holding the exhalations 1–5 counts with uddiyana bandha.

2. Classical Surya Namaskara
3 rounds, moving slowly and fluidly. Keep the gaze level with the horizon.

3. Surya Namaskara A
3 rounds, moving slowly and steadily. Rest in Tadasana 5 breaths.

4. Surya Namaskara B
1 round, then move from Adho Mukha Svanasana in exploring the next flow.

5. Dancing Warrior
1–5 rounds. Rest in Tadasana 5 breaths.

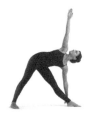

6. Utthita Trikonasana
5 breaths first side, then the next asana.

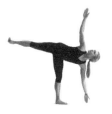

7. Ardha Chandrasana
5 breaths, then switch sides on asanas 6–7.

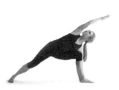

8. Utthita Parsvakonasana
5 breaths on each side, then slow vinyasa to Adho Mukha Svanasana.

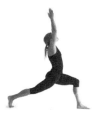

9. Ashta Chandrasana
1 breath in transition to the next asana.

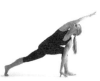

10. Parivrtta Ashta Chandrasana
5 breaths on the first side, then switch sides on asanas 13–14.

11. Balasana
5 breaths.

12. Setu Bandha Sarvangasana
Move dynamically in and out of the asana 5 times, then hold 5 breaths.

13. Urdhva Dhanurasana
1–3 times, 5 breaths each time.

14. Apanasana
5 breaths.

15. Virasana
2–3 minutes of sitali pranayama.

16. Bharadvajrasana A
5 breaths on each side.

Sequence 63: Pitta Balancing Class (continued)

21. Dandasana
5 breaths.

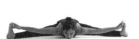

22. Upavista Konasana
10 breaths.

23. Parivrtta Janu Sirsasana
10 breaths on each side.

24. Baddha Konasana
1 minute.

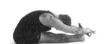

25. Paschimottanasana
1 minute.

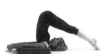

26. Halasana
5 breaths.

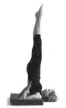

27. Salamba Sarvangasana
2–3 minutes.

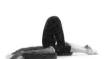

28. Karnapidasana
5 breaths.

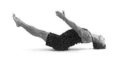

29. Uttana Padasana
5 breaths.

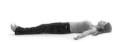

30. Savasana
5 minutes.

31. Sukhasana
2–3 minutes nadi shodhana pranayama, then meditation.

Kaphas, inclined as they are to lethargy and heaviness of movement, benefit most from a warming and flowing practice to stimulate their metabolism and circulation. Starting practice with a warming pranayama such as kapalabhati helps kaphas get their energy up for the asanas. Starting with simple flowing sequences to further warm the body and keep energy flowing, kaphas benefit from moving into sustained asana sequences requiring (and thereby cultivating) strength and stamina. Standing-pose sequences that involve heart-opening variations benefit kaphas by further stimulating circulation and the movement of mucus. Sustained back-bending sequences further stimulate circulation and the movement of energy in the chest and head, lending to more balanced energy and a clearer, more active mind.

Sequence 64: Kapha Balancing Class

1. Surya Namaskara A
3–5 times. Explore moving slightly faster each round.

2. Surya Namaskara B
3–5 times. Explore moving slightly faster each round.

3. Shishulasana
1 minute, then rest in Balasana.

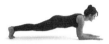

4. Shishula Phalakasana
1 minute while doing kapalabhati pranayama, transition to Adho Mukha Svanasana, then do Tail of the Dog in transitioning to Virabhadrasana II.

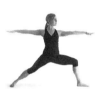

5. Virabhadrasana II
5–10 breaths on the first side.

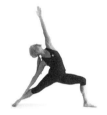

6. Parsva Virabhadrasana
1–5 breaths on the first side.

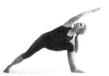

7. Utthita Parsvakonasana
1–2 minutes, then transition to Virabhadrasana II on the other side, repeat asanas 5–7, then vinyasa to Adho Mukha Svanasana.

8. Adho Mukha Svanasana
5–10 breaths (or rest in Balasana), then step or jump forward.

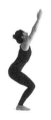

9. Utkatasana
5 breaths.

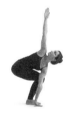

10. Parivrtta Utkatasana
5 breaths on each side, then stand in Tadasana for 5 breaths.

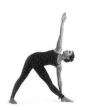

11. Utthita Trikonasana
5–10 breaths on each side.

12. Prasarita Padottanasana C
5 breaths.

13. Parsvottanasana
5 breaths on each side.

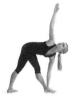

14. Parivrtta Trikonasana
5 breaths on each side, then transition to Tadasana.

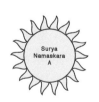

15. Surya Namaskara A
Hold Adho Mukha Svanasana 1 minute, then come to Dandasana.

16. Navasana
5 breaths, rest 3 breaths, and repeat 4 times before transitioning to Adho Mukha Svanasana and stepping the right foot forward.

Sequence 64: Kapha Balancing Class (continued)

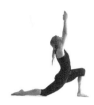

17. Anjaneyasana
5 breaths, then vinyasa,
switch sides, then lie supine.

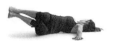

**18. Jathara
Parivartanasana**
1–2 minutes.

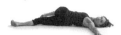

**19. Supta
Parivartanasana**
5–10 breaths on each side.

**20. Setu Bandha
Sarvangasana**
5–10 breaths; repeat 2–3
times, or do the
following asana.

**21. Urdhva
Dhanurasana**
5–10 breaths;
repeat 2–3 times.

22. Apanasana
5 breaths.

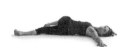

**23. Supta
Parivartanasana**
5–10 breaths on each side.

**24. Bharadvajrasana
A (or B)**
1 minute on each side.

25. Dandasana
5 breaths.

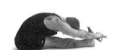

26. Paschimottanasana
1–2 minutes,
then transition to all fours.

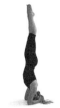

27. Salamba Sirsasana I
1–5 minutes, then either
do the following asana
or rest in Balasana.

28. Urdhva Dandasana
5–10 breaths, extend the
legs back up into Sirsasana I,
then Balasana.

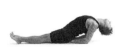

**29. Uttana
Padasana Prep**
5 breaths.

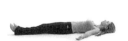

30. Savasana
5 minutes.

31. Sukhasana
1 minute of kapalabhati
pranayama, consider
repeating twice, then sit in
meditation.

Part Five

Bringing It All Together

Chapter Fifteen

Further Tips on Yoga Sequencing

It is for us to pray not for tasks equal to our powers,
but for powers equal to our tasks, to go forward with
a great desire forever beating at the door of our hearts
as we travel toward our distant goal.
—HELEN KELLER

Every yoga practice should flow like a good story, with a beginning, middle, and end that takes the class to a new and different awareness, experience, or ability (Ezraty 2006). As teachers, how we structure each class gives it a basic story line. The plot could be a theme or overarching intention, the principle characters the specific asanas, while the setting derives from the mood or vibe of the class. How we put this together to form a coherent class is "the art form of yoga practice" (Gannon and Life, 2002), which is inherently creative yet ideally based on an applied understanding of how asanas work in relationship to one another in the flow of the class. Each class should be planned and taught with a story line that takes students on a journey into themselves. The basic idea is to start from where students are and guide them to move consciously—in a special way—as they progress from simpler to more complex practices, gradually refining the bodymind and awakening

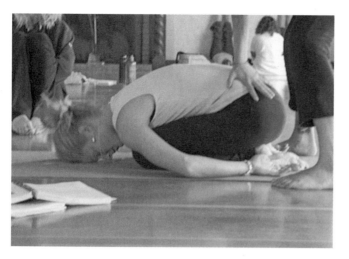

Being in the seat of the teacher

to a clearer self-awareness, sense of balance, and harmony in life—a more sattvic state of being. This is the heart of yoga sequencing, of vinyasa krama and parinamavada. This step-by-step process helps students to deepen their practice, gradually developing greater capacity for steadiness and ease amid the ever-increasing complexity and challenge of whatever they are doing, on or off the mat.

Yoga sequences are generally designed based on the style of yoga, the level and condition of students in the class, special themes, and your choice of peak asanas. Generally speaking, every class should offer a balanced practice that includes dynamic warming of the body, standing asanas that build further stamina and strength, a well-thought-out pathway to the peak asanas, time to fully explore the peak, and from there a calming and fully integrative pathway to Savasana (Corpse Pose or Final Relaxation Pose). Within each week and month of classes, variations in sequences should be offered that allow students to gradually move more deeply into their practice while still giving an overall balanced practice in each class.

Part of the challenge to you as a teacher is that student attendance is often uneven and inconsistent, with new students appearing each day and others disappearing. This makes it largely impractical to offer a highly structured curriculum in which you plan classes across a period of weeks or months around certain practice objectives.[1] Still, you can bring more coherence to the parinamavada process and the overall vinyasa krama of your classes by regularly alternating among different asana focus areas. This requires thinking about what you have recently taught, addressing tension that might have set in after previous classes, and introducing new asanas that encourage students to deepen and expand their practice. By applying basic principles of sequencing in planning your classes, you can offer students a rich variety of practices that are sustainable and self-transforming.

Pace and duration are important considerations in crafting and teaching classes, giving character to a class and making it more or less accessible or challenging. While we ultimately want to develop a personal practice in which we follow our inner teacher, pace and duration are two of the central qualities of any class and are essential in creating the space for students to refine their practice.

"Pace" refers to the temporal flow and intensity of a class, including the time and actions between asanas. In some Hatha yoga styles such as Ashtanga Vinyasa, the pace is partially given by a specific structure of the practice: each breath is connected to a movement in or out of an asana, most asanas are held for exactly five breaths, and many asanas are connected by the dynamic sequence that involves flowing through Chaturanga Dandasana (Four-Limbed Staff Pose) as part of the transition to the next asana. This is a very intense, essentially nonstop practice of connecting ujjayi pranayama to movement within and between the asanas until surrendering in Savasana. By contrast, in a restorative class, you might do as few as five or six asanas in ninety minutes, focusing on deep relaxation and integration. There are several factors to consider in pacing a class:

- *Basic considerations:* Start with basic elements—being present, staying with the breath, relaxing. Go only fast enough to maintain the integrity of these elements. With newer students and in basic classes, slow the pace to give more time for exploration, questions, and to allow students to feel the effects of each asana. It is okay if students in beginning classes take two or more breaths to complete a movement that might ordinarily be done with a single breath. In introductory classes, go even slower, frequently pausing to assess for understanding and encourage questions. With experienced students and flow-oriented classes, pace the class a little faster, yet slow enough to encourage attentiveness, expansive breathing, steadiness, and ease amid the greater physical exertion.

- *Class definition:* If a class is described on a schedule as "Level 1 Gentle Flow," this suggests a slower pace than one described as "Level 3 Power Yoga." The more basic class might also be scheduled for a shorter overall time period, perhaps an hour rather than ninety minutes or two hours.

- *Student ability:* With more experienced students, gradually maintain a steady pace free of breaks between asana sequences. Yet with even the most experienced students, you can create the space for deepening the practice inestimably by offering moments to pause, rest, feel, reflect, renew intention, and feel the full integration of the experience. Note that a common misunderstanding among teachers and students alike is the notion that a fast pace is somehow more challenging and "advanced." Moving slowly and consciously with smooth and spacious ujjayi pranayama is actually more physically (and mentally and emotionally) challenging than the extremely fast-paced "yoga-robics" type classes and allows the practice to go much deeper, both physically and energetically. Encourage all students to make the steady flow of the breath more important than getting right into an asana; encourage them to move with their breath, not your words—and to take as many breaths as needed for them to transition safely and comfortably.

- *Class theme:* If it is the summer solstice and you are teaching a heart-opening intensive, this suggests keeping the class moving to help students stay warm as you offer sequences to open the quads, hip flexors, spinal erectors, and shoulder girdle. A winter solstice class focusing on heart-openers could move much more slowly, tapping into deep release more than internal warmth to prepare the body for expansive back bends.

- *Time constraints:* Many classes offered at gyms are scheduled for less than an hour. In this situation you can either teach fewer asanas or increase the tempo. These are good classes to offer "homework" assignments, encouraging students to do certain sequences on their own outside of class. Regardless of the time you have, ensure that the pace feels comfortable to you and your students. Always save at least five minutes for Savasana.

"Duration" refers to the length of time and energetic intensity with which asanas are held. As with pace, temporal duration is prescribed in some Hatha yoga styles, including Iyengar yoga, which often gives a specific number of seconds or minutes for holding an asana. The effects of duration are inextricably intertwined with intentional actions in the held asana, including the relative degree of active or passive energetic engagement and where that energetic effort is consciously directed in the asana.[2] While duration itself is significant, what a student is actually doing while holding an asana—how one is playing the edge—is even more important. Another important variable is the extent to which the asana requires strength to hold, thus building strength when held longer.

When holding asanas that require significant physical strength, longer duration will build that strength while requiring greater physical exertion. Guiding students to stay with the overarching asana principle of steadiness and ease, you can offer a more strength-building sequence or class by holding certain asanas—primarily standing and arm balance asanas, and others such as Navasana (Boat Pose) that require core abdominal engagement—for longer. Encouraging students to stay with their intention (within a space where they can genuinely feel it is perfectly acceptable to come out of an asana whenever they want), you

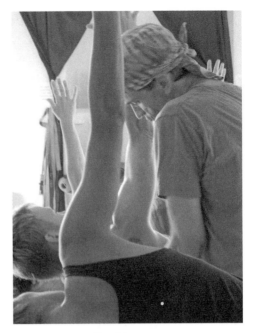

Teaching yoga

can play with varying durations, observing students to determine when it appears time to transition to another asana. As a general rule, when you observe some students showing instability or coming out of a long-held asana, reaffirm the importance of honoring one's personal intention in the practice, encouraging students to stay in or come out based on how they feel, not how they compare. This is a good time to affirm that the "no pain, no gain" mentality that pervades Western fitness culture is a risky proposition that more typically results in injury rather than health, wellness, or self-transformation. A similarly questionable notion is found in much of yoga culture, where "real yoga" is said to begin when one thinks one cannot hold an asana any longer. While it is important to self-assess when mental or emotional factors might lead us to avoid something that is challenging, the feedback of the body, heart, and mind is quite worth listening to and may make all the difference in cultivating a lifelong sustainable practice.

Holding asanas for relatively longer duration can allow deeper exploration of the practice. Depending on the asana and what is happening in one's body and life, long holds done with conscious breathing and subtle awareness of the movement of energy can release deeply held tension, bring awareness to dormant parts of the body, and stimulate insight into the inner dynamics of one's practice and life. When approaching feelings of discomfort in a long-held asana, there is an opportunity for students to discover anew the patterns and tendencies that manifest in their larger lives as obstacles to living with conscious openness and willful determination. Experiencing what one gravitates toward, resists, or finds enjoyable, frustrating, or perturbing in asanas can be a source of awakening to a clearer understanding of the deeper self. The more *tha* part of Hatha yoga—the more calming and integrative part of class—is a wonderful time to go into this aspect of practice, especially in forward bends, hip openers, twists, and supported inversions such as Salamba Sirsasana I (Headstand I), Salamba Sarvangasana (Supported Shoulder Stand), and Viparita Karani (Active Reversal Pose).

Particularly with beginning students, offer more dynamic movements in and out of an asana several times in rhythm with the breath.[3] Moving dynamically allows students to gradually feel the requirements and effects of an asana, contributing to their awareness of how to move in synchronization with the breath and how to use the breath as a tool connecting the body and mind. "A dynamic practice," Desikachar (1995, 29) says, "gives us greater possibilities for bringing breath to particular parts of the body and heightening the intensity of the effect." This, he intones, is beneficial to experienced practitioners who "often get caught in the habit of focusing their attention on fixing the posture somehow in static practice rather than really working in it and exploring its possibilities."

In creative flow classes, including vinyasa flow and its many branded expressions, there is an opportunity to be more playful as a teacher in exploring with your students the infinite possibilities for dynamic pacing and varied duration. Connected with the earth, flowing with the breath, the body expresses itself in flowing asanas that are expressions of spirit. It is here that you can introduce the "three friends: gravity, breath, and wave," as Vanda Scaravelli (1991, 24, 28) says, "that should be constantly with us."

While there are effective and ineffective ways to sequence asanas, there is not a singularly correct way to sequence asanas in creating complete classes. Rather, sequencing can tap into all the aspects of yoga along with your intention and creativity as a teacher to offer students a variety of experiences in the practice. Using the resources provided throughout this book, play around with designing sequences for different class levels, physical benefits, energetic effects, seasons, and other qualities that you find interesting and inspiring. Practice them on your own, share them with your fellow teachers, refine them as you teach them in classes, and observe how students respond. Continuously coming back to your own creative sensibilities, have fun with this while working to offer students the best classes you can for their needs and interests.

Keep breathing. Namaste.

Sequence 65: Soulful Vinyasa Yoga—An Integrated Level 1–2 Class

1. Sukhasana
Sitting for 5–7 minutes, do a few minutes of natural-breath-as-mantra mediation, set intention, chant "aum," and explore ujjayi pranayama.

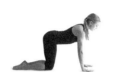

2. Bidalasana
5 rounds of Cat and Dog Tilts to awaken awareness and energy along the spine and to connect breath and movement.

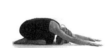

3. Utthita Balasana
Hold for 30 seconds with the knees wide apart so there's less tension in the lower back and knees. Then come back up to all fours.

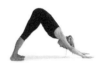

4. Adho Mukha Svanasana
1 minute, focusing on alignment of the hands and feet and the connection between roots and extension. Highlight alignment and energetic actions in the hands, arms, and shoulders.

5. Balasana
Hold for 30 seconds, allowing the shoulders to drop toward the floor.

6. Adho Mukha Svanasana
1 minute, again focusing on alignment of the hands and feet and the connection between roots and extension. Highlight alignment and energetic actions in the feet, legs, and pelvis. Walk forward and roll easily up to standing.

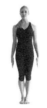

7. Tadasana
1 minute. Teach pada bandha, roots and extension, and renew the emphasis on heart-centered ujjayi pranayama.

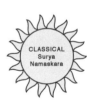

8. Classical Surya Namaskara
3 rounds. Pause in Anjaneyasana on the first round to explain pelvic neutrality in relation to the spine, moving dynamically into and out of the lunge before holding it for a few breaths. Pause in Salabhasana B on the third round to break down this asana and emphasize it as an alternative to Urdhva Mukha Svanasana whenever doing Surya Namaskaras.

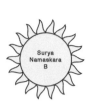

9. Surya Namaskara B
3 rounds. Pause in Virabha-drasana I on the first round to explain alignment and energetic actions in the legs, pelvic neutrality in relation to the spine, and neutral spinal extension and external rota-tion of the arms, then move dynamically into and out of the lunge before holding it for a few breaths.

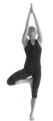

10. Vrksasana
After reconnecting with one's intention in Tadasana and reawakening pada bandha, hold each side for 1 minute.

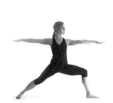

11. Virabhadrasana II
Set up from Prasarita stance and hold for 1 minute on the first side, then transi-tion to the next asana on that same side.

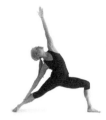

12. Parsva Virabhadrasana
3 breaths, then transition to the next asana on that same side.

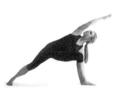

13. Utthita Parsvakonasana
Hold 1 minute. Encourage modifications and props to make it easier for students to find proper alignment, breathe deeply, and experi-ence spaciousness along the spine and around the chest and neck. Transition back up into Virabhadrasana II and switch sides on as asanas 11–13.

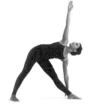

14. Utthita Trikonasana
5–15 breaths. If Ardha Chandrasana is acces-sible, hold for 5 breaths and transition to the next asana; otherwise stay in Utthita Trikonasana for 15 breaths.

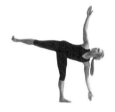

15. Ardha Chandrasana
5 breaths, then release slowly back into Utthita Trikonasana. Come back and switch sides on asanas 14–15.

16. Prasarita Padottanasana C
10 breaths. Encourage stu-dents with tight shoulders to use a strap between their hands.

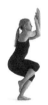

17. Garudasana
10 breaths on each side.

18. Parsvottanasana
5 breaths each side.

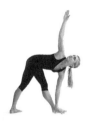

19. Parivrtta Trikonasana
5 breaths on each side.

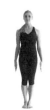

20. Tadasana
5 breaths.

Sequence 65: Soulful Vinyasa Yoga—An Integrated Level 1-2 Class (continued)

21. Surya Namaskara A
Flow through the Adho
Mukha Svanasana, then
transition to the next asanas
through Tail of the Dog.

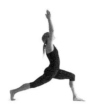

22. Ashta Chandrasana
5 breaths, then transition
to the next asana.

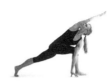

**23. Parivrtta Ashta
Chandrasana**
5 breaths, then vinyasa to
Adho Mukha Svanasana and
repeat asanas 22–23 on the
other side.

24. Balasana
1 minute.

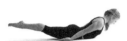

25. Salabhasana A
Move dynamically up
and completely down 5
times, each time a lifting a
little higher, then hold for
5 breaths with the fingers
interlaced behind the back
to leverage the expansion
of the heart center. Release
and turn over.

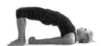

**26. Setu Bandha
Sarvangasana**
Do 3 times, holding each
tome for 5–10 breaths. As
an alternative to repeating,
do the next asana.

**27. Urdhva
Dhanurasana**
Do 2 times for
5–10 breaths.

28. Apanasana
1 minute, gently moving the
joined knees in circles to
release tension in the lower
back.

29. Ananda Balasana
5 breaths.

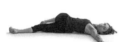

**30. Supta
Parivartanasana**
10 breaths on each side.

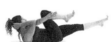

31. Yogic Bicycles
1 minute.

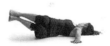

**32. Jathara
Parivartanasana**
Move to each side 5–7 times.
Keep the knees bent to take
it easier on the lower back;
extend the legs for more
core intensity.

33. Pelvic Tilts
10 times, then hold for
5 breaths.

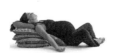

**34. Supta Baddha
Konasana**
1 minute, with arms draped
over in the same diamond
positioning as the legs.

35. Dandasana
5 breaths.

36. Gomukhasana
1–2 breaths each side.

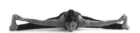

37. Upavista Konasana
2–3 minutes.

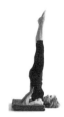

38. Parivrtta Janu Sirsasana
1 minute each side.

39. Baddha Konasana
2–3 minutes.

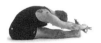

40. Paschimottanasana
1–2 minutes.

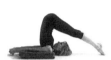

41. Halasana
5 breaths. Prop the shoulders on blankets to reduce flexion in the cervical spine and more easily open the heart center.

42. Salamba Sarvangasana
2–5 minutes. Play with leg variations.

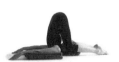

43. Karnapidasana
5 breaths.

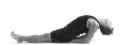

44. Uttana Padasana Prep
5 breaths.

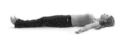

45. Savasana
5–7 minutes.

46. Sukhasana
5–25 minutes sitting meditation.

Sequence 66: Soulful Vinyasa Yoga—An Integrated Level 2-3 Class

1. Virasana
Sitting for 5 minutes (propped if necessary to relieve pressure in the knees), start with quiet breathing, then do 3 one-minute rounds of kapalabhati pranayama, the final round while raising the arms out and up overhead, then to the heart center, setting intention and sharing in the sound of aum.

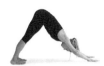

2. Adho Mukha Svanasana
2 minutes, bicycling the legs to release tension around the knees, gradually working more strongly into the asana.

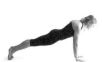

3. Phalakasana
5 breaths, then moving dynamically from Phalakasana to Adho Mukha Svanasana 5 times.

4. Tail of the Dog
5 breaths, opening the hip and bending the elevated leg to stretch more deeply into the thighs and groins, then transition to the next asana.

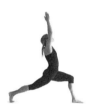

5. Ashta Chandrasana
Move from straight legs to successively deeper lunges 5 times, then hold for 5 breaths while feeding the back leg, maintaining pelvic neutrality and lifting up through the spine, shoulders, and arms. Repeat asana 4–5 on the other side, and then come to Tadasana.

6. Surya Namaskara A
3 times.

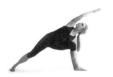

7. Surya Namaskara B
3 times.

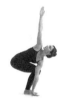

8. Parivrtta Utkatasana
5 breaths on each side.

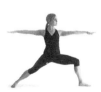

9. Virabhadrasana II
1–2 minutes, then transition to the next asana on the same side.

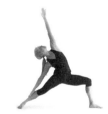

10. Parsva Virabhadrasana
5–8 breaths, then transition to the next asana on the same side.

11. Utthita Parsvakonasana
1–2 minutes, then transition back to Virabhadrasana II and switch sides on asanas 9–11. As an alternative transition, do the next two asanas on the path to Chaturanga (otherwise skip the next two asanas).

12. Eka Pada Koundinyasana A
Hold 2–3 breaths and either transition to the next asana or float back to Chaturanga. Repeat asanas 9–12.

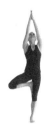

13. Astavakrasana
Hold 2–3 breaths, and then float back to Chaturanga. Repeat asanas 9–13, complete a vinyasa, and come to Tadasana.

14. Vrksasana
5 breaths each side.

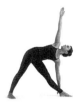

15. Utthita Hasta Padangusthasana A/B
5 breaths each position on each side. Then transition to Prasarita stance.

16. Utthita Trikonasana
10 breaths, then transition to the next asana on the same side.

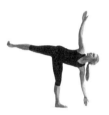

17. Ardha Chandrasana
10 breaths, offering variations, then release back to Utthita Trikonasana, switch sides on asanas 16–17, and then come to Tadasana.

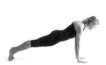

18. Surya Namaskara A
1 round, then from Adho Mukha Svanasana, come to the next asana.

19. Phalakasana
5 breaths.

20. Vasisthasana
5–10 breaths on each side. Start with both legs straight, then offer the Vrksasana transition to the fuller expression of the asana. Consider offering the Prep pose as an alternative. Complete a vinyasa, come back to Tadasana, and then to Prasarita stance.

21. Garudasana
1 minute each side.

22. Prasarita Padottanasana C
5–10 breaths.

23. Prasarita Padottanasana A
1–2 minutes. Offer more advanced students a Sirsasana II vinyasa with either Bakasana or Urdhva Kukkutasana.

24. Parsvottanasana
10 breaths each side.

Sequence 66: Soulful Vinyasa Yoga—An Integrated Level 2–3 Class (continued)

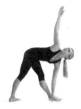

25. Parivrtta Trikonasana
10 breaths each side, then step to Tadasana.

26. Surya Namaskara A
1 round to Adho Mukha Svanasana, then transition to Virabhadrasana II, and then Utthita Parsvakonasana, wrapping and clasping in preparation for the following asana.

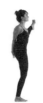

27. Svarga Dvijasana
1 minute, then transition back to the wrapped variation of Utthita Parsvakonasana, do a vinyasa, and switch sides, arriving back in Adho Mukha Svanasana.

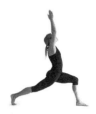

28. Ashta Chandrasana
5 breaths, then transition to the next asana.

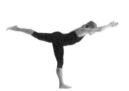

29. Virabhadrasana III
3–5 breaths, then transition to the next asana.

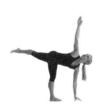

30. Parivrtta Ardha Chandrasana
10 breaths, then transition to the next asana, or skip it in transition to Adho Mukha Svanasana.

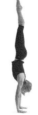

31. Adho Mukha Vrksasana
Hold for 1–5 breaths in transition to a vinyasa. Repeat asanas 28–31 on the other side.

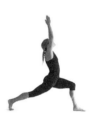

32. Ashta Chandrasana
5 breaths.

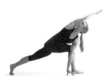

33. Parivrtta Ashta Chandrasana
1–2 minutes, then transition to the next asana in transition to a vinyasa, or skip it in transition to Adho Mukha Svanasana.

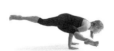

34. Eka Pada Koundinyasana B
1–2 breaths in transition to a vinyasa. Switch sides on asanas 32–34.

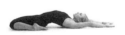

35. Supta Virasana
Hold 2–3 minutes, then transition to Adho Mukha Svanasana, bicycle out the legs, and come to standing on the knees.

36. Ustrasana
3 times for 5–10 breaths. On the second time, consider transitioning to the next asana instead.

Sequence 66: Soulful Vinyasa Yoga—An Integrated Level 2-3 Class (continued)

37. Laghu Vajrasana
Do 5 drop-backs, then hold for 5 breaths and either come up or transition to the next asana.

38. Kapotasana
5–10 breaths, then a vinyasa, and float through to a supine position.

39. Urdhva Dhanurasana
3–5 times, holding for 5–10 breaths each time.

40. Apanasana
1 minute.

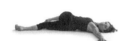

41. Supta Parivartanasana
10 breaths each side.

42. Bharadvajrasana B
10 breaths each side.

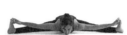

43. Dandasana
5 breaths.

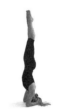

44. Upavista Konasana
1 minute.

45. Baddha Konasana
1 minute.

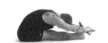

46. Paschimottanasana
1–2 minutes.

47. Gomukhasana
1 minute on each side.

48. Salamba Sirsasana A
2–3 minutes.

49. Urdhva Dandasana
5 breaths, then go back up to Sirsasana before releasing into Balasana for 5 breaths, then transition to lying supine.

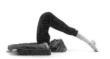

50. Halasana
5 breaths.

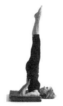

51. Salamba Sarvangasana
2–3 minutes, then fold the legs into Lotus position or release the knees towards the ears in Karnapidasana.

52. Urdhva Padmasana
5 breaths.

53. Pindasana
5 breaths.

54. Matsyasana
5 breaths.

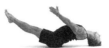

55. Uttana Padasana
5 breaths.

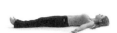

56. Savasana
5–10 minutes.

57. Padmasana
5–25 minutes meditation.

Sequence 67: Soulful Vinyasa Yoga—An Integrated Level 3+ Class

1. Padmasana
5 minutes meditation; set intention; share aum.

2. Surya Namaskara A
5 times. Explore moving slightly faster each round.

3. Surya Namaskara B
5 times. Hold Adho Mukha Svanasana on the 5th round.

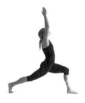

4. Ashta Chandrasana
Position the arms as for Prasarita Padottanasana C, fold forward for 5 breaths, then transition directly into the next asanas.

5. Eka Pada Koundin-yasana A
Hold for 5 breaths, then transition to Astavakrasana.

6. Astavakrasana
Hold for 5 breaths, then transition back into Eka Pada Koundinyasana A, float the Chaturanga, and flow to Adho Mukha Svanasana. Do asanas 4–6 on the other side, arriving back into Adho Mukha Svanasana.

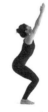

7. Utkatasana
Hold for 5 breaths, then transition to Parivrtta Utkatasana.

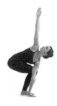

8. Parivrtta Utkatasana
Hold each side 5 breaths, then transition to the next asana.

9. Padangusthasana
5 breaths.

10. Pada Hastasana
5 breaths.

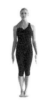

11. Tadasana
5 breaths, then hop to
Prasarita stance.

12. Utthita Trikonasana
10 breaths, then transition
to the next asana.

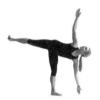

**13. Ardha
Chandrasana**
Hold for 1 minute, positioning the lifted hand on the
lifted foot as for Bhekasana
to stretch the quadriceps
muscles. Release back
to Utthita Trikonasana
and switch sides on
asanas 12–13.

14. Parsvottanasana
1 minute on each side.

**15. Parivrtta
Trikonasana**
1 minute, then transition to
the next asana.

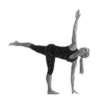

**16. Parivrtta Ardha
Chandrasana**
Hold for 1 minute, clasp-
ing the lifted foot with the
lifted hand to introduce a
twisted back bend. Release
to Parivrtta Trikonasana, and
transition to the other side on
asanas 14–16. Completing
the second side, transition
from Parivrtta Trikonasana to
the next asana.

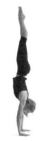

**17. Adho Mukha
Vrksasana**
Hold for 5 breaths, then
release to Chaturanga
and flow through to Adho
Mukha Svanasana in
preparation for the
next asana.

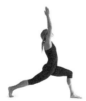

18. Ashta Chandrasana
5 breaths on the first side,
then transition to the
next asana.

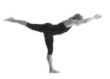

19. Virabhadrasana III
5–10 breaths on the first
side, then transition to
the next asana.

**20. Parivrtta Hasta
Padangusthasana**
5–10 breaths on the first
side, transition back to Virabhadrasana III for one breath,
then to Adho Mukha Svana-
sana in transition to a vinyasa
before switching sides on
asanas 18–20.

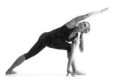

21. Parivrtta Parsvakonasana
10 breaths on the first side, then transition to the next asana.

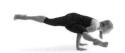

22. Eka Pada Koundinyasana B
10 breaths, then vinyasa and switch sides on asanas 21–22. Float through to Dandasana.

23. Agnistambhasana
1 minute each side.

24. Eka Pada Sirsasana
5–10 breaths on the first side, then transition to the next asana.

25. Chakorasana
5 breaths, then transition to the next asana.

26. Astavakrasana
5 breaths, then transition to the next asana.

27. Eka Pada Koundinyasana A
5 breaths, then vinyasa and switch sides on asanas 24–27.

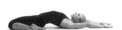

28. Supta Virasana
2 minutes.

29. Eka Pada Raj Kapotasana II
5–10 breaths on each side.

30. Urdhva Dhanurasana
2–3 times for 5–10 breaths. Explore the Eka Pada variation.

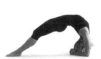

31. Viparita Dandasana
2–3 times for 5–10 breaths. Explore the Eka Pada variation, then spring up into Pincha Mayurasana in transition to a vinyasa and come to standing in Tadasana.

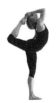

32. Natarajasana
2–3 times on each side for 5–10 breaths. Transition to Adho Mukha Svanasana.

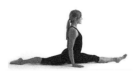

33. Hanumanasana
1–2 minutes each side. Explore forward and back bending variations.

34. Balasana
5 breaths.

35. Ardha Matsyendrasana
5–10 breaths each side.

36. Bharadvajrasana B
5–10 breaths each side.

Sequence 67: Soulful Vinyasa Yoga—An Integrated Level 3+ Class (continued)

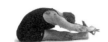

37. Paschimottanasana
2–3 minutes.

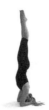

38. Salamba Sirsasana I
5–10 minutes. Explore leg variations, including Lotus positioning and twists, forward and back bending.

39. Urdhva Dandasana
5–10 breaths, then rest in Balasana, vinyasa, and float to lying supine.

40. Halasana
5 breaths.

41. Salamba Sarvangasana
2–3 minutes.

42. Urdhva Padmasana
5–10 breaths.

43. Pindasana
5–10 breaths.

44. Matsyasana
5 breaths.

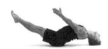

45. Uttana Padasana
5 breaths.

46. Baddha Padmasana
Hold for 1 minute.

47. Tolasana
Hold for 108 kapalabhati breaths.

48. Savasana
5–10 minutes.

49. Padmasana
5–25 minutes meditation.

Appendix A

Glossary

a-: Non-, as in *ahimsa*, "nonviolence."

abductor: Muscle that draws a bone away from the midline of the body.

adductor: Muscle that draws a bone toward the midline of the body.

adho: Downward.

adho mukha: Downward-facing.

afflictions: The five forms of suffering *(kleshas)*.

agni: Fire.

ahimsa: Nonviolence; not hurting.

ajna chakra: Third-eye chakra.

akarna: To the ear.

anahata chakra: Heart chakra.

ananda: Ecstasy; bliss; love.

anjali mudra: The gesture of *anjali*, palms together at the heart.

Anjaneya: The monkey god.

antara: Internal.

antara kumbhaka: Holding the breath after inhalation.

anterior: Forward; in front.

anuloma: With the grain. Refers to movement or breathing.

apana: Lower; downward.

Apanasana: Pelvic-floor poses; Wind-relieving Pose.

apana-vayu: Downward-moving *prana*.

aparigraha: Noncovetousness. One of the *yamas*.

ardha: Half.

asana: To take one's seat; a yoga pose; the third limb of Ashtanga yoga.

Astavakra: An Indian sage and Sanskrit scholar; the asana Astavakrasana is named for him.

asteya: Not stealing. One of the five *yamas*.

atman: The true self; consciousness.

aum: First described in the Upanishads as the originating and all-encompassing sound of the universe. Alternately spelled *om*.

avidya: Ignorance.

ayurveda: Ancient Indian "science of life"; traditional form of Indian medicine.

baddha: Bound.

bahya: External.

bahya kumbhaka: Suspension of the breath after complete exhalation.

baka: Crane.

bandha: To bind; energetic engagement.

bhadra: Peaceful or auspicious.

Bhagavad Gita: "Song of the Lord," a chapter in the epic Mahabharata and the most influential of all writings on yoga and spiritual philosophy.

bhakti: The practice of devotion.

Bharadvaj: An Indian sage.

Bharirava: An aspect of Shiva.

bhastrika: Bellows used in a furnace; type of *pranayama* where air is forcibly drawn in and out through the nostrils.

bhaya: Fear.

bheka: Frog.

bhuja: Arm or shoulder.

bhujanga: Cobra.

bhujapida: Pressure on the arm or shoulder.

Brahma: God; the supreme being; the creator; the first deity of the Hindu trinity.

brahmacharya: Celibacy; right use of sexual energy. One of the *yamas*.

brahman: Infinite consciousness.

buddhi: Intellect; seat of intelligence.

cervical spine: The vertebrae of the neck.

chakra: Subtle energy center.

chandra: Moon.

danda: Staff or stick.

dhanu: Bow.

dharana: Mental concentration; the sixth limb of Patanjali's Ashtanga yoga.

dharma: Virtuous duty.

dhyana: Meditation.

dristana: *Dristi* practice; the practice of gazing steadily at a single point in any given asana.

dristi: Gazing point.

dukha: Pain; sorrow; grief.

dwi: Two.

eka: One.

ekagrata: One-pointed mental focus.

eka pada: One-legged or one-footed.

extension: Movement of a joint whereby one part of the body is moved away from another.

external rotation: Rotation away from the center of the body.

flexion: Bending movement that decreases the angle between two points.

Galava: An Indian sage.

garuda: Eagle; name of the king of birds. Garuda is represented as a vehicle of Vishnu and as having a white face, an aquiline beak, red wings, and a golden body.

Gheranda: A sage, the author of the Gheranda Samhita, a classical work on Hatha yoga.

gomukha: Cow face.

guna: Literally "rope," it refers to something that binds; in reference to yoga, it refers to the three intertwined fundamental properties inherent in all phenomena: *sattva, rajas,* and *tamas.*

guru: A spiritual preceptor; one who illuminates the spiritual path; alternately, gee, you are you.

hala: Plough.

Hanuman: The monkey god, son of Anjaneya and Vayu.

hasta: Hand or arm.

Hatha yoga: Physical purification practices first described in written form in the fourteenth century CE in the Hatha Yoga Pradipika.

humerus: Upper arm bone.

hyperextension: Extension of a joint beyond 180 degrees.

ida: A *nadi* or channel of energy starting from the left nostril, moving to the crown of the head, and descending to the base of the spine.

insertion (of muscles): The end of a muscle that is more distant from the center of the body.

internal rotation: Rotation toward the midline of the body; synonymous with *medial rotation.*

Ishvara: The supreme being; Brahma with form.

isometric exercise: Exercise in which the muscles do not get shortened.

isotonic exercise: Exercise that involves shortening of a muscle.

jalandhara bandha: The chin lock where the chin is drawn toward the collarbones.

janu: Knee.

jathara: Belly.

jnana: Sacred knowledge derived from meditation on higher truths of religion and philosophy, which teaches people how to understand their own nature.

kapala: Skull.

kapalabhati: Skull cleansing, a *pranayama* technique.

kapha: One of the three ayurvedic humors.

kapota: Pigeon, dove.

karma: Action.

karma yoga: The yoga of action.

karna: Ear.

karnapida: Ears squeezed.

klesha: Suffering due to ignorance, egoism, desire, hatred, or fear.

kona: Angle.

Koundinya: A sage.

krama: Sequence of moments; succession of moments; stage.

Krishna: An incarnation of Vishnu; a form of God.

kriya: Action; also various purification practices.

krouncha: Heron.

kukkuta: Rooster.

kumbhaka: Breath retention after a complete inhalation or exhalation.

kundalini: Pranic energy, symbolized as a coiled and sleeping serpent lying dormant in the lowest nerve center at the base of the spinal column; a form of Hatha yoga practice.

kurma: Turtle.

kyphosis: Forward curvature of the spine.

laghu: Simple; little; small; handsome.

lateral: Sideways; away from the midline of the body.

lateral rotation: See *external rotation*.

laya: To merge.

lola: To swing or dangle.

lordosis: Backward curvature of the spine.

lumbar spine: The vertebrae of the lower back.

mahabandha: The great lock.

Mahabharata: A major Sanskrit epic of ancient India. Contains the Bhagavad Gita and major elements of Hindu mythology.

maha mudra: The great seal.

mala: Garland, wreath.

mandala: Spiritually significant concentric form used for meditation and rituals.

manduka: Frog.

manipura chakra: Navel chakra.

manos: The individual mind.

mantra: Sacred sound, thought, or prayer.

Marichi: A sage, one of the sons of Brahma.

Matsyendra: Lord of the fishes; a tantric adept.

maya: Illusion.

mayura: Peacock.

medial: Toward the midline of the body.

medial rotation: See *internal rotation*.

moksha: Liberation.

mudra: Seal; hand and finger positions; a specific combination of *asana, pranayama,* and *bandha.*

mukha: Face.

mula: Root, base.

mula bandha: Root lock; energetic engagement; sustained lifting of the perineum and levator ani.

muladhara chakra: Root chakra.

nadi: Literally "river"; energy channel.

nadi shodhana: Purification or cleansing of the *nadis; pranayama* technique for this purpose.

nakra: crocodile.

namaskara: Salutation; greeting.

nara: Man.

naravirala: Sphinx.

Nataraja: Dancing Shiva.

nauli: Physical purification technique involving churning the belly.

nava: Boat.

nidra: Sleep.

niyama: Second limb of Patanjali's eight-limbed path. Consists of *saucha*, *santosa*, *tapas*, *svadhyaya*, and *ishvarapranidhana*.

origin (of muscles): The end of a muscle that is closer to the body center.

pada: Foot or leg.

pada hasta: Hand(s) to feet.

padangustha: Big toe.

padma: Lotus.

parigha: Gate.

parigraha: Hoarding.

parinamavada: The constancy of change.

paripurna: Full.

parivrtta: Revolved; with a twist.

parsva: Side; flank; lateral.

paschimo: West; the back side of the body.

phalaka: Plank.

pincha: Chin; feather.

pinda: Fetus or embryo; body.

pingala: A *nadi* or channel of energy starting from the right nostril, moving to the crown of the head and downward to the base of the spine.

pitta: One of the three ayurvedic humors, sometimes translated as "bile."

posterior: Backward; opposite of anterior.

prakriti: Nature; the original source of the material world, consisting of *sattva*, *rajas*, and *tamas*.

prana: Life force; sometimes refers to the breath.

pranayama: Breath control; breath expansion; the fourth limb of Ashtanga yoga.

prasarana: Sweeping movement of the arms.

prasarita: Spread out; stretched out.

prasvasa: Expiration.

pratikriyasana: Counterpose.

pratiloma: Against the hair; against the grain.

pratyahara: Independence of the mind from sensory stimulation; the fifth limb of Ashtanga yoga.

prishta: Back.

puraka: Inhalation.

purna: Complete.

purva: East; the front of the body.

purvottana: Intense stretch of the front side of the body.

raga: Love; passion; anger.

raja: King, ruler.

raja kapota: King pigeon.

rajas: Impulsive or chaotic thought; the aspect of movement in nature; one of the three *gunas*.

rechaka: Exhalation, emptying of the lungs.

sadhana: Practice for achievement.

sahasrara chakra: Thousand-petaled lotus chakra, located in the cerebral cavity.

sahita: Aided.

sahita-kumbhaka: Intentional suspension of breath.

salabha: Locust.

salamba: With support.

sama: Equal; same.

samadhana: Mental peace.

samadhi: Bliss; meditative absorption.

samasthihi: A state of balance.

samskara: Subconscious imprint.

samyama: Combined application of *dharana, dhyana,* and *samadhi.*

santosa: Contentment.

sarvanga: The whole body.

sattva: Light, order; one of the three elements of *prakriti.*

satya: Truth; one of the five *yamas.*

saucha: Purity; cleanliness.

sava: Corpse.

setu bandha: Bridge.

Shakti: Life force, *prana;* consort of Shiva; divine feminine energy.

shishula: Dolphin.

Shiva: A form of God in Hinduism; the destroyer of illusion.

simha: Lion.

sirsa: Head.

sitali: A cooling form of *pranayama.*

Slumpasana: Habitual collapse of the heart center associated with lackadaisical slumping of the spine and torso.

sukham: Comfort; ease; pleasure.

supta: Supine; sleeping.

surya: The sun.

sushumna: Central energy channel, located in the spinal column.

svadhisthana chakra: Seat of vital force, situated above the reproductive organs.

svana: Dog.

svasa: Inspiration.

Swatmarama: Author of the Hatha Yoga Pradipika, the original book on Hatha yoga.

tada: Mountain.

tamas: Dullness; inertia; ignorance; one of the three *gunas.*

tantra: The practice of using all energies, including the mundane, for spiritual awakening.

tapa: Austerity.

tapas: Heat; burning effort that involves purification, self-discipline, and austerity.

thoracic spine: The vertebrae of the rib cage.

tibia: Shinbone.

tiriang mukha: Backward-facing.

tittibha: Firefly.

tola: Balance; scales.

tri: Three.

trikona: Triangle.

ubhaya: Both.

udana: A *prana vayu*.

uddiyana: Upward flying; a *bandha*.

uddiyana bandha: Drawing the lower abdominal core in and up.

ujjayi: Victorious.

ujjayi pranayama: Basic yogic breathing.

Upanishad: To sit down near; ancient philosophical texts considered an early source of Hinduism.

upavista: Seated with legs spread.

urdhva: Upward.

ustra: Camel.

utkata: Awkward; powerful; fierce.

utputahi: Lifting up.

uttana: Upright intense stretch.

Uttanasana: Forward bend.

utthita: Extended.

vajra: Thunderbolt.

vakra: Crooked.

Vasistha: A Vedic sage.

vata: One of the three ayurvedic humors, sometimes translated as "wind."

vayu: Wind; vital air current.

Vedanta: Literally "end of the Vedas"; the dominant Hindu philosophical tradition.

Vedas: Oldest sacred texts of humankind.

vidya: Knowledge; learning; lore; science.

viloma: Against the hair; against the order of things.

vinyasa: To place in a special way; the conscious connection of breath and movement.

viparita: Inverted; upside down.

vira: Hero; brave.

Virabhadra: A warrior.

Vishnu: A primary form of God in Hinduism; governs preservation, balance, sustainability.

vishuddha chakra: Pure chakra; situated in the pharyngeal region.

vrksa: Tree.

vrschika: Scorpion.

vyana: A *prana vayu*.

yama: Restraint; contain; the first of the eight limbs of Ashtanga yoga, consisting of *ahimsa, satya, brahmacharya, aparigraha,* and *asteya.*

yoga: From the root *yuj,* meaning "to join," "to yoke," "to make whole."

yoga-robics: Workout routines utilizing yoga asanas for purely physical exercise.

Appendix B

The Constituent Elements of Asanas

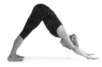 **Adho Mukha Svanasana**
Downward-Facing Dog Pose

Identifying Preparatory Asanas

Opening

What needs to be open: Calves, knee flexors, hip extensors, elbow flexors, shoulder extensors, shoulder retractors.

Asanas for opening: Ardha Uttanasana, Bidalasana, Uttanasana, Anahatasana. For arms and shoulders, these respective arm forms: Urdhva Hastasana, Gomukhasana, Garudasana.

Stabilizing

What needs to be stable: Intrinsic foot muscles, internal rotators of the leg, hip flexors and adductors, back extensors, transversus abdominis, shoulder stabilizers (emphasis protractors, flexors, extensors), external rotators of the arm, elbow extensors, wrist flexors.

Asanas for stabilizing: Anjaneyasana, Bidalasana, Phalakasana, Shishulasana, Tadasana, Uttanasana. Modify this pose with the hands placed hip height on a wall, hips at a right angle, torso neutral, and arms extended fully.

This asana prepares you for:

General conditioning pose; good prep for standing poses, arm balances, and full inversions, including Bakasana, Adho Mukha Vrksasana, Salamba Sirsasana I and II; Uttanasana.

Counterposes

Balasana, Apanasana, Supta Parivartanasana, Viparita Karani, Savasana.

Adho Mukha Vrksasana
Downward-Facing Tree Pose or Handstand

Identifying Preparatory Asanas

Opening

What needs to be open: Wrist flexors, shoulder extensors, back extensors, hip flexors, knee flexors.

Asanas for opening: Adho Mukha Svanasana, Bidalasana, Pincha Mayurasana, Tadasana, Phalakasana, Urdhva Dhanurasana. For arms and shoulders, these respective arm forms: Urdhva Hastasana, Gomukhasana, Garudasana.

Stabilizing

What needs to be stable: Wrist synergists, elbow synergists, shoulder stabilizers (emphasis flexors, protractors, retractors), obliques, abdominals, back extensors, hip flexors, adductors, and extensors, internal rotators of the leg, knee extensors.

Asanas for stabilizing: Adho/Urdhva Mukha Svanasana, Phalakasana, Pincha Mayurasana, Shishulasana, Urdhva Dhanurasana, Salamba Sirsasana, Navasana, Chaturanga Dandasana, Urdhva Hastasana, Vasisthasana.

This asana prepares you for:

Vrschikasana; Adho Mukha Vrksasana to Chaturanga Dandasana, or Urdhva Dhanurasana, Urdhva Kukkutasana; ticktocks, Salamba Sirsasana I and II, Pincha Mayurasana.

Counterposes

Balasana, Uttanasana, wrist therapy, Savasana.

Agnistambhasana
Two-Footed King Pigeon Pose or Fire Log Pose

Identifying Preparatory Asanas
Opening

What needs to be open: Hip adductors and extensors, internal rotators of the leg, back extensors, calves.

Asanas for opening: Ardha Baddha Padmottanasana Prep, Baddha Konasana, Eka Pada Raj Kapotasana Prep, Gomukhasana, Upavista Konasana.

Stabilizing

What needs to be stable: Pelvic floor, transversus abdominis, knee flexors, foot dorsiflexors.

Asanas for stabilizing: Ardha Chandrasana, Baddha Konasana, Balasana, Bidalasana, Malasana, Paschimottanasana, Prasarita Padottanasana A, B, and D.

This asana prepares you for:

Eka Pada Raj Kapotasana II, Natarajasana.

Counterposes

Simple twist followed by long forward bends.

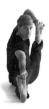

Akarna Dhanurasana
Shooting Bow Pose

Identifying Preparatory Asanas
Opening

What needs to be open: Grounded leg: calf, knee flexors. Gesture leg: hip adductors, internal rotators of the leg. Hip extensors, back extensors.

Asanas for opening: Ardha Baddha Padmottanasana, Baddha Konasana, Dandasana, Eka Pada Raj Kapotasana Prep, Janu Sirsasana, Marichyasana A, Padmasana, Uttana Prasithasana, Uttanasana.

Stabilizing

What needs to be stable: Extended leg: internal rotators of the leg, knee extensors, foot dorsiflexors. Raised leg: external rotators, knee flexors. Hip flexors, transversus abdominis, back extensors, obliques, shoulder retractors.

Asanas for stabilizing: Adho Mukha Svanasana, Ardha Baddha Padmottanasana Prep, Baddha Konasana, Dandasana, Malasana, Marichyasana A, Padangusthasana, Parsvottanasana, Supta Padangusthasana, Ubhaya Padangusthasana, Uttanasana, Utthita Parsvakonasana, Utthita Trikonasana.

This asana prepares you for:

Astavakrasana, Bhujapidasana, Malasana, Tittibhasana, Eka Pada Sirsasana series.

Counterposes

Apanasana, vinyasa series, Adho Mukha Svanasana.

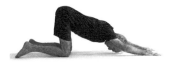

Anahatasana
Extended Puppy or Heart Chakra Pose

Identifying Preparatory Asanas

Opening

What needs to be open: Elbow flexors, shoulder extensors, retractors, and elevators. Chest, abdominals, hip extensors.

Asanas for opening: Adho Mukha Svanasana, Anjaneyasana, Ardha Uttanasana, Ashta Chandrasana, Balasana, Bidalasana, Garudasana, Gomukhasana, Urdhva Hastasana, Utkatasana.

Stabilizing

What needs to be stable: Knee flexors. Hip flexors and adductors. Back extensors, shoulder extensors, protractors, and retractors, external rotators of the arm, elbow extensors, wrist flexors.

Asanas for stabilizing: Adho Mukha Svanasana, Anjaneyasana, Ardha Uttanasana, Ashta Chandrasana, Balasana, Bidalasana, Shishulasana, Utkatasana, Malasana, Parsvottanasana.

This asana prepares you for:

Poses requiring open shoulders, external rotation of the arms: Adho Mukha Svanasana, Adho Mukha Vrksasana, Urdhva Dhanurasana; Gomukhasana arms.

Counterposes

Apanasana, Balasana, Savasana.

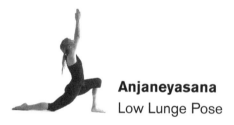

Anjaneyasana
Low Lunge Pose

Identifying Preparatory Asanas

Opening

What needs to be open: Back leg: knee flexors, hip flexors. Front leg: hip extensors. Abdominals, chest, shoulder elevators, shoulder extensors.

Asanas for opening: Adho/Urdhva Mukha Svanasana, Apanasana, Bhujangasana, Bidalasana,Urdhva Hastasana, Utkatasana. In itself an opening pose.

Stabilizing

What needs to be stable: Front leg: hip extensors, internal rotators of the leg. Rear leg: hip flexors, foot dorsiflexors. Intrinsic foot muscles, pelvic floor, hip abductors and adductors, transversus abdominis, shoulder flexors and protractors, external rotators of the arm, elbow extensors.

Asanas for stabilizing: Adho Mukha Svanasana, Ardha Uttanasana, Bhujangasana, Bidalasana, Phalakasana, Salabhasana A, B, and C, Utkatasana, Anahatasana, Uttanasana.

This asana prepares you for:

Back bends, arm balances with extended hips; Ashta Chandrasana, Eka Pada Adho Mukha Vrksasana, Hanumanasana, Supta Virasana, Virabhadrasana I and III, Virasana.

Counterposes

Adho Mukha Svanasana, Balasana, Uttanasana.

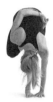

Ardha Baddha Padmottanasana
Half Bound Lotus Intense Stretch Pose

Identifying Preparatory Asanas

Opening

What needs to be open: Standing leg: knee flexors, hip extensors. Folded leg: knee extensors, hip adductors, internal rotators of the leg. Back extensors, shoulder extensors of bound arm.

Asanas for opening: Adho Mukha Svanasana, Agnistambhasana, Gomukhasana, Janu Sirsasana, Padmasana, Paschimottanasana, Uttanasana, Vrksasana.

Stabilizing

What needs to be stable: Standing leg: intrinsic muscles of foot, knee extensors, hip abductors, adductors and extensors, internal rotators of leg.

Asanas for stabilizing: Adho Mukha Svanasana, Ardha Uttanasana, Janu Sirsasana, Padmasana, Parsvottanasana, Paschimottanasana, Tadasana, Uttanasana, Vrksasana.

This asana prepares you for:

Other Padmasana poses: Kukkutasana, Ardha Baddha Padma

Paschimottanasana; Ardha Baddha Padma to Chaturanga Dandasana (keeping Half Lotus positioning), to Adho Mukha Svanasana, hop forward to Tadasana; Bharadvajrasana B.

Counterposes

Tadasana, vinyasa series, Urdhva Mukha Svanasana, Adho Mukha Svanasana.

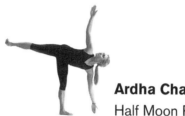

Ardha Chandrasana
Half Moon Pose

Identifying Preparatory Asanas

Opening

What needs to be open: Standing leg: knee flexors, hip extensors and adductors, internal rotators of the leg. Extended leg: knee flexors, hip flexors. Shoulder elevators, neck extensors and rotators.

Asanas for opening: Adho Mukha Svanasana, Utthita Hasta Padangusthasana, Prasarita Padottanasana D, Utthita Parsvakonasana, Utthita Trikonasana, Virabhadrasana II, Vrksasana.

Stabilizing

What needs to be stable: Standing leg: Intrinsic muscles of foot, hip abductors and adductors, external rotators of leg. Extended leg: hip abductors, external rotators of the leg, obliques, abdominals, back extensors, shoulder stabilizers (emphasis: protractors, retractors), elbow extensors, neck flexors and rotators.

Asanas for stabilizing: Adho Mukha Svanasana, Ardha Uttanasana, Parighasana, Phalakasana, Prasarita Padottanasana D, Tadasana, Utthita Parsvakonasana, Utthita Trikonasana, Vasisthasana, Virabhadrasana II, Vrksasana.

This asana prepares you for:

Grasp raised leg foot with same-side arm, Bakasana positioning; grasp foot with both hands; Vasisthasana. Do not transition directly to Virabhadrasana III or Parivrtta Ardha Chandrasana.

Counterposes

Balasana, Malasana, Prasarita Padottanasana A.

Ardha Matsyendrasana
Half Lord of the Fishes Pose

Identifying Preparatory Asanas
Opening
What needs to be open: Hip extensors, external rotators of the leg, obliques, back extensors, chest, internal rotators of the arm, neck rotators.

Asanas for opening: Baddha Konasana, Bharadvajrasana, Eka Pada Raj Kapotasana Prep A, Janu Sirsasana, Marichyasana C, Padmasana, Parivrtta Trikonasana, Parivrtta Utkatasana, Supta Parivartanasana, Virasana.

Stabilizing
What needs to be stable: Hip flexors, hip adductors, obliques, knee flexors, shoulder retractors and protractors.

Asanas for stabilizing: Adho Mukha Svanasana, Baddha Konasana, Balasana, Garudasana, Gomukhasana, Jathara Parivartanasana, Marichyasana A and C, Padmasana, Parivrtta Parsvakonasana, Parivrtta Trikonasana, Prasarita Padottanasana.

This asana prepares you for:
Deeper twists, Parsva Bakasana, Dwi Pada Koundinyasana, Eka Pada Koundinyasana, Astavakrasana.

Counterposes
Apanasana, Ananda Balasana, Dandasana, Paschimottanasana, Janu Sirsasana.

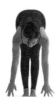

Ardha Uttanasana
Half Standing Forward Fold

Identifying Preparatory Asanas

Opening

What needs to be open: Calves, knee flexors, hip extensors, back extensors, chest, shoulder elevators.

Asanas for opening: Bhujangasana, Bidalasana, Dandasana, Tadasana, Supta Padangusthasana, Uttanasana.

Stabilizing

What needs to be stable: Intrinsic foot muscles, knee extensors, hip extensors, back extensors, transversus abdominis, shoulder retractors.

Asanas for stabilizing: Adho Mukha Svanasana, Bidalasana, Utkatasana, Uttanasana.

This asana prepares you for:

Uttanasana, Virabhadrasana III, Utkatasana, Paschimottanasana.

Counterposes

Balasana, Apanasana, Tadasana.

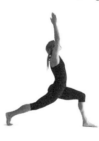

Ashta Chandrasana
High Lunge Pose or Crescent Pose

Identifying Preparatory Asanas

Opening

What needs to be open: Back leg: calf, knee flexors, hip flexors. Front leg: hip extensors. Abdominals, shoulder elevators, extensors, protractors.

Asanas for opening: Adho Mukha Svanasana, Anjaneyasana, Bidalasana, Utkatasana, Uttana Prasithasana.

What needs to be stable: Intrinsic foot muscles. Front leg: hip stabilizers (emphasis extensors, adductors) knee flexors. Back leg: foot dorsiflexors, hip flexors, knee extensors. Back extensors, transversus abdominis, shoulder retractors and protractors, external rotators of the arm, elbow extensors.

Asanas for stabilizing: Adho/Urdhva Mukha Svanasana, Anjaneyasana, Bidalasana, Bhujangasana, Garudasana, Prasarita Padottanasana, Tadasana, Urdhva Hastasana, Utkatasana, Uttanasana, Utthita Trikonasana, Virabhadrasana II.

This asana prepares you for:

Virabhadrasana I & III, Parivrtta Ashta Chandrasana, Parivrtta Parsvakonasana; transition into Virabhadrasana III, Parivritta Ardha Chandrasana, Adho Mukha Vrksasana and Parsvakonasana

Counterposes

Balasana, vinyasa series, Adho Mukha Svanasana.

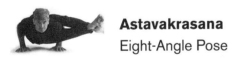

Astavakrasana
Eight-Angle Pose

Identifying Preparatory Asanas

Opening

What needs to be open: Wrist flexors, shoulder elevators and flexors, chest, obliques, knee flexors, hip extensors and abductors.
Asanas for opening: Adho/Urdhva Mukha Svanasana, Balasana, Jathara Parivartanasana, Marichyasana A and B, Parivrtta Parsvakonasana, Parivrtta Utkatasana, Uttanasana, Utthita Parsvakonasana.

Stabilizing

What needs to be stable: Wrist synergists, elbow synergists, rotators of the arm, chest, shoulder stabilizers (emphasis adductors, protractors, retractors) obliques, abdominals, hip adductors and flexors, knee extensors, foot dorsiflexors.

Asanas for stabilizing: Adho/Urdhva Mukha Svanasana, Bakasana, Bidalasana, Chaturanga Dandasana, Garudasana, Lolasana, Marichyasana A and C, Parivrtta Parsvakonasana, Parivrtta Utkatasana, Parsva Bakasana, Utkatasana.

This asana prepares you for:

Eka Pada Koundinyasana A to Chaturanga Dandasana, Dwi Pada Koundinyasana.

Counterposes

Vinyasa series, Urdhva Mukha Svanasana, Adho Mukha Svanasana, Supta Baddha Konasana, Balasana, wrist therapy.

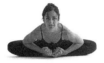

Baddha Konasana
Bound Angle Pose

Identifying Preparatory Asanas

Opening

What needs to be open: Hip adductors and extensors, internal rotators of the leg. Knee extensors, chest, shoulder elevators.

Asanas for opening: Agnistambhasana, Ananda Balasana, Eka Pada Raj Kapotasana Prep, Paschimottanasana, Supta Padangusthasana, Upavista Konasana.

Stabilizing

What needs to be stable: Pelvic floor, back extensors, transversus abdominis.

Asanas for stabilizing: Ardha Uttanasana, Dandasana, Gomukhasana, Malasana, Prasarita Padottanasana, Upavista Konasana.

This asana prepares you for:

Supta Baddha Konasana, Janu Sirsasana, Parivrtta Janu Sirsasana, Akarna Dhanurasana, Marichyasana A, Padmasana, Swastikasana.

Counterposes

Apanasana, Balasana, Adho Mukha Svanasana, Gomukhasana.

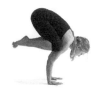

Bakasana
Crane Pose

Identifying Preparatory Asanas

Opening

What needs to be open: Wrist flexors, shoulder elevators and retractors, back extensors, hip extensors, ankle dorsiflexors.

Asanas for opening: Balasana, Bidalasana, Garudasana, Malasana, Marichyasana A, Prasarita Padottanasana A, Uttana Prasithasana, Uttanasana.

Stabilizing

What needs to be stable: Wrist synergists, elbow synergists, shoulder stabilizers (emphasis flexors, protractors), external rotators of the arm, chest, abdominals, hip adductors and flexors, pelvic floor, knee flexors.

Asanas for stabilizing: Adho Mukha Svanasana, Bidalasana, Chaturanga Dandasana, Garudasana, Malasana, Marichyasana A, Navasana, Phalakasana.

This asana prepares you for:

Tittibhasana, Parsva Bakasana, Eka Pada Koundinyasana, Sirsasana II series, transition to pose by hopping from Adho Mukha Svanasana.

Counterposes

Vinyasa series, Urdhva Mukha Svanasana, Adho Mukha Svanasana, wrist therapy, Balasana.

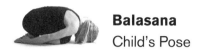

Balasana
Child's Pose

Identifying Preparatory Asanas

Opening

> **What needs to be open:** Foot dorsiflexors, knee flexors, hip extensors, back extensors.
>
> **Asanas for opening:** Apanasana. In itself an opening and restorative pose.

Stabilizing

> **What needs to be stable:** The floor—somewhat.
>
> **Asanas for stabilizing:** A preparatory or restorative to precede or follow any asana and practice.

This asana prepares you for:

> Utthita Balasana, Anahatasana, Virasana, Sasangasana.

Counterposes

> A deeply restorative pose, Savasana.

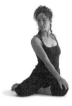

Bharadvajrasana A
Sage Bharadvaj's Pose A

Identifying Preparatory Asanas

Opening

> **What needs to be open:** Padma leg: hip adductors, internal rotators of the leg. Vira leg: external rotators of the leg, knee flexors, foot dorsiflexors. Hip extensors, obliques, chest. Bound arm: Shoulder flexors, external rotators of the arm. Shoulder elevators, neck rotators.
>
> **Asanas for opening:** Bidalasana, Gomukhasana arms, Jathara Parivarttanasana, Padmasana, Parivrtta Utkatasana, Virasana.

What needs to be stable: Pelvic floor, hip flexors, knee flexors, obliques, shoulder extensors.

Asanas for stabilizing: Baddha Konasana, Garudasana, Malasana, Parivrtta Hasta Padangusthasana, Parivrtta Parsvakonasana, Parivrtta Trikonasana, Parivrtta Utkatasana, Virasana.

This asana prepares you for:

Bharadvajrasana B, Swastikasana.

Counterposes

Dandasana, Paschimottanasana, Apanasana, Balasana.

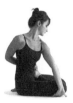

Bharadvajrasana B
Sage Bharadvaj's Pose B

Identifying Preparatory Asanas

Opening

What needs to be open: Padma leg: hip adductors, internal rotators of the leg. Vira leg: external rotators of the leg, knee flexors, foot dorsiflexors. Hip extensors, obliques, chest. Bound arm: Shoulder flexors, external rotators of the arm. Shoulder elevators, neck rotators.

Asanas for opening: Ardha Baddha Padmottanasana Prep, Bidalasana, Gomukhasana arms, Jathara Parivarttanasana, Padmasana, Parivrtta Utkatasana, Virasana.

Stabilizing

What needs to be stable: Pelvic floor, hip flexors, knee flexors, obliques, shoulder extensors.

Asanas for stabilizing: Ardha Matsyendrasana, Baddha Konasana, Padmasana, Parivrtta Hasta Padangusthasana, Parivrtta Parsvakonasana, Parivrtta Trikonasana, Parivrtta Utkatasana, Urdhva Mukha Svanasana, Virasana.

This asana prepares you for:

Tiriang Mukha Eka Pada Paschimottanasana, Krounchasana, Ardha Baddha Padma Paschimottanasana.

Counterposes

Urdhva Mukha Svanasana, Adho Mukha Svanasana, Dandasana, Paschimottanasana, Apanasana, Balasana.

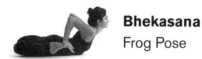

Bhekasana
Frog Pose

Identifying Preparatory Asanas
Opening

What needs to be open: Hip flexors, knee extensors, foot dorsiflexors, abdominals, chest, shoulder elevators and flexors, throat.
Asanas for opening: Bhujangasana, Dhanurasana, Naraviralasana, Prasarita Padottanasana C arms, Salabhasana A and C, Ustrasana, Virasana.

Stabilizing

What needs to be stable: Back extensors, transversus abdominis, pelvic floor, shoulders (emphasis flexors, protractors and adductors), neck.
Asanas for stabilizing: Bhujangasana, Dhanurasana, Pursvottanasana, Salabhasana A and C, Setu Bandha Sarvangasana, Urdhva Mukha Svanasana, Ustrasana.

This asana prepares you for:

Supta Virasana, Natarajasana, Eka Pada Raj Kapotasana, Urdhva Dhanurasana.

Counterposes

Balasana, Ardha Matsyendrasana, Adho Mukha Svanasana, Dandasana, Paschimottanasana.

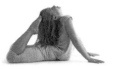

Bhujangasana
Cobra Pose

Identifying Preparatory Asanas

Opening

What needs to be open: Knee flexors, hip flexors, abdominals, chest, shoulder elevators and flexors, wrist flexors.

Asanas for opening: Bidalasana. In it's gradual expression, an opening pose for back bends.

Stabilizing

What needs to be stable: Wrist flexors, elbow flexors, rotators of the arm, chest, shoulder stabilizers (emphasis adductors, protractors, and retractors), transversus abdominis, spine extensors, hip extensors, knee extensors, calves.

Asanas for stabilizing: Bidalasana. In its gradual expression, a preparatory pose for back bends.

This asana prepares you for:

Urdhva Mukha Svanasana, Raj Kapotasana, Ustrasana, Bhekasana, Eka Pada Bakasana.

Counterposes

Adho Mukha Svanasana, Balasana, simple supine twist, Apanasana, Supta Baddha Konasana.

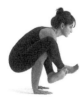

Bhujapidasana
Shoulder-Squeezing Pose

Identifying Preparatory Asanas

Opening

What needs to be open: Wrist flexors, shoulder retractors and elevators, hip extensors, back extensors, knee flexors.

Asanas for opening: Adho Mukha Svanasana, Bidalasana, Garudasana, Kurmasana, Malasana, Uttana Prasithasana, Prasarita Padottanasana A.

Stabilizing

What needs to be stable: Wrist synergists, elbow synergists, shoulder stabilizers (emphasis flexors, protractors), external rotators of the arm, chest, abdominals, hip adductors and flexors, pelvic floor, knee extensors, foot dorsiflexors.

Asanas for stabilizing: Adho Mukha Svanasana, Bakasana, Bidalasana, Chaturanga Dandasana, Garudasana, Marichyasana A, Navasana, Prasarita Padottanasana A.

This asana prepares you for:

Tittibhasana, Bakasana, Astavakrasana.

Counterposes

Adho Mukha Svanasana, Balasana, wrist therapy.

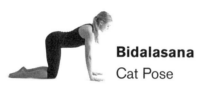

Bidalasana
Cat Pose

Identifying Preparatory Asanas

Opening

What needs to be open: Wrist flexors. Cat: Back extensors, shoulder extensors and retractors. Dog: Shoulder elevators, chest, abdominals, hip extensors.

Asanas for opening: In itself an opener for any asana practice.

Stabilizing

What needs to be stable: Wrist and hip synergists, abdominals, back extensors, chest, shoulder stabilizers (emphasis protractors), elbow extensors.

Asanas for stabilizing: A warming stabilizer that may precede any asana sequence.

This asana prepares you for:

Anahatasana, Phalakasana, Adho Mukha Svanasana.

Counterposes

Balasana, Savasana.

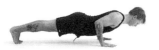

Chaturanga Dandasana
Four-Limbed Staff Pose

Identifying Preparatory Asanas

Opening

What needs to be open: Calves, wrist flexors, hip flexors, shoulder elevators.

Asanas for opening: Adho/Urdhva Mukha Svanasana, Phalakasana, Tadasana.

Stabilizing

What needs to be stable: Wrist flexors, elbow synergists, chest, shoulder stabilizers (emphasis protractors, retractors, adductors and flexors), abdominals, hip flexors, knee extensors, intrinsic foot muscles.

Asanas for stabilizing: Adho Mukha Svanasana, Ardha Uttanasana, Phalakasana, Samastihi, Tadasana, Urdhva Mukha Svanasana.

This asana prepares you for:

Surya Namaskara A and B, Nakrasana, Bakasana.

Counterposes

Adho Mukha Svanasana, Balasana, wrist therapy.

Dandasana
Staff Pose

Identifying Preparatory Asanas

Opening

What needs to be open: Calves, knee flexors, hip extensors, elbow flexors, shoulder elevators.

Asanas for opening: Adho Mukha Svanasana, Ardha Uttanasana, Supta Padangusthasana, Uttanasana.

Stabilizing

What needs to be stable: Hip flexors and adductors, internal rotators of the leg, knee extensors, foot dorsiflexors, back extensors, transversus abdominis, shoulder synergists (emphasis protractors, retractors, extensors), external rotators of the arm.

Asanas for stabilizing: Adho Mukha Svanasana, Ardha Uttanasana, Supta Padangusthasana, Uttanasana.

This asana prepares you for:

Seated forward bends, hip openers, and twists; Pursvottanasana.

Counterposes

Apanasana, Baddha Konasana, Supta Baddha Konasana, Viparita Karani, Savasana.

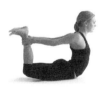

Dhanurasana
Bow Pose

Identifying Preparatory Asanas

Opening

What needs to be open: External rotators of the leg, hip flexors, abdominals, chest, shoulder protractors and extensors, internal rotators of the arm, elbow flexors, wrist flexors.

Asanas for opening: Anjaneyasana, Ashta Chandrasana, Bidalasana, Salabhasana A and C, Setu Bandha Sarvangasana, Urdhva Mukha Svanasana, Virasana.

Stabilizing

What needs to be stable: Back extensors, hip extensors and adductors, transversus abdominis, shoulder retractors, knee extensors, foot dorsiflexors.

Asanas for stabilizing: Bhujangasana, Pursvottanasana, Salabhasana A and C, Setu Bandha Sarvangasana.

This asana prepares you for:

Parsva Dhanurasana, Bhekasana, Raj Kapotasana, Ustrasana, Laghu Vajrasana.

Counterposes

Balasana, Apanasana, Ardha Matsyendrasana, Supta Parivartanasana.

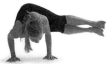

Dwi Pada Koundinyasana
Two-Leg Sage Koundinya's Pose

Identifying Preparatory Asanas

Opening

What needs to be open: Shoulder elevators, chest, obliques, back extensors, hip extensors, external rotators of the leg, knee flexors.

Asanas for opening: Adho Mukha Svanasana, Jathara Parivarttanasana, Marichyasana C, Parsva Bakasana, Parivrtta Parsvakonasana, Parivrtta Utkatasana, Uttanasana.

Stabilizing

What needs to be stable: Wrist synergists, elbow synergists, rotators of the arm, shoulder stabilizers (emphasis protractors, retractors, adductors, flexors), chest, obliques, abdominals, adductors, knee extensors, foot dorsiflexors.

Asanas for stabilizing: Adho Mukha Svanasana, Bidalasana, Bakasana, Chaturanga Dandasana, Garudasana, Parivrtta Parsvakonasana, Parivrtta Trikonasana, Parivrtta Utkatasana.

This asana prepares you for:

Transition to Eka Pada Koundinyasana A to Chaturanga Dandasana; add to Sirsasana II vinyasa.

Counterposes

Wrist therapy, Adho Mukha Svanasana, Balasana, vinyasa series.

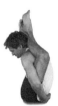

Dwi Pada Sirsasana
Two Legs behind Head Pose

Identifying Preparatory Asanas

Opening

What needs to be open: Hip adductors and extensors, internal rotators of the leg, back extensors, shoulder retractors and elevators.

Asanas for opening: Ananda Balasana, Ardha Baddha Padmottanasana, Ardha Baddha Padma Paschimottanasana, Agnistambhasana, Baddha Konasana, Baddha Padmasana, Bhujapidasana, Eka Pada Raj Kapotasana, Eka Pada Sirsasana, Gomukhasana, Karnapidasana, Kurmasana, Malasana, Marichyasana C, Pada Hastasana, Prasarita Padottanasana A, B, and D, Upavista Konasana, Uttana Prasithasana.

Stabilizing

What needs to be stable: Hip flexors and adductors, pelvic floor, abdominals, knee flexors, shoulder retractors and adductors.

Asanas for stabilizing: Agnistambhasana, Baddha Konasana, Eka Pada Raj Kapotasana, Eka Pada Sirsasana, Karnapidasana, Marichyasana A, Padmasana, Prasarita Padottanasana A, B, and D, Ubhaya Padangusthasana, Upavista Konasana, Urdhva Mukha Paschimottanasana, Uttana Prasithasana.

This asana prepares you for:

Supta Kurmasana, Chakorasana.

Counterposes

Apanasana, Balasana.

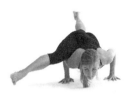

Eka Pada Koundinyasana A
One-Leg Sage Koundinya's Pose A

Identifying Preparatory Asanas

Opening

What needs to be open: Wrist flexors, shoulder elevators, chest, obliques, back extensors. Front leg: hip extensors, external rotators of the leg, knee flexors. Back leg: hip flexors, knee extensors.

Asanas for opening: Ardha Matsyendrasana, Jathara Parivartanasana, Marichyasana B, Parivrtta Parsvakonasana, Parivrtta Trikonasana, Parsva Bakasana, Parsvottanasana.

Stabilizing

What needs to be stable: Wrist synergists, elbow synergists, rotators of the arm, shoulder stabilizers (emphasis protractors, retractors, adductors, flexors), chest, obliques, abdominals, knee extensors, foot dorsiflexors. Lower leg: hip flexors and adductors. Upper leg: hip extensors.

Asanas for stabilizing: Adho/Urdhva Mukha Svanasana, Ardha Matsyendrasana, Bakasana, Chaturanga Dandasana, Parivrtta Ardha Chandrasana, Parivrtta Hasta Padangusthasana, Parivrtta Parsvakonasana, Parivrtta Trikonasana, Phalakasana.

This asana prepares you for:

Transition to Chaturanga Dandasana, add to Sirsasana II vinyasa, Dwi Pada Koundinyasana, Galavasana.

Counterposes

Wrist therapy, Adho Mukha Svanasana, Balasana.

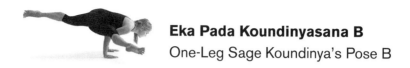

Eka Pada Koundinyasana B
One-Leg Sage Koundinya's Pose B

Identifying Preparatory Asanas

Opening

What needs to be open: Wrist flexors, shoulder elevators, chest, hip adductors. Front leg: hip extensors, internal rotators of the leg, knee flexors. Back leg: hip flexors, knee extensors.

Asanas for opening: Anjaneyasana, Prasarita Padottanasana A, Uttana Prasithasana, Utthita Parsvakonasana, Virabhadrasana II.

Stabilizing

What needs to be stable: Wrist synergists, elbow synergists, rotators of the arm, shoulder stabilizers (emphasis protractors, retractors, adductors, flexors), chest, obliques, abdominals, knee extensors, foot dorsiflexors. Propped leg: hip flexors and adductors. Back leg: hip extensors, knee extensors.

Asanas for stabilizing: Adho/Urdhva Mukha Svanasana, Ardha Chandrasana, Bakasana, Chaturanga Dandasana, Marichyasana A, Phalakasana, Prasarita Padottanasana A, Uttana Prasithasana, Utthita Parsvakonasana, Utthita Trikonasana, Vasisthasana, Virabhadrasana II.

This asana prepares you for:

Transition to Chaturanga Dandasana, Dwi Pada Koundinyasana, Eka Pada Koundinyasana A, Galavasana, add to Sirsasana II vinyasa.

Counterposes

Adho Mukha Svanasana, Balasana, vinyasa series, wrist therapy.

Eka Pada Raj Kapotasana
One-Leg King Pigeon Pose

Identifying Preparatory Asanas

Opening

What needs to be open: Front leg: hip adductors and extensors, internal rotators of the leg, knee extensors. Back leg: hip flexors, external rotators of the leg, knee flexors. Abdominals, chest, shoulder extensors, retractors and elevators, neck.

Asanas for opening: Adho/Urdhva Mukha Svanasana, Anjaneyasana, Ashta Chandrasana, Baddha Konasana, Bhujangasana, Garudasana arms, Gomukhasana, Shishulasana, Uttana Prasithasana, Virabhadrasana I.

Stabilizing

What needs to be stable: Pelvic floor. Front leg: hip flexors and abductors, knee flexors, foot dorsiflexors. Back leg: hip extensors and adductors, internal rotators of the leg, knee synergists. Transversus abdominis, back extensors, shoulder protractors and flexors, external rotators of the arm.

Asanas for stabilizing: Adho/Urdhva Mukha Svanasana, Anjaneyasana, Ashta Chandrasana, Bhujangasana, Parivrtta Parsvakonasana, Salabhasana B, Virabhadrasana I.

This asana prepares you for:

Eka Pada Raj Kapotasana II, Natarajasana, Eka Pada Sirsasana series, Hanumanasana, Kapotasana, Raj Kapotasana.

Counterposes

Vinyasa series, simple twists, Balasana.

Eka Pada Sirsasana

One Leg behind Head Pose

Identifying Preparatory Asanas

Opening

What needs to be open: Grounded leg: hip synergists, external rotators of the leg, knee flexors, calf. Sirsa leg: hip adductors and extensors, internal rotators of the leg. Back extensors, shoulder elevators, chest.

Asanas for opening: Adho/Urdhva Mukha Svanasana, Agnistambhasana, Akarna Dhanurasana, Anjaneyasana, Ardha Baddha Padmottanasana, Ashta Chandrasana, Baddha Konasana, Bhujangasana, Gomukhasana, Malasana, Uttana Prasithasana, Virabhadrasana I.

Stabilizing

What needs to be stable: Hip flexors and adductors. Grounded leg: internal rotators of the leg, knee extensors, foot dorsiflexors. Gesture leg: external rotators, knee flexors. Transversus abdominis, back extensors, obliques, shoulder retractors.

Asanas for stabilizing: Akarna Dhanurasana, Eka Pada Raj Kapotasana Prep, Gomukhasana, Karnapidasana, Malasana, Marichyasana A, Uttanasana, Uttana Prasithasana, Utthita Parsvakonasana.

This asana prepares you for:

Chakorasana, Dwi Pada Sirsasana, Yoganidrasana.

Counterposes

Vinyasa series, simple twists, Balasana.

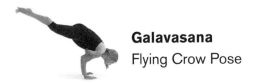

Galavasana
Flying Crow Pose

Identifying Preparatory Asanas

Opening

What needs to be open: Wrist flexors, shoulder elevators, retractors. Folded leg: hip extensors and adductors, internal rotators of the leg. Extended leg: hip flexors, knee flexors.

Asanas for opening: Bakasana and its Prep poses, Eka Pada Raj Kapotasana I and its Prep poses, Utkatasana.

Stabilizing

What needs to be stable: Wrist synergists, elbow synergists, shoulder stabilizers (emphasis flexors, protractors), external rotators of the arm, abdominal core. Grounded leg: external rotators, hip flexors, knee flexors. Extended leg: hip extensors, knee extensors, foot dorsiflexors.

Asanas for stabilizing: Adho Mukha Svanasana, Agnistambhasana, Bakasana, Eka Pada Raj Kapotasana, I and II, Gomukhasana, Padmasana.

This asana prepares you for:

Uttana Prasithasana, Eka Pada Bakasana.

Counterposes

Vinyasa series, Balasana, wrist therapy, Balasana.

Garbha Pindasana
Embryo in the Womb Pose

Identifying Preparatory Asanas

Opening

What needs to be open: Hip adductors and extensors, internal rotators of the leg, back extensors, shoulder retractors and elevators.

Asanas for opening: Adho Mukha Svanasana, Agnistambhasana, Ardha

Baddha Padmottanasana, Baddha Konasana, Balasana, Malasana, Marichyasana A, Padangusthasana, Padmasana, Paschimottanasana, Pindasana, Prasarita Padottanasana A and D, Urdhva Mukha Paschimottanasana, Uttanasana.

Stabilizing

What needs to be stable: Hip flexors, external rotators of the leg, pelvic floor, abdominals, back extensors, knee flexors, shoulder retractors and adductors, elbow flexors.

Asanas for stabilizing: Agnistambhasana, Baddha Konasana, Kurmasana, Malasana, Padmasana, Prasarita Padottanasana A, Ubhaya Padangusthasana, Upavista Konasana, Uttana Prasithasana, Uttanasana.

This asana prepares you for:

Pindasana, Matsyasana.

Counterposes

Matsyasana Prep, Uttana Padasana, Savasana.

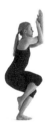

Garudasana
Eagle Pose

Identifying Preparatory Asanas

Opening

What needs to be open: Calf of standing leg, hip extensors, external rotators of the leg, shoulder retractors, extensors, and elevators, internal rotators of the arm.

Asanas for opening: Gomukhasana, Tadasana, Utkatasana, Vrksasana Bidalasana.

Stabilizing

What needs to be stable: Grounded leg: intrinsic foot muscles. Both legs: knee and hip synergists. Hip adductors, internal rotators of the leg, back extensors, transversus abdominis, shoulder flexors, protractors, adductors, and depressors. Internal rotators of the arm, elbow flexors.

Asanas for stabilizing: Ashta Chandrasana, Gomukhasana, Tadasana, Utkatasana, Virabhadrasana III, Vrksasana.

This asana prepares you for:

Gomukhasana, Bharadvajrasana, Virasana.

Counterposes

Tadasana, Uttanasana, Adho Mukha Svanasana, Baddha Konasana.

Gomukhasana
Cow Face Pose

Identifying Preparatory Asanas

Opening

What needs to be open: Hip adductors, extensors, and internal rotators. Back extensors, shoulder retractors and elevators. Top arm: shoulder and elbow extensors. Bottom arm: shoulder flexors, external rotators of the arm.

Asanas for opening: Ardha Matsyendrasana, Marichyasana C, Parivrtta Janu Sirsasana, Paschimottanasana, Virasana.

Stabilizing

What needs to be stable: Hip flexors and adductors, external rotators of the leg, pelvic floor, transversus abdominis, knee flexors. Lower arm: internal rotators, shoulder extensors. Upper Arm: shoulder flexors, protractors, and adductors, elbow flexors.

Asanas for stabilizing: Ardha Matsyendrasana, Baddha Konasana, Bidalasana, Dandasana, Janu Sirsasana, Uttana Prasithasana, Uttanasana.

This asana prepares you for:

Eka Pada Raj Kapotasana, Bharadvajrasana A and B.

Counterposes

Dandasana, Baddha Konasana, Upavista Konasana, Adho Mukha Svanasana.

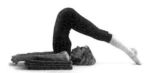

Halasana
Plow Pose

Identifying Preparatory Asanas

Opening

What needs to be open: Foot dorsiflexors, knee extensors, hip extensors, back extensors.

Asanas for opening: Dandasana, Prasarita Padottanasana C, Salamba Sarvangasana, Setu Bandha Sarvangasana.

Stabilizing

What needs to be stable: Shoulder stabilizers (emphasis retractors, adductors, extensors), back extensors, hip extensors and adductors, internal rotators of the leg, knee extensors, foot dorsiflexors.

Asanas for stabilizing: Adho Mukha Svanasana, Ardha Uttanasana, Bidalasana, Dandasana, Prasarita Padottanasana C arms, Salamba Sarvangasana, Setu Bandha Sarvangasana, Uttanasana.

This asana prepares you for:

Karnapidasana, Salamba Sarvangasana.

Counterposes

Uttana Padasana, simple twists, Adho Mukha Svanasana, Viparita Karani, Savasana.

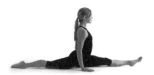

Hanumanasana
Divine Monkey Pose

Identifying Preparatory Asanas

Opening

What needs to be open: Front leg: calf, knee flexors, hip extensors. Back leg: knee flexors, hip flexors. Abdominals, shoulder retractors, elevators, and extensors, elbow flexors.

Asanas for opening: Anjaneyasana, Janu Sirsasana, Supta Padangusthasana, Supta Virasana, Upavista Konasana, Virabhadrasana I.

Stabilizing

What needs to be stable: Pelvic floor, back extensors, transversus abdominis, hip stabilizers (emphasis flexors, adductors, and rear leg hip extensors), internal rotators of the leg, shoulder flexors, protractors, internal rotators and adductors of the arm, elbow extensors.

Asanas for stabilizing: Anjaneyasana, Ardha Uttanasana, Ashta Chandrasana, Bhujangasana, Eka Pada Raj Kapotasana I and II, Supta Padangusthasana, Tiriang Mukha Eka Pada Paschimottanasana, Urdhva Mukha Svanasana, Utthita Hasta Padangusthasana, Virabhadrasana III.

This asana prepares you for:

Eka Pada Raj Kapotasana I and II, Hanumanasana back-bend variation, Natarajasana.

Counterposes

Balasana, Setu Bandha Sarvangasana.

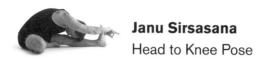

Janu Sirsasana
Head to Knee Pose

Identifying Preparatory Asanas

Opening

What needs to be open: Extended leg: calf, knee flexors, hip extensors. Folded leg: knee extensors, hip adductors, rotators, and extensors. Back extensors, shoulder retractors and elevators.

Asanas for opening: Baddha Konasana, Dandasana, Paschimottanasana, Supta Padangusthasana, Vrksasana.

Stabilizing

What needs to be stable: Hip flexors. Extended leg: internal rotators, knee extensors, foot dorsiflexors. Folded leg: external rotators, knee flexors. Transversus abdominis, back extensors, obliques, shoulder depressors.

Asanas for stabilizing: Baddha Konasana, Dandasana, Prasarita Padottanasana A, B, and D, Upavista Konasana, Uttanasana.

This asana prepares you for:

Parivrtta Janu Sirsasana, Upavista Konasana, Tiriang Mukha Eka Pada Paschimottanasana.

Counterposes

Apanasana, Setu Bandha Sarvangasana, Gomukhasana.

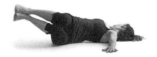

Jathara Parivartanasana
Revolving Twist Pose

Identifying Preparatory Asanas

Opening

What needs to be open: Back extensors, obliques, top hip adductors, chest, shoulder elevators, knee flexors, calves.

Asanas for opening: Ardha Matsyendrasana, Apanasana, Dandasana, Marichyasana C, Yogic Bicycles.

Stabilizing

What needs to be stable: Shoulder extensors, depressors, and retractors, obliques, hip flexors and adductors, knee extensors, calves.

Asanas for stabilizing: Adho Mukha Svanasana, Dandasana, Navasana, Parivrtta Ardha Chandrasana, Parivrtta Hasta Padangusthasana, Parivrtta Parsvakonasana, Parivrtta Trikonasana, Parivrtta Utkatasana, Ubhaya Padangusthasana, Uttanasana.

This asana prepares you for:

Arm balances, neutral and twisting; Salamba Sirsasana II vinyasa.

Counterposes

Apanasana, Ananda Balasana, Supta Baddha Konasana.

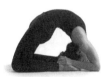

Kapotasana
Pigeon Pose

Identifying Preparatory Asanas

Opening

What needs to be open: Knee extensors, hip flexors, abdominals, chest, shoulder extensors, elbow extensors.

Asanas for opening: Eka Pada Raj Kapotasana II, Gomukhasana, Laghu Vajrasana, Urdhva Dhanurasana, Ustrasana.

Stabilizing

What needs to be stable: Knee extensors, hip adductors and extensors, internal rotators of the leg, back extensors, transversus abdominis, shoulder stabilizers (emphasis retractors/protractors, flexors), external rotators of the arm, elbow extensors.

Asanas for stabilizing: Anjaneyasana, Ashta Chandrasana, Bhekasana, Bhujangasana, Dhanurasana, Eka Pada Raj Kapotasana, I and II,

Salabhasana A, B, and C, Setu Bandha Sarvangasana, Shishulasana arms, Supta Virasana, Urdhva Dhanurasana, Urdhva Mukha Svanasana, Ustrasana, Viparita Dandasana, Virabhadrasana I.

This asana prepares you for:

Eka Pada Raj Kapotasana II, Natarajasana, Laghu Vajrasana.

Counterposes

Simple twist followed by long forward bends.

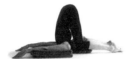

Karnapidasana
Ear-Squeezing Pose

Identifying Preparatory Asanas

Opening

What needs to be open: Elbow flexors, shoulder flexors, back extensors, hip extensors.

Asanas for opening: Balasana, Dandasana, Halasana, Paschimottanasana.

Stabilizing

What needs to be stable: Shoulder stabilizers (emphasis retractors, adductors, extensors), elbow extensors, back extensors, hip flexors, internal rotators of the leg, knee extensors, foot dorsiflexors.

Asanas for stabilizing: Agnistambhasana, Halasana, Marichyasana A, Parivrtta Utkatasana, Paschimottanasana, Prasarita Padottanasana C, Tiriang Mukha Eka Pada Paschimottanasana, Urdhva Padmasana, Uttana Prasithasana, Uttanasana.

This asana prepares you for:

Pindasana, long-held forward bends.

Counterposes

Uttana Padasana, simple twists, Adho Mukha Svanasana, Viparita Karani, Savasana.

Krounchasana
Heron Pose

Identifying Preparatory Asanas

Opening

What needs to be open: Virasana leg: foot dorsiflexors, knee extensors. Extended leg: hip extensors, knee flexors. Shoulder elevators.

Asanas for opening: Dandasana, Paschimottanasana, Tiriang Eka Pada Paschimottanasana, Virasana.

Stabilizing

What needs to be stable: Hip flexors and adductors, internal rotators of the leg, back extensors, abdominals, shoulder depressors and flexors. Extended leg: knee extensors, calf.

Asanas for stabilizing: Adho Mukha Svanasana, Balasana, Dandasana, Marichyasana A, Pada Hastasana, Parsvottanasana, Paschimottanasana, Tiriang Mukha Eka Pada Paschimottanasana, Virasana, Ubhaya Padangusthasana.

This asana prepares you for:

Pick up and float back to Chaturanga Dandasana, Eka Pada Sirsasana to Chakorasana vinyasa; Ubhaya Padangusthasana, Urdhva Mukha Paschimottanasana.

Counterposes

Vinyasa series, Balasana.

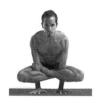

Kukkutasana
Rooster Pose

Identifying Preparatory Asanas

Opening

What needs to be open: Hip adductors and extensors, internal rotators of the leg. Back extensors, chest, shoulder retractors and elevators, elbow flexors.

Asanas for opening: Bakasana, Padmasana and its Prep poses.

Stabilizing

What needs to be stable: Wrist synergists, elbow synergists, shoulder stabilizers (emphasis flexors, protractors), external rotators of the arm, chest abdominals, hip adductors and flexors, pelvic floor, knee flexors, foot dorsiflexors.

Asanas for stabilizing: Adho Mukha Svanasana, Agnistambhasana, Ardha Baddha Padmottanasana, Bakasana, Bhujapidasana, Chaturanga Dandasana, Garbha Pindasana, Janu Sirsasana, Kurmasana, Lolasana, Malasana, Prasarita Padottanasana A, Tittibhasana, Tolasana, Urdhva Kukkutasana, Uttana Prasithasana.

This asana prepares you for:

Urdhva Kukkutasana.

Counterposes

Dandasana, Paschimottanasana, Gomukhasana, Balasana.

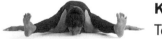

Kurmasana
Tortoise Pose

Identifying Preparatory Asanas

Opening

What needs to be open: Hip adductors and extensors, internal rotators of the leg. Back extensors, shoulder retractors and elevators.

Asanas for opening: Baddha Konasana, Dandasana, Paschimottanasana, Upavista Konasana.

Stabilizing

What needs to be stable: Hip synergists, external rotators of the leg, back extensors, abdominals, shoulder stabilizers (emphasis depressors, protractors), internal rotators of the arm, elbow extensors.

Asanas for stabilizing: Dandasana, Eka Pada Sirsasana, Janu Sirsasana, Malasana, Marichyasana A, Paschimottanasana, Prasarita Padottanasana, Uttanasana.

This asana prepares you for:

Tittibhasana, Eka Pada Sirsasana, Supta Kurmasana.

Counterposes

Simple twists, Setu Bandha Sarvangasana, Apanasana, Balasana.

Laghu Vajrasana
Little Thunderbolt Pose

Identifying Preparatory Asanas

Opening

What needs to be open: Knee extensors, hip flexors, abdominals, shoulder extensors, elbow extensors, chest, throat.

Asanas for opening: Supta Virasana, Ustrasana and its Prep poses, Virasana.

Stabilizing

What needs to be stable: Knee extensors, hip adductors and extensors, internal rotators of the leg, back extensors, transversus abdominis, shoulder stabilizers (emphasis retractors/protractors, extensors), internal rotators of the arm, elbow flexors.

Asanas for stabilizing: Anjaneyasana, Ashta Chandrasana, Bhekasana,

Bhujangasana, Bidalasana, Dhanurasana, Eka Pada Raj Kapotasana II, Raj Kapotasana, Setu Bandha Sarvangasana, Salabhasana B,Supta Virasana, Urdhva Dhanurasana, Urdhva Mukha Svanasana, Ustrasana, Viparita Dandasana.

This asana prepares you for:

Kapotasana, drop-backs, Natarajasana, ticktocks.

Counterposes

Balasana, simple twists, Supta Baddha Konasana, seated forward bends.

Lolasana
Dangling Earring Pose

Identifying Preparatory Asanas

Opening

What needs to be open: Wrist flexors, elbow flexors, shoulder flexors and elevators, back extensors, hip extensors, knee extensors.
Asanas for opening: Bakasana and its Prep poses, Tolasana.

Stabilizing

What needs to be stable: Wrist synergists, elbow synergists, shoulder stabilizers (emphasis flexors, protractors), external rotators of the arm, chest, abdominals, hip adductors and flexors, pelvic floor, knee flexors, calves.
Asanas for stabilizing: Adho Mukha Svanasana, Balasana, Bidalasana, Chaturanga Dandasana, Garudasana, Gomukhasana, Malasana, Marichyasana A, Navasana, Prasarita Padottanasana A, Salamba Sirsasana II, Utkatasana, Uttana Prasithasana.

This asana prepares you for:

Transition through Dandasana, Tolasana, Lolasana to Chaturanga Dandasana; transition to Bakasana or Adho Mukha Vrksasana.

Counterposes

Apanasana, Ananda Balasana, Supta Baddha Konasana, Gomukhasana, Adho Mukha Svanasana.

Malasana
Garland Pose

Identifying Preparatory Asanas

Opening

What needs to be open: Calves, knee extensors, hip extensors and adductors, internal rotators of the leg, back extensors, chest, shoulder elevators and retractors.

Asanas for opening: Baddha Konasana, Marichyasana A, Upavista Konasana, Virasana.

Stabilizing

What needs to be stable: Intrinsic foot muscles, knee flexors, hip flexors and adductors, external rotators of the leg, pelvic floor, abdominals, back extensors, shoulder retractors and extensors, elbow flexors, wrist flexors.

Asanas for stabilizing: Ardha Uttanasana, Baddha Konasana, Balasana, Uttanasana, Virabhadrasana II.

This asana prepares you for:

Akarna Dandasana, Bakasana, Bhujapidasana, Tittibhasana.

Counterposes

Balasana, Paschimottanasana, Adho Mukha Svanasana, simple twists, Uttanasana.

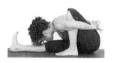

Marichyasana A

Sage Marichi's Pose

Identifying Preparatory Asanas

Opening

What needs to be open: Grounded leg: calf, knee flexors. Gesture leg: knee extensors, external rotators. Hip extensors, back extensors, shoulder retractors, elevators.

Asanas for opening: Anjaneyasana, Ardha Baddha Padmottanasana, Dandasana, Paschimottanasana.

Stabilizing

What needs to be stable: Hip flexors and adductors. Extended leg: internal rotators, knee extensors, foot dorsiflexors. Folded leg: internal rotators, knee flexors. Abdominals, back extensors, obliques, shoulder depressors and extensors, elbow flexors.

Asanas for stabilizing: Adho Mukha Svanasana, Agnistambhasana, Dandasana, Eka Pada Sirsasana, Prasarita Padottanasana A, Uttana Prasithasana, Uttanasana.

This asana prepares you for:

Akarna Dandasana, Bakasana, Bhujapidasana, Malasana, Tittibhasana, Eka Pada Sirsasana, Tiriang Mukha Eka Pada Paschimottanasana.

Counterposes

Apanasana, Supta Baddha Konasana, Supta Parivartanasana, Ananda Balasana.

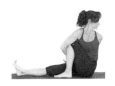

Marichyasana C
Sage Marichi's Pose C

Identifying Preparatory Asanas

Opening

What needs to be open: Grounded leg: calf, knee flexors. Gesture leg: knee extensors, external rotators. Hip extensors, back extensors, obliques, chest, shoulder retractors and elevators, throat.

Asanas for opening: Marichyasana A and its Prep poses, Ardha Matsyendrasana.

Stabilizing

What needs to be stable: Hip flexors and adductors. Extended leg: internal rotators, knee extensors, foot dorsiflexors. Folded leg: hip abductors, knee flexors. Abdominals, back extensors, obliques, shoulder depressors and extensors, elbow flexors.

Asanas for stabilizing: Adho Mukha Svanasana, Ardha Matsyendrasana, Ardha Uttanasana, Dandasana, Parivrtta Hasta Padangusthasana, Parivrtta Parsvakonasana, Parivrtta Utkatasana, Uttana Prasithasana.

This asana prepares you for:

Ardha Matsyendrasana, Bharadvajrasana B, Parsva Bakasana, Eka Pada Koundinyasana B.

Counterposes

Symmetrical forward bends, Baddha Konasana, Upavista Konasana, Supta Baddha Konasana.

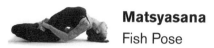

Matsyasana
Fish Pose

Identifying Preparatory Asanas
Opening

What needs to be open: Knee extensors, hip adductors and extensors, internal rotators of the leg. Abdominals, chest, shoulder flexors, throat.

Asanas for opening: Padmasana and its Prep poses, Setu Bandha Sarvangasana, Uttana Padasana.

Stabilizing

What needs to be stable: Hip flexors, adductors, internal rotators of the leg, knee extensors, foot dorsiflexors, back extensors, transversus abdominis, shoulder retractors and extensors, elbow extensors, neck.

Asanas for stabilizing: Adho Mukha Svanasana, Anjaneyasana, Ardha Uttanasana, Ashta Chandrasana, Dandasana, Dhanurasana, Navasana, Salabhasana A and C, Supta Virasana, Urdhva Mukha Svanasana, Ustrasana.

This asana prepares you for:

Transition to Uttana Padasana, Chakorasana.

Counterposes

Apanasana, Ananda Balasana, Savasana.

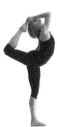

Natarajasana
King Dancer Pose

Identifying Preparatory Asanas
Opening

What needs to be open: Standing leg: knee flexors. Gesture leg: hip flexors, external rotators, foot dorsiflexors. Abdominals, chest, shoulder extensors and elevators, throat.

Asanas for opening: Adho Mukha Svanasana, Anjaneyasana, Eka Pada Raj Kapotasana II, Gomukhasana, Shishulasana, Supta Virasana, Tadasana, Urdhva Dhanurasana, Utthita Hasta Padangusthasana, Virabhadrasana I and III.

Stabilizing

What needs to be stable: Standing leg: intrinsic foot muscles, knee extensors. Pelvic floor, back extensors, transversus abdominis, hip stabilizers (emphasis flexors, adductors, and rear leg hip extensors), internal rotators of the leg, shoulder flexors, protractors. Bound arm: internal rotators, elbow extensors.

Asanas for stabilizing: Adho Mukha Svanasana, Anjaneyasana, Ardha Uttanasana, Ashta Chandrasana, Bhujangasana, Bhekasana, Dhanurasana, Eka Pada Raj Kapotasana I and II, Laghu Vajrasana, Raj Kapotasana, Salabhasana A, B, and C, Urdhva Mukha Svanasana, Virabhadrasana III, Vrksasana.

This asana prepares you for:

Drop Backs, Eka Pada Raj Kapotasana.

Counterposes

Ardha Uttanasana, Apanasana, Supta Parivartanasana, simple twists, Paschimottanasana, Viparita Karani, Salamba Sarvangasana, Savasana.

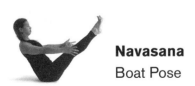

Navasana
Boat Pose

Identifying Preparatory Asanas

Opening

What needs to be open: Hip extensors, knee flexors, back extensors, chest, shoulder retractors and elevators.

Asanas for opening: Adho Mukha Svanasana, Ardha Uttanasana,

Bidalasana, Chaturanga Dandasana, Dandasana, Supta Padangusthasana, Uttanasana.

Stabilizing

What needs to be stable: Hip flexors, adductors, internal rotators of the leg, knee extensors, calves, back extensors, transversus abdominis, shoulder protractors and retractors, external rotators of the arm.

Asanas for stabilizing: Adho Mukha Svanasana, Ardha Uttanasana, Bidalasana, Dandasana, Supta Padangusthasana, Uttanasana, Utthita Hasta Padangusthasana I, Yogic Bicycles.

This asana prepares you for:

Transition to Ardha Navasana with kapalabhati pranayama, then back up; press into Lolasana between rounds; Tolasana, Ubhaya Padangusthasana, Urdhva Mukha Paschimottanasana.

Counterposes

Simple twists, Setu Bandha Sarvangasana, Apanasana, Balasana, Supta Baddha Konasana, Supta Konasana, Adho Mukha Svanasana.

Pada Hastasana
Hand to Foot Pose

Identifying Preparatory Asanas

Opening

What needs to be open: Calves, knee flexors, hip extensors, back extensors, shoulder elevators, wrist extensors.

Asanas for opening: Padangusthasana and its Prep poses.

Stabilizing

What needs to be stable: Hip flexors, internal rotators of the leg, rotators, knee extensors, intrinsic foot muscles, transversus abdominis, back extensors, shoulder depressors.

Asanas for stabilizing: Adho Mukha Svanasana, Ardha Uttanasana,

Bidalasana, Prasarita Padottanasana D, Supta Padangusthasana, Uttanasana.

This asana prepares you for:

Padangusthasana, Paschimottanasana, Supta Padangusthasana, Upavista Konasana, Utthita Hasta Padangusthasana.

Counterposes

Tadasana, Adho Mukha Svanasana, Balasana, simple twists.

Padangusthasana
Big Toe Pose

Identifying Preparatory Asanas

Opening

What needs to be open: Calves, knee flexors, hip extensors, back extensors, shoulder elevators.

Asanas for opening: Tadasana, Uttanasana.

Stabilizing

What needs to be stable: Hip flexors, internal rotators of the leg, knee extensors, intrinsic foot muscles, transversus abdominis, back extensors, shoulder depressors.

Asanas for stabilizing: Adho Mukha Svanasana, Ardha Uttanasana, Bidalasana, Prasarita Padottanasana D, Supta Padangusthasana, Uttanasana.

This asana prepares you for:

Pada Hastasana, Paschimottanasana, Supta Padangusthasana, Upavista Konasana, Utthita Hasta Padangusthasana.

Counterposes

Tadasana, Adho Mukha Svanasana, Balasana, simple twists.

Padmasana
Lotus Pose

Identifying Preparatory Asanas

Opening

What needs to be open: Hip adductors and extensors, internal rotators of the leg, knee extensors.

Asanas for opening: Baddha Konasana, Dandasana, Eka Pada Raj Kapotasana I and its Prep poses, Gomukhasana, Sukhasana, Virasana.

Stabilizing

What needs to be stable: Hip flexors, external rotators of the leg, pelvic floor, transversus abdominis, back extensors, knee flexors, shoulder retractors and protractors.

Asanas for stabilizing: Agnistambhasana, Ardha Baddha Padmottanasana, Baddha Konasana, Bharadvajrasana A and B, Gomukhasana, Malasana, Prasarita Padottanasana, Upavista Konasana, Uttanasana.

This asana prepares you for:

Tolasana, Matsyasana, Urdhva Padmasana, Urdhva Kukkutasana, yoga mudra.

Counterposes

Dandasana, Supta Padangusthasana, Adho Mukha Svanasana.

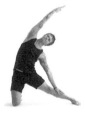

Parighasana
Gate Pose

Identifying Preparatory Asanas

Opening

What needs to be open: Extended leg: hip adductors, knee flexors. Virasana leg: hip extensors, knee extensors. Virasana side of torso:

abdominals, ribs, obliques, shoulder extensors and elevators.

Asanas for opening: Baddha Konasana, Janu Sirsasana, Supta Padangusthasana, Upavista Konasana, Utthita Trikonasana, Virasana.

Stabilizing

What needs to be stable: Bent leg: knee synergists. Extended leg: knee extensors. Hip synergists (emphasis adductors, extensors), internal rotators of the leg, abdominals, obliques, shoulder stabilizers (emphasis retractors, protractors). Top arm: external rotators, shoulder extensors, elbow extensors.

Asanas for stabilizing: In itself a prep for side bending and inner thigh stabilization. Anjaneyasana, Ashta Chandrasana, Prasarita Padottanasana, Tadasana, Vasisthasana Prep, Virabhadrasana II.

This asana prepares you for:

Parivrtta Janu Sirsasana, Utthita Trikonasana, Utthita Parsvakonasana.

Counterposes

Symmetrical forward bends, Adho Mukha Svanasana, Balasana.

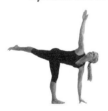

Parivrtta Ardha Chandrasana
Revolved Half Moon Pose

Identifying Preparatory Asanas

Opening

What needs to be open: Standing leg: calf, knee flexors, hip extensors, external rotators of the leg. Gesture leg: foot dorsiflexors, knee flexors, hip flexors. Obliques, chest, shoulder retractors and elevators.

Asanas for opening: Parivrtta Trikonasana and its Prep poses, Virabhadrasana III and its Prep poses.

Stabilizing

What needs to be stable: Standing leg: intrinsic foot muscles, hip stabilizers (emphasis flexors, adductors). Extended leg: hip extensors. Knee extensors, back extensors, transversus abdominis, obliques, shoulder retractors and protractors, elbow extensors, neck.

Asanas for stabilizing: Adho Mukha Svanasana, Ardha Uttanasana, Ashta Chandrasana, Parivrtta Hasta Padangusthasana, Parivrtta Parsvakonasana, Parivrtta Trikonasana, Parivrtta Utkatasana, Parsvottanasana, Utthita Hasta Padangusthasana I, Virabhadrasana III, Vrksasana.

This asana prepares you for:

Clasp lifted-side foot with lifted hand, transition to Virabhadrasana III, Adho Mukha Vrksasana, then Chaturanga Dandasana. Do not transition directly to Ardha Chandrasana.

Counterposes

Uttanasana, Adho Mukha Svanasana, Balasana, Gomukhasana.

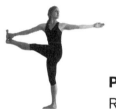

Parivrtta Hasta Padangusthasana
Revolved Hand to Big Toe Pose

Identifying Preparatory Asanas

Opening

What needs to be open: Standing leg: calf, knee flexors, hip flexors. Gesture leg: calf, knee flexors, hip extensors, external rotators of the leg. Obliques, chest, shoulder retractors and elevators.

Asanas for opening: Parivrtta Trikonasana and its Prep poses, Utthita Hasta Padangusthasana and its Prep poses, Virabhadrasana III and its Prep poses.

Stabilizing

What needs to be stable: Standing leg: intrinsic foot muscles. Hip stabilizers, knee extensors, (emphasis adductors, internal rotators of the leg). Extended leg: hip flexors. Back extensors, transversus abdominis, obliques, shoulder retractors, protractors, and abductors, internal rotators of Hasta Pada arm, elbow extensors.

Asanas for stabilizing: Adho Mukha Svanasana, Ardha Uttanasana, Ashta Chandrasana, Dandasana, Parivrtta Parsvakonasana, Parivrtta Trikonasana, Parivrtta Utkatasana, Parsvottanasana, Virabhadrasana III, Vrksasana.

This asana prepares you for:

Transition to Utthita Hasta Padangusthasana, Virabhadrasana III, Adho Mukha Vrksasana, then Chaturanga Dandasana.

Counterposes

Uttanasana, Adho Mukha Svanasana, Balasana, Gomukhasana.

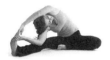 **Parivrtta Janu Sirsasana**
Revolved Head to Knee Pose

Identifying Preparatory Asanas

Opening

What needs to be open: Extended leg: calf, knee flexors. Folded leg: knee extensors. Hip extensors and adductors, internal rotators of the leg. Folded leg side of torso: obliques, ribs, abdominals, back extensors, shoulder extensors and elevators.

Asanas for opening: Baddha Konasana, Janu Sirsasana, Upavista Konasana, Utthita Parsvakonasana, Vrksasana.

Stabilizing

What needs to be stable: Hip flexors. Extended leg: rotators, knee extensors, foot dorsiflexors. Folded leg: external rotators, knee flexors. Transversus abdominis, back extensors, obliques, shoulder retractors and protractors, top shoulder adductors, bottom shoulder abductors.

Asanas for stabilizing: Adho Mukha Svanasana, Agnistambhasana, Ardha Baddha Padmottanasana.

This asana prepares you for:

Upavista Konasana, Baddha Konasana, Kurmasana.

Counterposes

Symmetrical forward bends, Supta Baddha Konasana, Apanasana.

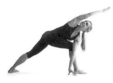

Parivrtta Parsvakonasana
Revolved Extended Side Angle Pose

Identifying Preparatory Asanas

Opening

What needs to be open: Front leg: calf, hip extensors, external rotators of the leg. Back leg: calf, knee flexors, hip flexors. Obliques, chest. Gesture arm: shoulder flexors. Grounded arm: shoulder elevators.

Asanas for opening: Anjaneyasana, Ashta Chandrasana, Gomukhasana, Parivrtta Trikonasana, Parivrtta Utkatasana, Virabhadrasana I.

Stabilizing

What needs to be stable: Intrinsic foot muscles. Front leg: hip stabilizers (emphasis flexors, adductors), knee flexors. Back leg: hip extensors, knee extensors, back extensors, transversus abdominis, obliques, shoulder retractors and protractors, neck.

Asanas for stabilizing: Adho Mukha Svanasana, Anjaneyasana, Ardha Matsyendrasana, Ashta Chandrasana, Marichyasana C, Parivrtta Hasta Padangusthasana, Parivrtta Utkatasana, Uttana Prasithasana, Virabhadrasana I and III.

This asana prepares you for:

Transition to Eka Pada Koundinyasana B, hold five breaths, then Chaturanga Dandasana; Bharadvajrasana, Marichyasana C.

Counterposes

Vinyasa series, Urdhva Mukha Svanasana, Adho Mukha Svanasana, Balasana, Supta Baddha Konasana.

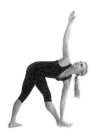

Parivrtta Trikonasana
Revolved Triangle Pose

Identifying Preparatory Asanas

Opening

What needs to be open: Front leg: calf, knee extensors, hip adductors and extensors, internal rotators of the leg. Back leg: calf, knee flexors, hip abductors and flexors, internal rotators of the leg. Obliques, chest, shoulder retractors and elevators, neck.

Asanas for opening: Parivrtta Ashta Chandrasana, Parivrtta Utkatasana, Parsvottanasana, Prasarita Padottanasana, Utthita Trikonasana.

Stabilizing

What needs to be stable: Intrinsic foot muscles. Front leg: hip stabilizers (emphasis flexors, adductors), knee extensors. Back leg: hip extensors, knee extensors, back extensors, transversus abdominis, obliques, shoulder retractors and protractors, elbow extensors, neck.

Asanas for stabilizing: Adho Mukha Svanasana, Ardha Uttanasana, Ashta Chandrasana, Parivrtta Ardha Chandrasana, Parivrtta Hasta Padangusthasana, Parivrtta Parsvakonasana, Parivrtta Utkatasana, Parsvottanasana, Prasarita Padottanasana.

This asana prepares you for:

Transition to Parivrtta Ardha Chandrasana.

Counterposes

Tadasana, Uttanasana, Vinyasa series, Adho Mukha Svanasana, Balasana, Supta Baddha Konasana, Ardha Matsyendrasana, Marichyasana C.

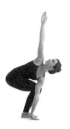

Parivrtta Utkatasana
Revolved Chair Pose

Identifying Preparatory Asanas

Opening

What needs to be open: Hip extensors and abductors, external rotators of the leg. Obliques, chest. Shoulder elevators, back of the neck.

Asanas for opening: Adho Mukha Svanasana, Anjaneyasana, Ardha Uttanasana. In itself a preparatory twist; may be modified by using a chair.

Stabilizing

What needs to be stable: Intrinsic foot muscles, knee synergists, hip adductors, flexors, and extensors, back extensors, transversus abdominis, shoulder protractors, retractors, and depressors, shoulder extensor of lower arm.

Asanas for stabilizing: Adho Mukha Svanasana, Anjaneyasana, Ashta Chandrasana, Garudasana, Parivrtta Hasta Padangusthasana, Tadasana, Utkatasana, Uttanasana.

This asana prepares you for:

Other twisting poses; Astavakrasana, Eka Pada Koundinyasana A, Parivrtta Ardha Chandrasana, Parivrtta Hasta Padangusthasana, Parivrtta Janu Sirsasana, Parivrtta Parsvakonasana, Parivrtta Trikonasana, Parsva Bakasana.

Counterposes

Adho Mukha Svanasana, Balasana, Uttanasana, Vinyasa series.

Parsva Bakasana
Side Crane Pose

Identifying Preparatory Asanas

Opening

What needs to be open: Wrist flexors, shoulder elevators, obliques, hip extensors.

Asanas for opening: Bakasana, Marichyasana A and C.

Stabilizing

What needs to be stable: Wrist synergists, elbow synergists, rotators of the arm, shoulder stabilizers (emphasis protractors, retractors, flexors), chest, obliques, abdominals, hip flexors, knee flexors, foot dorsiflexors.

Asanas for stabilizing: Adho Mukha Svanasana, Anjaneyasana, Ardha Matsyendrasana, Ardha Uttanasana, Ashta Chandrasana, Bakasana, Chaturanga Dandasana, Garudasana, Marichyasana C, Parivrtta Ardha Chandrasana, Parivrtta Parsvakonasana, Parivrtta Trikonasana, Parivrtta Utkatasana, Phalakasana, Utkatasana, Uttana Prasithasana, Uttanasana.

This asana prepares you for:

Transition to Dwi Pada Koundinyasana, Eka Pada Koundinyasana A, then Chaturanga Dandasana; as part of Salamba Sirsasana II vinyasa.

Counterposes

Wrist therapy, Balasana, Supta Baddha Konasana, Uttanasana, Viparita Karani.

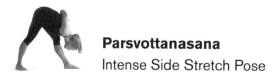

Parsvottanasana

Intense Side Stretch Pose

Identifying Preparatory Asanas

Opening

What needs to be open: Knee flexors, hip extensors, internal rotators of the leg, back extensors, chest, external rotators of the arm, shoulder flexors and elevators, wrist flexors.

Asanas for opening: Adho Mukha Svanasana, Ardha Uttanasana, Gomukhasana, Prasarita Padottanasana, Uttanasana, Utthita Trikonasana.

Stabilizing

What needs to be stable: Intrinsic foot muscles. Front leg: hip stabilizers (emphasis flexors, adductors), knee extensors. Back leg: hip extensors, knee extensors, back extensors, abdominals, obliques, shoulder retractors and protractors, internal rotators of the arm, elbow flexors.

Asanas for stabilizing: Adho Mukha Svanasana, Ardha Uttanasana, Ashta Chandrasana, Parivrtta Ardha Chandrasana, Parivrtta Parsvakonasana, Paschimottanasana, Prasarita Padottanasana C, Supta Padangusthasana.

This asana prepares you for:

Transition to Parivrtta Trikonasana and Prep poses for Hanumanasana, Virabhadrasana I and III.

Counterposes

Tadasana, Balasana, Apanasana, Supta Baddha Konasana, Supta Padangusthasana.

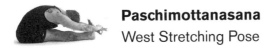

Paschimottanasana
West Stretching Pose

Identifying Preparatory Asanas

Opening

What needs to be open: Calves, knee flexors, hip extensors, back extensors, shoulder retractors and elevators, chest, shoulder extensors.

Asanas for opening: Adho Mukha Svanasana, Balasana, Dandasana, Janu Sirsasana, Supta Padangusthasana.

Stabilizing

What needs to be stable: Hip flexors, internal rotators of the leg, knee extensors, foot dorsiflexors, transversus abdominis, back extensors, shoulder depressors.

Asanas for stabilizing: Adho Mukha Svanasana, Agnistambhasana, Ardha Uttanasana, Balasana, Dandasana, Halasana, Karnapidasana, Pada Hastasana, Padangusthasana, Parsvottanasana, Prasarita Padottanasana D, Supta Padangusthasana, Upavista Konasana, Uttanasana.

This asana prepares you for:

Transition to Halasana, Salamba Sarvangasana, Karnapidasana; Upavista Konasana, Tiriang Mukha Eka Pada Paschimottanasana, Krounchasana, Kurmasana, Ubhaya Padangusthasana, Urdhva Mukha Paschimottanasana.

Counterposes

Simple seated and supine twists, Supta Baddha Konasana, Apanasana, Savasana.

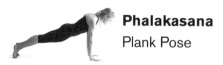

Phalakasana
Plank Pose

Identifying Preparatory Asanas

Opening

What needs to be open: Calves, hip flexors, shoulder elevators and retractors, wrist flexors.

Asanas for opening: Adho Mukha Svanasana, Bidalasana, ashtanga pranam sequence.

Stabilizing

What needs to be stable: Foot dorsiflexors, knee extensors, hip adductors and flexors, internal rotators of the leg, abdominals, chest, external rotators of the arm, shoulder stabilizers (emphasis depressors, protractors), elbow extensors, wrist flexors.

Asanas for stabilizing: Adho Mukha Svanasana, Ardha Uttanasana, Bhujangasana, Shishulasana, Tadasana.

This asana prepares you for:

Transition to Chaturanga Dandasana; press back to Adho Mukha Svanasana; transition to Vasisthasana; lower to Shishula Phalakasana, and do kapalabhati pranayama.

Counterposes

Adho Mukha Svanasana, Balasana, wrist therapy.

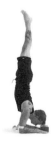

Pincha Mayurasana
Feathered Peacock Pose

Identifying Preparatory Asanas

Opening

What needs to be open: Internal rotators of the arm, shoulder elevators and retractors, hip flexors, knee flexors.

Asanas for opening: Adho Mukha Svanasana, Adho Mukha Vrksasana, Anjaneyasana, Gomukhasana arms, Shishulasana, Supta Virasana, Virabhadrasana I.

Stabilizing

What needs to be stable: Wrist flexor/extensors, elbow flexors, shoulder stabilizers (emphasis protractors, flexors), internal rotators of the arm, abdominals, back extensors, hip stabilizers, internal rotators of the leg, knee extensors, calves.

Asanas for stabilizing: Adho Mukha Svanasana, Adho Mukha Vrksasana, Anjaneyasana, Ashta Chandrasana, Bhujangasana, Chaturanga Dandasana, Dandasana, Garudasana, Phalakasana, Pursvottanasana, Salabhasana A and C, Salamba Sirsasana I, Shishulasana.

This asana prepares you for:

Vrschikasana, Adho Mukha Vrksasana, transition to Viparita Dandasana (feet all the way down to the floor, extend legs).

Counterposes

Balasana, Garudasana arms, simple or supine twists.

Pindasana
Embryo Pose

Identifying Preparatory Asanas

Opening

What needs to be open: Hip adductors and extensors, internal rotators of the leg, back extensors, shoulder retractors and elevators.

Asanas for opening: Urdhva Padmasana and its Prep poses.

Stabilizing

What needs to be stable: Shoulder stabilizers (emphasis retractors, adductors), back extensors, hip extensors, abdominals.

Asanas for stabilizing: Adho Mukha Svanasana, Ardha Baddha Padmottanasana, Baddha Konasana, Bhujapidasana, Garbha Pindasana, Halasana, Karnapidasana, Kurmasana, Marichyasana A, Padmasana, Paschimottanasana, Salamba Sarvangasana, Upavista Konasana, Urdhva Padmasana, Uttanasana.

This asana prepares you for:

Transition to Matsyasana, to Uttana Padasana, to Chakorasana.

Counterposes

Matsyasana Prep, Uttana Padasana, Savasana.

Prasarita Padottanasana A
Spread-Leg Forward Fold Pose A

Identifying Preparatory Asanas

Opening

What needs to be open: All variations: hip adductors and extensors, back extensors, shoulder elevators. C: shoulder flexors, elbow flexors.
Asanas for opening: Adho Mukha Svanasana, Supta Baddha Konasana, Supta Padangusthasana, Uttanasana, Utthita Trikonasana.

Stabilizing

What needs to be stable: Intrinsic foot muscles, knee extensors, hip stabilizers (emphasis flexors, adductors), transversus abdominis, back extensors, shoulder depressors. C: shoulder flexors.
Asanas for stabilizing: Adho Mukha Svanasana, Anjaneyasana Ardha Uttanasana, Ashta Chandrasana, Baddha Konasana, Dandasana, Malasana, Parsvottanasana, Uttana Prasithasana, Uttanasana, Utthita Parsvakonasana, Utthita Trikonasana, Virabhadrasana I and II.

This asana prepares you for:

Uttanasana, Salamba Sirsasana I, transition to Sirsasana II arm balance vinyasa, Upavista Konasana, Bakasana.

Counterposes

Malasana, Uttanasana, Adho Mukha Svanasana, Balasana.

Prasarita Padottanasana B
Spread-Leg Forward Fold Pose B

Identifying Preparatory Asanas

Opening

What needs to be open: All variations: hip adductors and extensors, back extensors, shoulder elevators. C: shoulder flexors, elbow flexors.
Asanas for opening: Adho Mukha Svanasana, Supta Baddha Konasana, Supta Padangusthasana, Uttanasana, Utthita Trikonasana.

Stabilizing

What needs to be stable: Intrinsic foot muscles, knee extensors, hip stabilizers (emphasis flexors, adductors), transversus abdominis, back extensors, shoulder depressors. C: shoulder flexors.
Asanas for stabilizing: Adho Mukha Svanasana, Anjaneyasana Ardha Uttanasana, Ashta Chandrasana, Baddha Konasana, Dandasana, Malasana, Parsvottanasana, Uttana Prasithasana, Uttanasana, Utthita Parsvakonasana, Utthita Trikonasana, Virabhadrasana I and II.

This asana prepares you for:

Uttanasana, Upavista Konasana, Bakasana.

Counterposes

Malasana, Uttanasana, Adho Mukha Svanasana, Balasana.

Prasarita Padottanasana C
Spread-Leg Forward Fold Pose C

Identifying Preparatory Asanas

Opening

What needs to be open: All variations: hip adductors and extensors, back extensors, shoulder elevators. C: shoulder flexors, elbow flexors.

Asanas for opening: Adho Mukha Svanasana, Supta Baddha Konasana, Supta Padangusthasana, Uttanasana, Utthita Trikonasana.

Stabilizing

What needs to be stable: intrinsic foot muscles, knee extensors, hip stabilizers (emphasis flexors, adductors), transversus abdominis, back extensors, shoulder depressors. C: shoulder flexors.

Asanas for stabilizing: Adho Mukha Svanasana, Anjaneyasana Ardha Uttanasana, Ashta Chandrasana, Baddha Konasana, Dandasana, Malasana, Parsvottanasana, Uttana Prasithasana, Uttanasana, Utthita Parsvakonasana, Utthita Trikonasana, Virabhadrasana I and II.

This asana prepares you for:

Bakasana, Pursvottanasana, Setu Bandha Sarvangasana, Salamba Sarvangasana.

Counterposes

Malasana, Garudasana, Uttanasana, Adho Mukha Svanasana, Balasana.

Prasarita Padottanasana D
Spread-Leg Forward Fold Pose D

Identifying Preparatory Asanas

Opening

What needs to be open: All variations: hip adductors and extensors, back extensors, shoulder elevators. C: shoulder flexors, elbow flexors.

Asanas for opening: Adho Mukha Svanasana, Supta Baddha Konasana, Supta Padangusthasana, Uttanasana, Utthita Trikonasana.

Stabilizing

What needs to be stable: Intrinsic foot muscles, knee extensors, hip stabilizers (emphasis flexors, adductors), transversus abdominis, back extensors, shoulder depressors. C: shoulder flexors.

Asanas for stabilizing: Adho Mukha Svanasana, Anjaneyasana Ardha Uttanasana, Ashta Chandrasana, Baddha Konasana, Dandasana, Malasana, Pada Hastasana, Padangusthasana, Parsvottanasana, Uttana Prasithasana, Uttanasana, Utthita Parsvakonasana, Utthita Trikonasana, Virabhadrasana I and II.

This asana prepares you for:

Bakasana, Uttanasana, Upavista Konasana.

Counterposes

Malasana, Uttanasana, Adho Mukha Svanasana, Balasana.

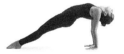

Pursvottanasana
Upward-Facing Plank Pose or East Intense Stretch Pose

Identifying Preparatory Asanas

Opening

What needs to be open: Foot dorsiflexors, hip flexors, abdominals, chest, shoulder flexors and elevators, throat.

Asanas for opening: Anjaneyasana, Prasarita Padottanasana C, Setu Bandha Sarvangasana, Ustrasana, Virasana.

Stabilizing

What needs to be stable: Wrist synergists, internal rotators of the arm, shoulder stabilizers (emphasis retractors, depressors), throat, back extensors, transversus abdominis, hip extensors and adductors, calves.

Asanas for stabilizing: Adho Mukha Svanasana, Ardha Uttanasana,

Chaturanga Dandasana, Dandasana, Matsyasana, Navasana, Phalakasana, Salabhasana A and C, Salamba Sarvangasana, Setu Bandha Sarvangasana, Supta Virasana, Tadasana, Urdhva Dhanurasana, Urdhva Mukha Svanasana, Ustrasana, Vasisthasana.

Counterposes

Adho Mukha Svanasana, wrist therapy, Balasana, Supta Parivartanasana, seated forward bends.

 Kapotasana
Pigeon Pose

Identifying Preparatory Asanas

Opening

What needs to be open: Knee flexors, hip flexors, foot dorsiflexors, abdominals, chest, shoulder elevators and flexors, upper back muscles, wrist flexors.

Asanas for opening: Bhujangasana, Dhanurasana, Laghu Vajrasana, Naraviralasana, Salabhasana A, B, and C, Urdhva Mukha Svanasana, Ustrasana.

Stabilizing

What needs to be stable: Wrist synergists, elbow flexors, external rotators of the arm, chest, shoulder stabilizers (emphasis adductors, protractors, and retractors), neck, transversus abdominis, back extensors, hip adductors and flexors, knee flexors, calves.

Asanas for stabilizing: Anjaneyasana, Ashta Chandrasana, Bhekasana, Bhujangasana, Bidalasana, Dhanurasana, Eka Pada Raj Kapotasana II, Setu Bandha Sarvangasana, Salabhasana B, Supta Virasana, Urdhva Dhanurasana, Urdhva Mukha Svanasana, Ustrasana.

This asana prepares you for:

Eka Pada Raj Kapotasana, Natarajasana.

Counterposes

Prone Savasana, simple twists, vinyasa series, Balasana, Savasana.

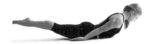 **Salabhasana A, B, C**
Locust Pose

Identifying Preparatory Asanas

Opening

What needs to be open: All: abdominals, hip flexors, knee flexors, foot dorsiflexors, chest, shoulder elevators, neck. A and C: shoulder flexors. B: shoulder extensors.

Asanas for opening: All simple twists, Balasana, Supta Baddha Konasana.

Stabilizing

What needs to be stable: Back extensors, hip extensors and adductors, transversus abdominis, shoulder retractors, neck, knee extensors, foot dorsiflexors. A: shoulder extensors, elbow flexors, wrist synergists. B: Shoulder flexors, external rotators of the arm, elbow extensors. C: Shoulder extensors and adductors, wrist synergists.

Asanas for stabilizing: Bidalasana. The Salabhasana poses are themselves prep for general practice and all back bends.

This asana prepares you for:

Transition through A, B, and C, Dhanurasana, Bhekasana, Bhujangasana, Setu Bandha Sarvangasana.

Counterposes

Balasana, simple twists, Supta Baddha Konasana, seated forward bends.

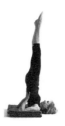

Salamba Sarvangasana
Supported Shoulder Stand

Identifying Preparatory Asanas
Opening

What needs to be open: Neck, chest, shoulder flexors, back extensors, hip flexors.

Asanas for opening: Anjaneyasana, Halasana, Prasarita Padottanasana C, Setu Bandha Sarvangasana, Viparita Karani, Virasana.

Stabilizing

What needs to be stable: Shoulder stabilizers (emphasis retractors, adductors, extensors), elbow flexors, wrist flexors, back extensors, hip extensors and adductors, internal rotators of the leg, knee extensors, foot dorsiflexors.

Asanas for stabilizing: Adho Mukha Svanasana, Ardha Uttanasana, Bidalasana, Prasarita Padottanasana C arms, Phalakasana, Pursvottanasana, Setu Bandha Sarvangasana, Tadasana, Uttanasana.

This asana prepares you for:

Urdhva Padmasana, transition one leg at a time to Setu Bandha Sarvangasana, Chakorasana.

Counterposes

Balasana, Halasana, neck therapy, Savasana, Matsyasana Prep, Uttana Padasana.

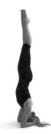

Salamba Sirsasana I
Supported Headstand I

Identifying Preparatory Asanas
Opening

What needs to be open: Shoulder extensors and retractors.

Asanas for opening: Adho Mukha Svanasana, Pincha Mayurasana, Phalakasana, Salamba Sirsasana II, Shishulasana, Uttanasana; abdominal core work.

Stabilizing

What needs to be stable: Elbow synergists, shoulder stabilizers (emphasis flexors, protractors, retractors), neck, obliques, abdominals, back extensors, hip flexors, adductors, and extensors, internal rotators of the leg, knee extensors.

Asanas for stabilizing: Adho Mukha Svanasana, Adho Mukha Vrksasana, Ardha Uttanasana, Ashta Chandrasana, Chaturanga Dandasana, Navasana, Phalakasana, Shishulasana, Urdhva Dhanurasana, Urdhva Hastasana, Uttanasana.

This asana prepares you for:

Twist to each side; fold legs into Padmasana position, Parsvaikapada Sirsasana, Urdhva Dandasana.

Counterposes

Balasana, Adho Mukha Svanasana: relax neck, let head hang, neck therapy, Salamba Sarvangasana.

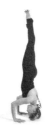

Salamba Sirsasana II
Supported Headstand II

Identifying Preparatory Asanas

Opening

What needs to be open: Shoulder retractors.

Asanas for opening: Prasarita Padottanasana B, Setu Bandha Sarvangasana, Salamba Sirsasana I and its Prep poses.

Stabilizing

What needs to be stable: Wrist synergists, elbow synergists, shoulder stabilizers (emphasis flexors, protractors, retractors), external rotators of the arm, neck, obliques, abdominals, back extensors, hip flexors, adductors, and extensors, internal rotators of the leg, knee extensors.

Asanas for stabilizing: Adho Mukha Svanasana, Adho Mukha Vrksasana, Ardha Uttanasana, Ashta Chandrasana, Bakasana, Chaturanga Dandasana, Navasana, Phalakasana, Prasarita Padottanasana A, Shishulasana, Urdhva Dhanurasana, Urdhva Hastasana, Uttanasana.

This asana prepares you for:

Arm balance vinyasa: Prasarita Padottanasana to Salamba Sirsasana II to Bakasana and back; transition to Chaturanga Dandasana.

Counterposes

Balasana, Adho Mukha Svanasana: relax neck, let head hang, neck nherapy, Salamba Sarvangasana.

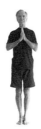

Samastihi
Balanced Standing Pose

Identifying Preparatory Asanas

Opening

What needs to be open: Chest, shoulder elevators, mind.
Asanas for opening: Tadasana.

Stabilizing

What needs to be stable: Intrinsic foot muscles, knee extensors, hip synergists, transversus abdominis, back extensors, shoulder depressors, neck.
Asanas for stabilizing: Bidalasana, Tadasana.

This asana prepares you for:

Standing poses, Utkatasana, Vrksasana.

Counterposes

Uttanasana, Ardha Uttanasana, Adho Mukha Svanasana, Balasana.

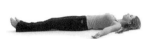

Savasana
Corpse Pose

Identifying Preparatory Asanas

Opening

What needs to be open: Everything.

Asanas for opening: For integration following practice.

Stabilizing

What needs to be stable: The floor—somewhat.

Asanas for stabilizing: Final restorative after any practice.

This asana prepares you for:

Often sequenced as the final pose of the practice; restorative pose, slowly transition up to sitting.

Counterposes

At the end of practice, allow at least five minutes in this asana; practice a shorter hold within an asana practice.

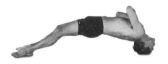

Setu Bandhasana
Supported Bridge Pose

Identifying Preparatory Asanas

Opening

What needs to be open: Foot dorsiflexors, knee flexors, hip flexors, abdominals, chest, shoulder retractors, throat.

Asanas for opening: Matsyasana, Salabhasana A, B, and C, Salamba Sirsasana II, Urdhva Dhanurasana, Urdhva Mukha Svanasana, Viparita Dandasana.

Stabilizing

What needs to be stable: Neck, shoulder protractors, retractors, and adductors, back extensors, transversus abdominis, hip extensors and adductors, internal rotators of the leg, knee extensors, foot dorsiflexors.

Asanas for stabilizing: Anjaneyasana, Ashta Chandrasana, Bhekasana, Bhujangasana, Bidalasana, Dhanurasana, Eka Pada Raj Kapotasana II, Raj Kapotasana, Setu Bandha Sarvangasana, Salabhasana A and C, Salamba Sirsasana I and II, Supta Virasana, Urdhva Dhanurasana, Urdhva Mukha Svanasana, Ustrasana, Viparita Dandasana.

This asana prepares you for:

This is a peak pose!

Counterposes

Adho Mukha Svanasana: relax neck, let head hang, neck therapy, Salamba Sarvangasana, Savasana.

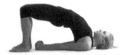 ## Setu Bandha Sarvangasana
Bridge Pose

Identifying Preparatory Asanas

Opening

What needs to be open: Elbow flexors, shoulder flexors and elevators, chest, hip flexors, external rotators of the leg.

Asanas for opening: Bhekasana, Bhujangasana, Dhanurasana, Salabhasana A, C, Setu Bandha Sarvangasana, Supta Virasana, Urdhva Mukha Svanasana, Ustrasana.

Stabilizing

What needs to be stable: Shoulder stabilizers (emphasis retractors, adductors, extensors), back extensors, hip extensors and adductors, internal rotators of the leg, intrinsic foot muscles.

Asanas for stabilizing: Bhujangasana, Dhanurasana, Eka Pada Raj Kapotasana I, Salamba Sarvangasana, Setu Bandha Sarvangasana, Supta Virasana, Urdhva Mukha Svanasana, Ustrasana.

This asana prepares you for:

Deeper back bends, such as Urdhva Dhanurasana, Bhujangasana, Eka Pada variation, transition up to Salamba Sarvangasana.

Counterposes

Apanasana, simple twists, Supta Baddha Konasana, Ananda Balasana, Balasana, seated forward bends.

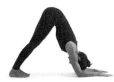

Shishulasana
Dolphin Pose

Identifying Preparatory Asanas

Opening

What needs to be open: Calves, knee flexors, hip extensors, shoulder extensors and retractors, internal rotators of the arm.

Asanas for opening: Anahatasana, Ardha Uttanasana, Bidalasana, Phalakasana, Uttanasana, Anahatasana. For arms and shoulders these respective arm forms: Urdhva Hastasana, Gomukhasana, Garudasana.

Stabilizing

What needs to be stable: Intrinsic foot muscles, internal rotators of the leg, hip flexors and adductors, back extensors, transversus abdominis, shoulder stabilizers (emphasis protractors, flexors), external rotators of the arm, elbow flexors, wrist flexors.

Asanas for stabilizing: Adho Mukha Svanasana, Ardha Uttanasana, Bidalasana, Chaturanga Dandasana, Garudasana, Phalakasana, Uttanasana.

This asana prepares you for:

Other back bends, such as Bhujangasana, Bhekasana, Dhanurasana, Kapotasana, Laghu Vajrasana, Raj Kapotasana, Urdhva Dhanurasana.

Counterposes

Balasana, seated forward bends, simple twists, Supta Baddha Konasana.

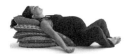

Supta Baddha Konasana
Reclined Bound Angle Pose

Identifying Preparatory Asanas

Opening

What needs to be open: Hip adductors, internal rotators of the leg, abdominals, chest.

Asanas for opening: Baddha Konasana and its Prep poses, Supta Padangusthasana, Supta Virasana, Utthita Trikonasana, Virabhadrasana II.

Stabilizing

What needs to be stable: The strap and bolster.

Asanas for stabilizing: In itself a restorative that can be practiced independently or after any practice.

This asana prepares you for:

Practice with a block under the sacrum or along the spine between shoulder blades; place sandbags on the thighs, or bolster along the spine.

Counterposes

Apanasana, Ananda Balasana, Supta Parivartanasana, Viparita Karani, Savasana.

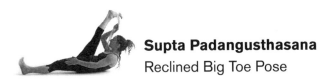

Supta Padangusthasana
Reclined Big Toe Pose

Identifying Preparatory Asanas

Opening

What needs to be open: Grounded leg: foot dorsiflexors, knee flexors, hip flexors. Gesture leg: hip extensors, knee flexors. Back extensors, shoulder elevators, neck.

Asanas for opening: Adho Mukha Svanasana, Apanasana, Baddha Konasana.

Stabilizing

What needs to be stable: Grounded leg: hip extensors and adductors. Extended leg: hip flexors. Internal rotators of the leg, knee extensors, foot dorsiflexors, obliques, transversus abdominis, shoulder retractors.

Asanas for stabilizing: In itself a preparation and restorative for opening hip extensors and calves. Adho Mukha Svanasana, Dandasana, Tadasana, Uttana Prasithasana.

This asana prepares you for:

Supta Konasana, Upavista Konasana, Kurmasana, Ubhaya Padangusthasana, Urdhva Mukha Paschimottanasana, Utthita Hasta Padangusthasana.

Counterposes

Apanasana, Supta Parivartanasana, Viparita Karani, Savasana.

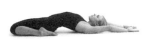

Supta Virasana
Reclined Hero Pose

Identifying Preparatory Asanas

Opening

What needs to be open: Foot dorsiflexors, knee flexors, hip abductors and flexors, abdominals, chest, shoulder extensors.

Asanas for opening: Anjaneyasana, Setu Bandha Sarvangasana, Ustrasana, Virasana.

Stabilizing

What needs to be stable: Hip extensors, internal rotators of the leg, knee flexors, transversus abdominis, shoulder retractors and flexors, elbow extensors.

Asanas for stabilizing: Anjaneyasana, Ashta Chandrasana, Balasana, Bharadvajrasana A and B, Bhekasana, Bhujangasana, Bidalasana, Dhanurasana, Garudasana, Matsyasana, Parivrtta Parsvakonasana, Parivrtta Utkatasana, Raj Kapotasana, Setu Bandha Sarvangasana, Urdhva Mukha Svanasana, Ustrasana, Virasana.

This asana prepares you for:

Laghu Vajrasana, Kapotasana, Raj Kapotasana, curl toes under for Prapada Paryankasana

Counterposes

Bidalasana, Adho Mukha Svanasana, Balasana, Ananda Balasana, simple twists, Supta Baddha Konasana, seated forward bends.

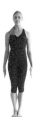

Tadasana
Mountain Pose

Identifying Preparatory Asanas

Opening

What needs to be open: Shoulder elevators.

Asanas for opening: Savasana, Bidalasana.

Stabilizing

What needs to be stable: Intrinsic foot muscles, knee extensors, hip synergists, transversus abdominis, back extensors, shoulder depressors, external rotators of the arm, neck.

Asanas for stabilizing: In itself a prep pose for any practice.

This asana prepares you for:

Vrksasana and other standing asanas, Utkatasana.

Counterposes

Uttanasana, Ardha Uttanasana, Adho Mukha Svanasana, Balasana.

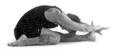 **Tiriang Mukha Eka Pada Paschimottanasana**
Three Limbs Facing One Foot West Stretching Pose

Identifying Preparatory Asanas

Opening

What needs to be open: Virasana leg: foot dorsiflexors, knee extensors. Extended leg: calf, knee flexors. Hip extensors, back extensors, shoulder extensors, retractors, and elevators.

Asanas for opening: Dandasana, Janu Sirsasana, Paschimottanasana, Virasana.

Stabilizing

What needs to be stable: Hip flexors. Extended leg: internal rotators, knee extensors, foot dorsiflexors. Folded leg: internal rotators, knee flexors. Hip adductors, transversus abdominis, back extensors, obliques, shoulder depressors.

Asanas for stabilizing: Adho Mukha Svanasana, Bharadvajrasana A and B, Balasana, Dandasana, Garudasana, Marichyasana A and C, Pada Hastasana, Padangusthasana, Parivrtta Utkatasana, Paschimottanasana, Virasana.

This asana prepares you for:

Krounchasana, Ubhaya Padangusthasana, Urdhva Mukha Paschimottanasana.

Counterposes

Urdhva Mukha Svanasana, Adho Mukha Svanasana, Apanasana, Ananda Balasana, Supta Parivartanasana.

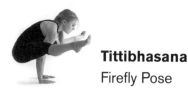

Tittibhasana

Firefly Pose

Identifying Preparatory Asanas

Opening

What needs to be open: Wrist flexors, elbow flexors, shoulder flexors, back extensors, hip adductors and extensors, knee flexors, ankle dorsiflexors.

Asanas for opening: Adho Mukha Svanasana, Baddha Konasana, Bakasana, Bhujapidasana, Garudasana, Malasana, Prasarita Padottanasana A, Upavista Konasana, Utthita Trikonasana.

Stabilizing

What needs to be stable: Wrist synergists, elbow synergists, shoulder stabilizers (emphasis flexors, protractors), external rotators of the arm, chest, abdominals, hip adductors and flexors, pelvic floor, knee extensors, calves.

Asanas for stabilizing: Adho Mukha Svanasana, Bakasana, Balasana, Bidalasana, Chaturanga Dandasana, Eka Pada Koundinyasana B, Kurmasana, Malasana, Marichyasana A, Navasana, Parivrtta Janu Sirsasana, Prasarita Padottanasana A, Salamba Sirsasana II, Upavista Konasana, Urdhva Kukkutasana, Uttana Prasithasana.

This asana prepares you for:

Transition to Bakasana then Chaturanga Dandasana, Bhujapidasana.

Counterposes

Vinyasa series, Urdhva Mukha Svanasana, Adho Mukha Svanasana, wrist therapy, Balasana.

Tolasana
Scales Pose

Identifying Preparatory Asanas

Opening

What needs to be open: Wrist flexors, elbow flexors, shoulder elevators, retractors, and flexors, back extensors, hip adductors and extensors, internal rotators of the leg, knee extensors.

Asanas for opening: Padmasana and its Prep poses, abdominal core work.

Stabilizing

What needs to be stable: Wrist synergists, elbow synergists, shoulder stabilizers (emphasis flexors, protractors), external rotators of the arm, chest, abdominals, hip adductors and flexors, external rotators of the leg, pelvic floor, knee flexors, foot dorsiflexors.

Asanas for stabilizing: Adho Mukha Svanasana, Agnistambhasana, Ardha Baddha Padmottanasana, Baddha Konasana, Bakasana, Chaturanga Dandasana, Malasana, Padmasana, Phalakasana, Urdhva Mukha Svanasana

This asana prepares you for:

Transition to Lolasana or Urdhva Kukkutasana.

Counterposes

Dandasana, Pursvottanasana, Urdhva Mukha Svanasana, Adho Mukha Svanasana, Balasana, wrist therapy.

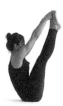

Ubhaya Padangusthasana
Both Big Toes Pose

Identifying Preparatory Asanas

Opening

What needs to be open: Hip extensors, back extensors, shoulder retractors, chest, shoulder elevators, knee flexors, foot dorsiflexors.

Asanas for opening: Adho Mukha Svanasana, Bidalasana, Chaturanga Dandasana, Dandasana, Navasana, Padangusthasana, Parsvottanasana, Phalakasana, Prasarita Padottanasana D, Supta Padangusthasana, Tadasana, Upavista Konasana, Uttanasana, Utthita Hasta Padangusthasana I and II.

Stabilizing

What needs to be stable: Hip flexors, adductors, internal rotators of the leg, knee extensors, foot dorsiflexors, back extensors, abdominals, shoulder protractors and retractors, elbow extensors.

Asanas for stabilizing: Adho Mukha Svanasana, Ardha Uttanasana, Balasana, Dandasana, Marichyasana A, Navasana, Padangusthasana, Parsvottanasana, Prasarita Padottanasana D, Upavista Konasana, Utthita Hasta Padangusthasana I and II.

This asana prepares you for:

Urdhva Mukha Paschimottanasana, transition to Paripurna Navasana and back.

Counterposes

Simple seated and supine twists, Supta Baddha Konasana, Apanasana, Savasana.

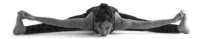

Upavista Konasana
Wide-Angle Forward Fold Pose

Identifying Preparatory Asanas

Opening

What needs to be open: Hip adductors and extensors, internal rotators of the leg, knee flexors, calves, back extensors, chest, elbow flexors.

Asanas for opening: Baddha Konasana, Dandasana, Paschimottanasana, Prasarita Padottanasana A, Supta Padangusthasana, Utthita Trikonasana.

Stabilizing

What needs to be stable: Hip flexors, external rotators of the leg, knee extensors, foot dorsiflexors, transversus abdominis, back extensors, shoulder retractors and adductors.

Asanas for stabilizing: Adho Mukha Svanasana, Agnistambhasana, Ardha Uttanasana, Baddha Konasana, Balasana, Bidalasana, Dandasana, Malasana, Padangusthasana, Paschimottanasana, Prasarita Padottanasana D, Supta Padangusthasana, Uttana Prasithasana, Utthita Hasta Padangusthasana I and II, Utthita Trikonasana, Virabhadrasana II.

This asana prepares you for:

Kurmasana, transition to Tittibhasana and Bhujapidasana, rock back to Supta Konasana, and up again.

Counterposes

Dhanurasana, Marichyasana C, Virasana, Gomukhasana, Adho Mukha Svanasana, Balasana.

Urdhva Dhanurasana
Upward-Facing Bow Pose, Wheel Pose

Identifying Preparatory Asanas

Opening

What needs to be open: Hip flexors, external rotators of the leg, abdominals, chest, shoulder elevators, retractors and extensors, wrist flexors.

Asanas for opening: Bhujangasana, ashtanga pranam, Chaturanga Dandasana, Anjaneyasana, Phalakasana.

Stabilizing

What needs to be stable: Wrist synergists, elbow extensors, external rotators of the arm, shoulder stabilizers (emphasis retractors, protractors, flexors), back extensors, transversus abdominis, hip extensors and adductors, intrinsic foot muscles.

Asanas for stabilizing: Adho Mukha Svanasana, Adho Mukha

Vrksasana, Anjaneyasana, Ashta Chandrasana, Bhujangasana, Bidalasana, Chaturanga Dandasana, Dhanurasana, Garudasana arms, Setu Bandha Sarvangasana, Supta Virasana, Urdhva Mukha Svanasana, Virabhadrasana I.

This asana prepares you for:

Maintaining parallel positioning of the feet, move hands closer to the feet; Eka Pada Urdhva Dhanurasana, Viparita Dandasana, drop-backs, ticktocks.

Counterposes

Apanasana, simple twists, Supta Baddha Konasana, Ananda Balasana, Balasana, seated forward bends.

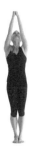

Urdhva Hastasana
Upward Hands Pose

Identifying Preparatory Asanas

Opening

What needs to be open: Abdominal muscles, elbow flexors, hip extensors, shoulder extensors and elevators, chest, elbow flexors.

Asanas for opening: Tadasana; in itself a preparatory for all poses requiring shoulder flexion and external rotation of the arm.

Stabilizing

What needs to be stable: Intrinsic foot muscles, knee extensors, hip synergists, transversus abdominis, back extensors, shoulder depressors and protractors, external rotators of the arm, elbow extensors.

Asanas for stabilizing: Itself a prep pose for all practice requiring shoulder flexion, external rotation of the arm, and elbow extension. Adho Mukha Svanasana, Shishulasana.

This asana prepares you for:

Stretch to one side, then the other; standing back bend with hands on lower back, Surya Namaskara all types.

Counterposes

Tadasana, Uttanasana, Balasana.

Urdhva Kukkutasana
Upward Rooster Pose

Identifying Preparatory Asanas
Opening
What needs to be open: Wrist flexors, elbow flexors, shoulder elevators and retractors, back extensors, hip adductors and extensors, internal rotators of the leg, knee extensors.

Asanas for opening: Bakasana and its Prep poses, Padmasana and its Prep poses, Salamba Sirsasana II.

Stabilizing
What needs to be stable: Wrist synergists, elbow synergists, shoulder stabilizers (emphasis flexors, protractors), external rotators of the arm, chest abdominals, hip adductors and flexors, pelvic floor, knee flexors, foot dorsiflexors.

Asanas for stabilizing: Adho Mukha Svanasana, Agnistambhasana, Ardha Baddha Padmottanasana, Bakasana, Bhujapidasana, Chaturanga Dandasana, Janu Sirsasana, Kurmasana, Lolasana, Malasana, Prasarita Padottanasana A, Tittibhasana, Tolasana, Uttana Prasithasana.

This asana prepares you for:

Add to Salamba Sirsasana I vinyasa; transition into asana from Adho Mukha Vrksasana.

Counterposes

Vinyasa series, Balasana, Supta Baddha Konasana, wrist therapy.

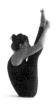

Urdhva Mukha Paschimottanasana
Upward-Facing West Intense Stretch Pose

Identifying Preparatory Asanas

Opening

What needs to be open: Hip extensors, back extensors, shoulder retractors, chest, shoulder elevators, knee flexors, foot dorsiflexors.

Asanas for opening: Adho Mukha Svanasana, Bidalasana, Chaturanga Dandasana, Dandasana, Navasana, Pada Hastasana, Padangusthasana, Parsvottanasana, Phalakasana, Prasarita Padottanasana D, Supta Padangusthasana, Tadasana, Upavista Konasana, Uttanasana, Utthita Hasta Padangusthasana I and II.

Stabilizing

What needs to be stable: Hip flexors, adductors, internal rotators of the leg, knee extensors, calves, back extensors, abdominals, shoulder protractors and retractors, elbow extensors.

Asanas for stabilizing: Adho Mukha Svanasana, Ardha Uttanasana, Balasana, Dandasana, Marichyasana A, Navasana, Padangusthasana, Parsvottanasana, Prasarita Padottanasana D, Paschimottanasana, Upavista Konasana, Utthita Hasta Padangusthasana I and II.

This asana prepares you for:

Transition to Paripurna Navasana and back.

Counterposes

Urdhva Mukha Svanasana, Adho Mukha Svanasana, Apanasana, Ananda Balasana, Supta Parivartanasana.

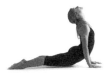

Urdhva Mukha Svanasana
Upward-Facing Dog Pose

Identifying Preparatory Asanas

Opening

What needs to be open: Wrist flexors, elbow flexors, shoulder elevators and retractors, throat, chest, abdominals, hip flexors, knee flexors, calves.

Asanas for opening: Bhujangasana, Chaturanga Dandasana, Naraviralasana, Phalakasana, Salabhasana A and B, Setu Bandha Sarvangasana.

Stabilizing

What needs to be stable: Wrist synergists, elbow synergists, external rotators of the arm, chest, shoulder stabilizers (emphasis adductors, protractors, and retractors), transversus abdominis, back extensors, hip flexors, knee extensors, calves.

Asanas for stabilizing: Adho Mukha Svanasana, Anjaneyasana, Ardha Uttanasana, Ashta Chandrasana, Bhujangasana, Bidalasana, Chaturanga Dandasana, Salabhasana A.

This asana prepares you for:

Bhujangasana, Raj Kapotasana.

Counterposes

Adho Mukha Svanasana, Ardha Matsyendrasana, Apanasana, Balasana.

Urdhva Padmasana
Upward Lotus Pose

Identifying Preparatory Asanas

Opening

What needs to be open: Neck, hip adductors and extensors, internal rotators of the leg, knee extensors.

Asanas for opening: Baddha Konasana, Padmasana and its Prep poses, Salamba Sarvangasana.

Stabilizing

What needs to be stable: Shoulder stabilizers (emphasis retractors, adductors), neck, elbow extensors, back extensors, hip extensors, abdominals.

Asanas for stabilizing: Adho Mukha Svanasana, Ardha Baddha Padmottanasana, Ardha Uttanasana, Baddha Konasana, Halasana, Karnapidasana, Malasana, Padmasana, Paschimottanasana, Phalakasana, Salamba Sarvangasana, Upavista Konasana, Uttanasana.

This asana prepares you for:

In Salamba Sarvangasana: transition to Pindasana, or lift knees up to extend Lotus and revolve to one side, then the other (one hand to sacrum); transition to Mayurasana.

Counterposes

Matsyasana, Uttana Padasana, Supta Parivartanasana, Savasana.

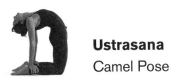

Ustrasana
Camel Pose

Identifying Preparatory Asanas

Opening

What needs to be open: Foot dorsiflexors, knee extensors, abdominals, chest, throat, elbow flexors.

Asanas for opening: Anjaneyasana, Salabhasana, Setu Bandha Sarvangasana, Supta Virasana, Virabhadrasana I.

Stabilizing

What needs to be stable: Knee extensors, hip adductors and extensors, internal rotators of the leg, back extensors, abdominals, shoulder stabilizers (emphasis retractors, extensors), external rotators of the arm, elbow flexors.

Asanas for stabilizing: Anjaneyasana, Ashta Chandrasana, Bhekasana, Bhujangasana, Bidalasana, Dhanurasana, Eka Pada Raj Kapotasana II, Raj Kapotasana, Setu Bandha Sarvangasana, Salabhasana B, Supta Virasana, Urdhva Dhanurasana, Urdhva Mukha Svanasana.

This asana prepares you for:

Pursvottanasana, Laghu Vajrasana, Kapotasana, Urdhva Dhanurasana.

Counterposes

Balasana, simple twists, Supta Baddha Konasana, seated forward bends.

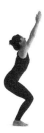

Utkatasana
Chair Pose

Identifying Preparatory Asanas

Opening

What needs to be open: Calves, hip extensors, shoulder elevators, extensors, and retractors.

Asanas for opening: Adho Mukha Svanasana, Salabhasana B, Tadasana, Virasana.

Stabilizing

What needs to be stable: Intrinsic foot muscles, knee flexors, hip flexors and extensors, back extensors, transversus abdominis, shoulder protractors and flexors, internal rotators of the arm, elbow extensors.

Asanas for stabilizing: Adho Mukha Svanasana, Anjaneyasana, Ardha Uttanasana, Ashta Chandrasana, Bidalasana, Tadasana, Uttanasana.

This asana prepares you for:

Parivrtta Utkatasana, Parivrtta Ashta Chandrasana; transition to sitting on the heels.

Counterposes

Uttanasana, Adho Mukha Svanasana, Balasana.

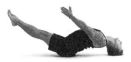

Uttana Padasana
Extended Leg Pose or Flying Fish Pose

Identifying Preparatory Asanas

Opening

What needs to be open: Abdominals, chest, throat, shoulder elevators, knee flexors, foot dorsiflexors.

Asanas for opening: Dandasana, Paripurna Navasana, Setu Bandha Sarvangasana, Virasana.

Stabilizing

What needs to be stable: Hip flexors, adductors, internal rotators of the leg, knee extensors, foot dorsiflexors, back extensors, transversus abdominis, shoulder retractors, protractors, and flexors, elbow extensors, neck.

Asanas for stabilizing: Adho Mukha Svanasana, Anjaneyasana, Ardha Uttanasana, Ashta Chandrasana, Bhujangasana, Bidalasana, Chaturanga Dandasana, Dandasana, Navasana, Salabhasana B, Urdhva Mukha Svanasana, Ustrasana, Utkatasana.

This asana prepares you for:

Setu Bandhasana.

Counterposes

Apanasana, simple twists, Savasana.

Uttana Prasithasana
Flying Lizard Pose

Identifying Preparatory Asanas

Opening

What needs to be open: Wrist flexors, shoulder elevators and flexors, obliques, hip extensors. Folded leg: hip adductors, internal rotators of the leg. Extended leg: knee flexors foot dorsiflexors.

Asanas for opening: Arkarna Dandasana, Astavakrasana, Bakasana, Eka Pada Raj Kapotasana Prep poses, Galavasana, Marichyasana A and C.

Stabilizing

What needs to be stable: Extended leg: hip adductors and extensors, internal rotators of the leg, knee synergists. Folded leg: internal rotators of the leg, knee flexors. Abdominals, transversus abdominis, chest, shoulder stabilizers (emphasis protractors, flexors), external rotators of the arm, elbow synergists, wrist flexors.

Asanas for stabilizing: Anjaneyasana, Ashta Chandrasana, Balasana,

Bidalasana, Phalakasana, Uttanasana, Utthita Parsvakonasana, Virabhadrasana I.

This asana prepares you for:

A peak pose! Transition to Chaturanga Dandasana.

Counterposes

Upavista Konasana, Supta Baddha Konasana, Apanasana, Balasana, wrist therapy.

Uttanasana
Standing Forward Bend Pose

Identifying Preparatory Asanas

Opening

What needs to be open: Calves, knee flexors, hip extensors, back extensors, shoulder elevators.
Asanas for opening: Adho Mukha Svanasana, Ardha Uttanasana, Supta Padangusthasana, Tadasana.

Stabilizing

What needs to be stable: Intrinsic foot muscles, knee extensors, hip flexors and extensors, back extensors, transversus abdominis, shoulder depressors.
Asanas for stabilizing: Adho Mukha Svanasana, Ardha Uttanasana, Balasana, Bidalasana, Prasarita Padottanasana A and B, Tadasana, Utkatasana.

This asana prepares you for:

Padangusthasana, Pada Hastasana, Eka Pada Adho Mukha Vrksasana, Paschimottanasana.

Counterposes

Malasana, Supta Baddha Konasana, Apanasana, Balasana, Savasana.

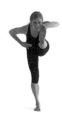

Utthita Hasta Padangusthasana I, II
Extended Hand to Foot Pose

Identifying Preparatory Asanas

Opening

What needs to be open: Standing leg: hip flexors. Gesture leg: hip adductors and extensors, internal rotators of the leg, shoulder retractors, chest, neck.

Asanas for opening: Supta Padangusthasana, Tadasana, Utthita Parsvakonasana, Utthita Trikonasana, Vrksasana.

Stabilizing

What needs to be stable: Standing leg: intrinsic foot muscles. Hip stabilizers, (emphasis adductors, internal rotators of the leg). Extended leg: hip flexors. Knee extensors, back extensors, transversus abdominis, obliques. Hasta arm: shoulder retractors, protractors, elbow extensors.

Asanas for stabilizing: Adho Mukha Svanasana, Anjaneyasana, Ardha Uttanasana, Ashta Chandrasana, Garudasana, Padangusthasana, Parsvottanasana, Paschimottanasana, Prasarita Padottanasana D, Supta Padangusthasana, Tadasana, Ubhaya Padangusthasana, Utkatasana, Virabhadrasana III.

This asana prepares you for:

Draw lifted leg higher without compromising alignment; release clasp of foot, hold lifted leg 5 breaths; Parvritta variation.

Counterposes

Tadasana, Garudasana, vinyasa series, Urdhva Mukha Svanasana, Adho Mukha Svanasana, Balasana.

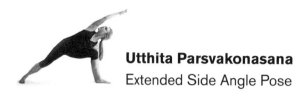

Utthita Parsvakonasana
Extended Side Angle Pose

Identifying Preparatory Asanas

Opening

What needs to be open: Front leg: hip extensors and adductors, internal rotators of the leg. Back leg: knee flexors, hip flexors. Grounded elbow: flexors. Gesture elbow: flexors, shoulder extensors. Abdominals, chest, shoulder elevators.

Asanas for opening: Malasana, Supta Padangusthasana, Tadasana, Urdhva Hastasana, Utthita Trikonasana, Vrksasana.

Stabilizing

What needs to be stable: Intrinsic foot muscles. Front leg: hip stabilizers (emphasis flexors, adductors), external rotators of the leg, knee flexors. Back leg: hip extensors, knee extensors, back extensors, transversus abdominis, obliques, shoulder retractors and protractors. Top arm: external rotators. Bottom arm: wrist synergists. Elbow extensors, neck.

Asanas for stabilizing: Adho Mukha Svanasana, Anjaneyasana, Ardha Uttanasana, Ashta Chandrasana, Parsvottanasana, Prasarita Padottanasana B, Salabhasana B, Virabhadrasana I and II.

This asana prepares you for:

Wrap upper arm behind and lower arm under front leg, clasp wrist of upper arm, transition to Eka Pada Koundinyasana A or Svarga Dvijasana.

Counterposes

Vinyasa series, Urdhva Mukha Svanasana, Adho Mukha Svanasana, Prasarita Padottanasana C, Apanasana, Balasana.

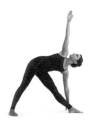

Utthita Trikonasana
Extended Triangle Pose

Identifying Preparatory Asanas

Opening

What needs to be open: Front leg: hip adductors and extensors, internal rotators of the leg, knee flexors. Back leg: hip flexors, knee flexors. Obliques, chest, shoulder elevators and retractors, neck.

Asanas for opening: Adho Mukha Svanasana, Supta Padangusthasana, Tadasana, Virabhadrasana II, Vrksasana.

Stabilizing

What needs to be stable: Intrinsic foot muscles. Front leg: hip stabilizers (emphasis flexors, adductors), external rotators of the leg. Back leg: hip extensors. Knee extensors, back extensors, transversus abdominis, obliques, shoulder abductors, retractors, and protractors, elbow extensors, neck.

Asanas for stabilizing: Adho Mukha Svanasana, Ardha Uttanasana, Ashta Chandrasana, Bidalasana, Prasarita Padottanasana B and D, Utthita Parsvakonasana, Vasisthasana, Virabhadrasana I and II.

This asana prepares you for:

Transition to Ardha Chandrasana, keeping alignment of standing foot and hip.

Counterposes

Tadasana, Adho Mukha Svanasana, Garudasana, Gomukhasana, Balasana.

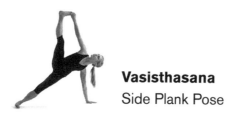

Vasisthasana
Side Plank Pose

Identifying Preparatory Asanas

Opening

What needs to be open: Shoulder elevators and retractors, chest.
Asanas for opening: Adho Mukha Svanasana, Ardha Chandrasana, Phalakasana, Prasarita Padottanasana B and D, Supta Padangusthasana, Utthita Hasta Padangusthasana, Utthita Trikonasana, Vrksasana.

Stabilizing

What needs to be stable: Grounded leg: intrinsic foot muscles. Hip stabilizers, (emphasis abductors, external rotators of the leg). Extended leg: external rotators, hip flexors. Knee extensors, back extensors, transversus abdominis, obliques. Grounded arm: wrist synergists. Top arm: shoulder retractors, protractors, and flexors. Elbow extensors.
Asanas for stabilizing: Adho Mukha Svanasana, Ardha Chandrasana, Ardha Uttanasana, Ashta Chandrasana, Chaturanga Dandasana, Parighasana, Phalakasana, Tadasana, Utthita Parsvakonasana, Utthita Trikonasana, Virabhadrasana II.

This asana prepares you for:

Transition to Visvamitrasana or Eka Pada Koundinyasana A.

Counterposes

Vinyasa series, Urdhva Mukha Svanasana, Adho Mukha Svanasana, Gomukhasana, wrist therapy, Balasana.

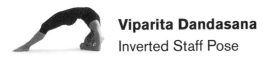 **Viparita Dandasana**
Inverted Staff Pose

Identifying Preparatory Asanas

Opening

What needs to be open: Shoulder elevators, extensors, and retractors, chest, abdominals, hip flexors, knee flexors, foot dorsiflexors.

Asanas for opening: Adho Mukha Svanasana, Anjaneyasana, Gomukhasana, Pursvottanasana, Setu Bandha Sarvangasana, Shishulasana, Supta Virasana, Urdhva Dhanurasana, Virabhadrasana I.

Stabilizing

What needs to be stable: Wrist flexors, elbow flexors, external rotators of the arm, shoulder stabilizers (emphasis retractors, protractors, flexors), back extensors, transversus abdominis, hip extensors and adductors, intrinsic foot muscles.

Asanas for stabilizing: Adho Mukha Vrksasana, Anjaneyasana, Ashta Chandrasana, Bhujangasana, Bidalasana, Dhanurasana, Eka Pada Raj Kapotasana I and II, Garudasana, Matsyasana, Pincha Mayurasana, Salamba Sirsasana I, Supta Virasana, Urdhva Mukha Svanasana, Ustrasana.

This asana prepares you for:

Eka Pada variation; walk feet in and transition to Pincha Mayurasana.

Counterposes

Apanasana, Simple twists, Supta Baddha Konasana, Ananda Balasana, Balasana, seated forward bends.

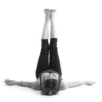

Viparita Karani
Active Reversal Pose

Identifying Preparatory Asanas

Opening

What needs to be open: Hip extensors, knee flexors.

Asanas for opening: A deeply restorative asana that can be practiced on its own or after any sequence.

Stabilizing

What needs to be stable: Hip adductors.

Asanas for stabilizing: In itself a restorative that can be practiced independently or after any practice.

This asana prepares you for:

Strap thighs together, place sandbag over feet; explore wall-supported Ardha Salamba Sarvangasana or Supta Konasana.

Counterposes

Apanasana, Supta Baddha Konasana, Savasana.

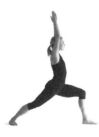

Virabhadrasana I
Warrior I Pose

Identifying Preparatory Asanas

Opening

What needs to be open: Front leg: hip extensors, knee extensors. Back leg: calf, hip flexors, internal rotators of the leg, knee flexors. Abdominals, chest, shoulder retractors, extensors, and elevators.

Asanas for opening: Adho Mukha Svanasana, Anjaneyasana, Ashta Chandrasana, Gomukhasana, Tadasana, Virabhadrasana II, Virasana.

Stabilizing

What needs to be stable: Intrinsic foot muscles. Front leg: hip stabilizers (emphasis extensors, adductors), knee flexors. Back leg: foot dorsiflexors, hip flexors, knee extensors, back extensors, transversus abdominis, shoulder retractors and protractors, external rotators of the arm.

Asanas for stabilizing: Adho Mukha Svanasana, Anjaneyasana, Ardha Uttanasana, Ashta Chandrasana, Bhujangasana, Bidalasana, Tadasana, Urdhva Hastasana, Urdhva Mukha Svanasana, Utkatasana, Uttana Prasithasana.

This asana prepares you for:

Dancing Warrior series, transition into other standing asanas, use alternate arm positions: Garudasana or Gomukhasana arms, Parivrtta Ashta Chandrasana, Parivrtta Parsvakonasana, Virabhadrasana III.

Counterposes

Vinyasa series, Urdhva Mukha Svanasana, Adho Mukha Svanasana, Supta Padangusthasana, Supta Baddha Konasana, Apanasana, Ananda Balasana, Balasana.

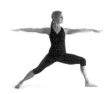

Virabhadrasana II
Warrior II Pose

Identifying Preparatory Asanas

Opening

What needs to be open: Front leg: hip extensors, adductors, and internal rotators. Back leg: calf, knee flexors, hip adductors. Shoulder elevators and retractors, chest.

Asanas for opening: Anjaneyasana, Ashta Chandrasana, Baddha Konasana, Supta Padangusthasana, Tadasana, Utthita Trikonasana, Vrksasana.

Stabilizing

What needs to be stable: Intrinsic foot muscles. Front leg: hip stabilizers (emphasis extensors, adductors), external rotators of the leg, knee flexors. Back leg: hip extensors, knee extensors, foot dorsiflexors. Back extensors, transversus abdominis, obliques, shoulder abductors, retractors, and protractors, elbow extensors.

Asanas for stabilizing: Adho Mukha Svanasana, Anjaneyasana, Ardha Uttanasana, Ashta Chandrasana, Bidalasana, Prasarita Padottanasana D, Tadasana, Vasisthasana.

This asana prepares you for:

Reverse Warrior, Utthita Parsvakonasana, Utthita Trikonasana, Ardha Chandrasana, Svarga Dvijasana, Dancing Warrior series.

Counterposes

Vinyasa series, Urdhva Mukha Svanasana, Adho Mukha Svanasana, Gomukhasana, Paschimottanasana, Balasana.

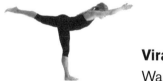

Virabhadrasana III
Warrior III Pose

Identifying Preparatory Asanas

Opening

What needs to be open: Standing leg: calf, knee, flexors, hip extensors. Gesture leg: foot dorsiflexors, knee flexors, hip flexors. Shoulder extensors, elevators, and retractors.

Asanas for opening: Anjaneyasana, Ashta Chandrasana, Supta Padangusthasana, Tadasana, Uttanasana, Virabhadrasana I, Vrksasana.

Stabilizing

What needs to be stable: Standing leg: intrinsic foot muscles, knee extensors. Back extensors, transversus abdominis, hip stabilizers (emphasis extensors, adductors, standing hip flexors), internal rotators of the leg, shoulder flexors, protractors, elbow extensors.

Asanas for stabilizing: Adho Mukha Svanasana, Anjaneyasana, Ardha Uttanasana, Ashta Chandrasana, Bhujangasana, Bidalasana,

Garudasana, Parsvottanasana, Phalakasana, Urdhva Hastasana, Utkatasana, Utthita Hasta Padangusthasana I and II, Virabhadrasana I, Vrksasana.

This asana prepares you for:

Parivrtta Ardha Chandrasana, Parivrtta Hasta Padangusthasana, Natarajasana, Adho Mukha Vrksasana. Do not transition directly into Ardha Chandrasana.

Counterposes

Malasana, Garudasana, Supta Baddha Konasana, Balasana.

Virasana
Hero Pose

Identifying Preparatory Asanas

Opening

What needs to be open: Foot dorsiflexors, knee extensors, hip abductors and flexors.

Asanas for opening: Apanasana, Baddha Konasana, Balasana, Gomukhasana.

Stabilizing

What needs to be stable: Hip flexors, internal rotators of the leg, knee flexors, transversus abdominis, shoulder retractors and protractors, elbow extensors.

Asanas for stabilizing: Adho Mukha Svanasana, Anjaneyasana, Ardha Uttanasana, Ashta Chandrasana, Balasana, Bharadvajrasana A and B, Bidalasana, Garudasana, Utkatasana.

This asana prepares you for:

Supta Virasana, Bhekasana, Tiriang Mukha Eka Pada Paschimottanasana.

Counterposes

Phalakasana, Adho Mukha Svanasana.

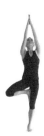

Vrksasana
Tree Pose

Identifying Preparatory Asanas

Opening

What needs to be open: Standing leg: hip flexors. Gesture leg: hip adductors, internal rotators of the leg. Knee extensors, shoulder elevators, extensors, and retractors, elbow flexors.

Asanas for opening: Baddha Konasana, Supta Padangusthasana, Tadasana, Utthita Trikonasana, Virabhadrasana II.

Stabilizing

What needs to be stable: Grounded leg: intrinsic foot muscles, hip stabilizers, (emphasis adductors, internal rotators of the leg). Folded leg: hip flexors and external rotators, knee flexors, calf. Back extensors, transversus abdominis, shoulder retractors and protractors, external rotators of the arm, elbow extensors.

Asanas for stabilizing: Adho Mukha Svanasana, Adho Mukha Vrksasana, Anjaneyasana, Ardha Uttanasana, Ashta Chandrasana, Baddha Konasana, Bidalasana, Garudasana, Malasana, Phalakasana, Prasarita Padottanasana B and D, Salamba Sirsasana I and II, Tadasana, Urdhva Hastasana, Virabhadrasana II.

This asana prepares you for:

Transition to Utthita Hasta Padangusthasana, explore with eyes closed, Vasisthasana with top leg in Vrksasana positioning.

Counterposes

Tadasana, Ardha Uttanasana, Uttanasana, Garudasana, Balasana.

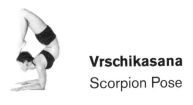

Vrschikasana

Scorpion Pose

Identifying Preparatory Asanas

Opening

What needs to be open: Wrist flexors, shoulder elevators and retractors, throat, chest, abdominals, hip flexors.

Asanas for opening: Adho Mukha Vrksasana, Shishulasana, Pincha Mayurasana, Adho Mukha svanasana, Bhujangasana, Eka Pada Raj Kapotasana II.

Stabilizing

What needs to be stable: Wrist flexors, elbow flexors, external rotators of the arm, shoulder stabilizers (emphasis retractors, protractors, flexors), back extensors, transversus abdominis, hip flexors and adductors.

Asanas for stabilizing: Adho Mukha Svanasana, Adho Mukha Vrksasana, Anjaneyasana, Ashta Chandrasana, Bhekasana, Bhujangasana, Bidalasana, Chaturanga Dandasana, Dhanurasana, Eka Pada Raj Kapotasana I and II, Pincha Mayurasana, Garudasana, Phalakasana, Raj Kapotasana, Salabhasana B, Salamba Sirsasana I, Shishulasana, Urdhva Dhanurasana, Urdhva Hastasana, Urdhva Mukha Svanasana, Ustrasana, Virabhadrasana I.

This asana prepares you for:

With Adho Mukha Vrksasana arms: Drop into Urdhva Dhanurasana, ticktocks.

Counterposes

Simple twists, Apanasana, Balasana.

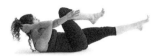 **Yogic Bicycles**
Dvicakravahanasana

Identifying Preparatory Asanas

Opening

What needs to be open: Shoulder elevators, hip extensors.
Asanas for opening: Ardha Matsyendrasana, Jathara Parivartanasana, Marichyasana C, Paripurna Navasana.

Stabilizing

What needs to be stable: Abdominals, obliques, shoulder protractors and retractors, hip flexors and adductors, internal rotators of the leg.
Asanas for stabilizing: All twists, Adho Mukha Svanasana, Bakasana, Bidalasana, Chaturanga Dandasana, Dandasana, Lolasana, Navasana, Ubhaya Padangusthasana, Urdhva Mukha Paschimottanasana.

This asana prepares you for:

Other abdominal core movements, Paripurna Navasana to Ardha Navasana and back, Jathara Parivartanasana, Tolasana, Lolasana.

Counterposes

Apanasana, Supta Parivartanasana, Ananda Balasana, Supta Baddha Konasana.

Appendix C

Yoga Class Sequencing Worksheet

General Class Elements

Type of Class: _____ Level: _____ Season: _____

Class Theme: _____

Peak Asana(s): _____

_____

What needs to be open? _____

_____

What needs to be stable? _____

_____

How is the yogic process initiated?   Time: 5–10 minutes

_____

_____

_____

How is the body generally warmed?   Time: 5–20 minutes

_____

_____

_____

What is the further pathway to the peak?   Time: 15–30 minutes
Anticipatory elements: _____

_____

_____

_____

_____

_____

_____

_____

_____

_____

_____

Preparatory Asanas	Relationship to Previous and Subsequent Asanas
1. _____	_____
2. _____	_____
3. _____	_____
4. _____	_____
5. _____	_____
6. _____	_____
7. _____	_____
8. _____	_____
9. _____	_____
10. _____	_____

How is the peak explored?   Time: 5–15 minutes

_____
_____
_____
_____
_____
_____

How is the practice integrated?   Time: 15–30 minutes

Peak Pratikriyasana: _____
_____
_____
_____
_____
_____

General Deeper Release: _____
_____
_____
_____
_____

Pranayama?   Time: (1–45 minutes)

_____

_____

_____

_____

_____

_____

Meditation?   Time: 3–60 minutes (or longer)

_____

_____

_____

_____

_____

_____

Other Class Elements?   Time: _____?

_____

_____

_____

_____

_____

_____

_____

_____

_____

_____

_____

_____

_____

_____

Appendix D

Popular Hatha Yoga Sequences

The following sequences offer a glimpse at the diverse ways that different yoga styles, brands, and lineages design yoga classes. Explore applying the essential yoga sequencing principles to your assessment and appreciation of each sequence. What do you think? Then explore each sequence in practice. How do you feel? How does someone whose intention, physical, or mental condition differs from yours feel after each sequence? Keep asking the basic question of yoga sequencing: "Why this then that?"

Table D.1. Anusara Sequence—Basic Template

1. Sitting and centering: meditation and/or breathing	9. Abdominals
2. Warm-up exercises	10. Supta Virasana
3. Adho Mukha Svanasana	11. Inversions/Salamba Sirsasana and variations
4. Surya Namaskara	12. Back bends
5. Adho Mukha Vrksasana and/or Pincha Mayurasana	13. Sarvangasana
6. Standing asanas	14. Twists and Forward Bends
7. Basic hip openers	15. Meditation
8. Hand-balancing	16. Savasana

Table D.2. Ashtanga Vinyasa Sequence (Primary Series)

1. Tadasana/Samasthihi	26. Kurmasana
2. Surya Namaskara A (5 times)	27. Supta Kurmasana
3. Surya Namaskara B (5 times)	28. Garbha Pindasana
4. Padangusthasana	29. Kukkutasana
5. Pada Hastasana	30. Baddha Konasana A, B
6. Utthita Trikonasana (from Prasarita stance)	31. Upavista Konasana A, B
7. Parivrtta Trikonasana	32. Supta Konasana
8. Utthita Parsvakonasana	33. Supta Padangusthasana A, B, C
9. Parivrtta Parsvakonasana	34. Ubhaya Padangusthasana
10. Prasarita Padottanasana A, B, C, D	35. Urdhva Mukha Paschimottanasana
11. Parsvottanasana	36. Setu Bandhasana
12. Utthita Hasta Padangusthasana A, B, C, D	37. Urdhva Dhanurasana
13. Ardha Baddha Padmottanasana	38. Paschimottanasana
14. Utkatasana (from vinyasa)	39. Salamba Sarvangasana
15. Virabhadrasana I	40. Halasana
16. Virabhadrasana II	41. Karnapidasana
17. Dandasana	42. Urdhva Padmasana
18. Paschimottanasana A/B	43. Pindasana
19. Pursvottanasana	44. Matsyasana
20. Ardha Baddha Padma Paschimottanasana	45. Uttana Padasana
21. Tiriang Mukha Eka Pada Paschimottanasana	46. Salamba Sirsasana I
22. Janu Sirsasana A, B, C	47. Baddha Padmasana

(Continued on following page.)

Table D.2. Ashtanga Vinyasa Sequence (Primary Series) (continued)

23. Marichyasana ABCD	48. Padmasana
24. Paripurna Navasana	49. Tolasana
25. Bhujapidasana	50. Savasana

Note: The vinyasa of Chaturanga Dandasana–Urdhva Mukha Svanasana–Adho Mukha Svanasana–Dandasana is performed between all of the asanas from numbers 20 through 36, including between each side of asanas that have two sides (such as Janu Sirsasana A), as well as after several asanas following number 38.

Table D.3. Bikram Sequence—Beginning Class

1. Pranayama series	14. Pavanamuktasana
2. Ardha Chandrasana with Pada Hastasana	15. Sit up
3. Utkatasana	16. Bhujangasana
4. Garudasana	17. Salabhasana
5. Dandayamana–Janu Sirsasana	18. Poorna–Salabhasana
6. Dandayamana–Dhanurasana	19. Dhanurasana
7. Tuladandasana (Balancing Stick Pose)	20. Supta–Vajrasana
8. Dandayamana–Bibhaktapada–Paschimottanasana	21. Ardha–Kurmasana
9. Utthita Trikonasana	22. Ustrasana
10. Dandayamana–Bibhaktapada–Janu Sirsasana	23. Sasangasana
11. Tadasana	24. Janus Sirsasana with Paschimottanasana
12. Padangusthasana	25. Ardha–Matsyendrasana
13. Savasana	26. Kapalabhati pranayama

Note: This sequence of asanas is performed in a room heated to 105 degrees Fahrenheit. Each asana is performed twice.

Table D.4. Iyengar Sequence—Basic Class

1. Tadasana (with various arm positions)	14. Upavista Konasana
2. Utthita Trikonasana	15. Adho Mukha Virasana
3. Utthita Parsvakonasana	16. Adho Mukha Swastikasana
4. Virabhadrasana I	17. Paschimottanasana
5. Virabhadrasana II	18. Janu Sirsasana
6. Adho Mukha Svanasana	19. Paschimottanasana
7. Prasarita Padottanasana	20. Bharadvajrasana
8. Uttanasana	21. Marichyasana C
9. Dandasana	22. Parsva Virasana
10. Virasana	23. Supta Baddha Konasana
11. Janu Sirsasana (upward-facing—i.e., without folding forward)	24. Supta Padangusthasana
12. Swastikasana	25. Setu Bandha Sarvangasana
13. Baddha Konasana	26. Savasana

Table D.5. Kripalu Sequence—Sun Flow

1. Mountain Pose and centering	11. Half Curl Up
2. Standing Twists	12. Serpent
3. Monkey Stretch	13. Half Locust
4. Forward Fold	14. Child
5. Sun Salutation	15. Great Seal
6. Breath of Joy	16. Half Circle
7. Warrior	17. Spinal Twist
8. Triangle	18. Dead Bug
9. Standing Angle	19. Deep Relaxation in Corpse
10. Crane	

Table D.6. Power Yoga Sequence

1. Balasana	24. Ustrasana
2. Adho Mukha Svanasana	25. Setu Bandha Sarvangasana
3. Uttanasana	26. Urdhva Dhanurasana
4. Sun Salutation A, 3–5 repetitions	27. Supta Baddha Konasana
5. Sun Salutation B	28. Leg Lifts
6. Anjaneyasana	29. Supta Baddha Konasana
7. Parivrtta Ashta Chandrasana	30. Yogic Bicycles
8. Utthita Parsvakonasana	31. Supta Baddha Konasana
9. Vasisthasana	32. Navasana
10. Parivrtta Utkatasana	33. Supta Baddha Konasana
11. Pada Hastasana	34. Salamba Sarvangasana
12. Bakasana	35. Halasana
13. Garudasana	36. Karnapidasana
14. Utthita Hasta Padangusthasana A, B	37. Adho Mukha Eka Pada Raj Kapotasana
15. Virabhadrasana III	38. Dwi Pada Raj Kapotasana
16. Natarajasana	39. Bekasana
17. Vrksasana	40. Janu Sirsasana A
18. Trikonasana	41. Paschimottanasana
19. Parivrtta Trikonasana	42. Pursvottanasana
20. Prasarita Padottanasana A	43. Matsyasana
21. Parsvottanasana	44. Ananda Balasana
22. Salabhasana	45. Supta Parivaratasana
23. Dhanurasana	46. Savasana

Table D.7. Prana Flow Sequence for Natarajasana

1. Opening Meditation: Chanting "aum" with Spiral Arm Movement from Anahata Chakra to Hasta Mudra	21. Hanumanasana Lunge with Gomukhasana arms
2. Namaskara Opening: Dancing Warrior variation	22. Dhanurasana variation with strap
3. Anahatasana	23. Parsvottanasana
4. Pincha Mayurasana Prep	24. Virabhadrasana III
5. Adho Mukha Svanasana to lift leg	25. Hanumanasana Lunge with Gomukhasana arms
6. Utthita Trikonasana	26. Anahatasana with twist
7. Ardha Chandrasana with quad opening	27. Pincha Mayurasana
8. Utthita Trikonasana	28. Parivrtta Trikonasana
9. Ardha Hanumanasana	29. Parivrtta Ardha Chandrasana
10. Ardha Dhanurasana on knees (both sides)	30. Standing Split to Standing Natarajasana with strap
11. Adho Mukha Svanasana	31. Parivrtta Trikonasana
12. Adho Mukha Svanasana to lift leg	32. Parivrtta Ardha Chandrasana
13. Utthita Trikonasana	33. Setu Bandhasana Prep
14. Ardha Chandrasana with quad opening	34. Urdhva Dhanurasna Prep
15. Utthita Trikonasana	35. Setu Bandhasana
16. Ardha Hanumanasana	36. Urdhva Dhanurasana
17. Anahatasana	37. Ardha Matsyendrasana
18. Pincha Mayurasana Prep with one leg up	38. Gomukhasana
19. Parsvottanasana	39. Salamba Sarvangasana
20. Virabhadrasana III	40. Savasana

Table D.8. Sivananda Sequence

1. Savasana (2–3 minutes)	10. Matsyasana
2. Seated position—pranayama	11. Paschimottanasana
3. Neck, shoulder, and eye exercises	12. Bhujangasana
4. Classical Surya Namaskara (using Cobra in place of Locust)	13. Salabhasana
5. Leg raises	14. Dhanurasana
6. Salamba Sirsasana I	15. Ardha Matsyendrasana
7. Salamba Sarvangasana	16. Bakasana
8. Halasana	17. Utthita Trikonasana
9. Setu Bandha Sarvangasana	18. Savasana

Table D.9. White Lotus Sequence

1. Warm-up sequence: 4 each A, B, C Salutations	16. Bridge (Setu Bandha Sarvangasana) or Wheel (Urdhva Dhanurasana)
2. Transition: 1 A series salutation, including: hold 5 breaths in each of these poses:	17. A Salutations to Half Forward Fold (Janu Sirsasana)
3. Up Dog, Down Dog, Forward Fold, Half Fold	18. Forward Fold (Paschimottanasana)
4. Continue A series into: Triangle (Trikonasana)	19. Hip openers Cobbler (Baddha Konasana)
5. Warrior Pose (Virabhadrasana II)	20. Straddle Splits (Upavista Konasana)
6. Extended Warrior (Utthita Parsvakonasana)	21. Rock the Baby
7. Half Moon (Ardha Chandrasana)	22. Twisting Seated Spinal Twist (Ardha Matsyendrasana)
8. Forward Warrior (Virabhadrasana I)	23. Inversions Optional: Handstand (Adho Mukha Vrksasana)
9. Warrior Balance (Virabhadrasana III)	24. Headstand (Sirsasana) or Dolphin 30–100 breaths
10. Standing Straddle Fold Twist, or Twisting Triangle (Parivrtta Trikonasana)	25. Shoulder Stand Cycle (Sarvangasana) 30–100 breaths
11. Downward-Facing Dog (Adho Mukha Svanasana) + twice the number of breaths	26. Fish (Matsyasana) 20 breaths

(Continued on following page.)

Table D.9. White Lotus Sequence (continued)

12. Jump through to: Upward-Facing Boat (Navasana) + twice the number of breaths	27. Pranayama Lotus, or sit erect for 10–20 Complete breaths
13. Optional: sit-ups and leg lifts	28. Final Relaxation Corpse Pose (Savasana) 5–15 minutes
14. Back Bends (no Salutations)—Standing Supported Arch—2–3 rounds each pose:	
15. Hold, rest, repeat Camel (Ustrasana)	

Appendix E

Additional Resources

The Teaching Yoga Resource Center is an online service provided by Mark Stephens where you will find:

- Extensive curriculum materials designed for use in Yoga Teacher Trainings in conjunction with this book and with *Teaching Yoga: Essential Foundations and Techniques.*

- An instructional yoga video library containing over one hundred three- to five-minute videos showing how to guide students in beginning to advanced asanas.

- Videos showing each of the sixty-seven sequences described in this book.

- A gallery of slide shows giving step-by-step guidance on how to do over seventy-five asanas.

- Articles on asanas, pranayama, meditation, the yoga profession, the yoga studio business, and more.

- Detailed information on Yoga Teacher Certification programs with Mark Stephens, including 200-hour Foundational Teacher Training, 500-hour Advanced Teacher Training, and 1,000-hour Teacher Trainer Certification.

- A calendar of workshops, retreats, and yoga teacher certification courses.

- Links to additional resources on the Internet and at yoga centers, institutes, and conferences worldwide.

Teaching Yoga Resource Center

http://www.markstephensyoga.com/resources

Notes

Introduction: The Art and Science of Yoga Sequencing

1. Cope (1999 and 2006) offers a beautiful exploration of the fullness of yoga practice. For contrasting perspectives that bear directly on yoga sequencing, see Eliade (1958), Ghosh (1914), Grilley (2002), Iyengar (2009), Jois (2002), Prabhavananda (1944), Ramaswami (2005), Scaravelli (1991), Schiffmann (1996), Stryker (2011), and G. White (2007).

Chapter One: Philosophy and Principles of Sequencing

1. Hatha yoga comprises all forms of physical yoga in which asanas are the primary tool for self-exploration and self-transformation, regardless of style or brand, from Anusara and Ashtanga to Bikram and Power to Yin and Vinyasa. It is to be distinguished from *bhakti* (devotional), *karma* (service), and *jnana* (mental) yoga, even if these more ancient practices are incorporated into the Hatha practices. The *raja yoga* of Patanjali is essentially a form of jnana yoga. Early Hatha yoga was first described as a path to the more challenging practices of raja yoga (Swatmarama 2004). See Stephens (2010) for further discussion.

2. For a basic introduction to the Yoga Sutras of Patanjali, see Stephens (2010, 6–13). To explore further, see Bouanchaud (1999).

3. This eightfold path—the original ashtanga yoga—is given in Sutra II:29–32 (Bouanchaud 1999, 109–13).

4. While a number of teachers, gurus, books, and other sources continue to say that yogis were doing lots of different asanas thousands of years ago, the mythical nature of this assertion is becoming increasingly clear. Many still insist that their style of asana practice dates back thousands of years, despite overwhelming historical evidence to the contrary. For a scholarly discussion of the development of modern asana practice, see Singleton (2010).

5. Bodymind? Body-mind? Or body and mind? The view taken here is that the mind arises from, yet is not reducible to, the brain, which is clearly part of the body. The qualities of mind (thought, memory) manifesting throughout the body through the body's neurological network are thus further embodied.

Much of what we are doing in yoga is awakening and developing this fuller somatic intelligence. When referring to this integrated being, we use the term *bodymind*.

6. This can be expressed through the kosha model of subtle (or esoteric) anatomy: the pranamaya kosha is the essential medium integrating the annamaya and manomaya koshas. See Stephens (2010, 48–50) for further discussion of the kosha model in teaching yoga.

7. Shiva Rea first posited the qualities of "effective, beautiful, and integrated" with respect to sequencing; the elaboration here is mine.

8. Erich Schiffmann has brought the concept of moving into stillness alive in his now classic book, *Yoga: The Spirit and Practice of Moving into Stillness* (1996).

Chapter Two: The Arc Structure of Yoga Classes

1. This point is emphasized by Farhi (1999), who stresses that "each asana acts as a container for subtle and dynamic inner movement."

2. The practice of mindfulness is found in a variety of spiritual disciplines, most notably in Zen Buddhism; see Hanh (1975). For an eclectic resource on cultivating being present in the moment, see Watts (1980). More recently, Eckhart Tolle has helped popularized the practice of being in the moment through his writings and talks, including *The Power of Now* (1999); Powers (2008) explores mindfulness and asana practice.

3. *Aum* is mentioned in all of the Upanishads, where it is set forth as a profound object of spiritual meditation, its sound equated with Brahma. It is discussed extensively in the Chandogya Upanishad, Taittiriya Upanishad, and Mandukya Upanishad. See the Katha Upanishad (1.2.15) for a simple definition of *aum* as "the highest" syllable, the "aim of all human desire," which in knowing the support of this sound, its meaning, makes one "adored in the world of Brahma."

4. Regarding both *kapalabhati* and *bhastrika,* Iyengar (1985, 180) tells us, "if people perform them because they believe that they awaken the kundalini, disaster to body, nerves, and brain may result." Yet the Hatha Yoga Pradipika, Iyengar's primary source, says that this pranayama "quickly arouses kundalini. It is pleasant and beneficial, and removes obstruction due to excess mucus accumulated at the entrance to brahma nadi" (Hatha Yoga Pradipika II.66).

5. Resilient buoyancy is where we find the space for refinement in a held asana. It can be contrasted with being right up against the final edge of maximum possibility in an asana.

6. Traditional Hatha yoga texts counsel doing six *satkarma* (internal cleansing) practices before attempting pranayama. The six practices are *dhauti* (essentially flossing the esophagus, stomach, and small intestines), *neti* (warm saline nasal irrigation), *nauli* (muscular abdominal churning), *basti* (essentially a warm water enema), *trataka* (clipping the skin at the back base of the tongue, then bringing the tip of the tongue to the third eye and gazing in that direction), and *kapalabhati pranayama* (skull-cleansing pranayama). Here we will offer guidance on kapalabhati only. For detailed discussion of shatkarma, see Swatmarama (2004).

7. The concept of yoga chikitsa is recognition that yoga is a process for healing that involves transforming the conditioned patterns that influence every aspect of one's life. It is also the name given to the primary series of Ashtanga Vinyasa yoga, one of the overarching aspects of therapeutic yoga, and is at the center of Iyengar's practice and teachings.

Chapter Three: Sequencing Within and Across Asana Families

1. For details on the anatomy of pada bandha, see the discussion of the feet in Chapter Four. For more on balance in the feet, see Holleman and Sen-Gupta (1999) and Little (2001).

2. This is a popular sequence that some students will be able to practice safely throughout their lives. However, it presents serious risks to most students, with injury typically occurring before the bodymind recognizes the problem.

3. See Stephens (2010), Chapter 11, on contraindications for each trimester of pregnancy.

4. For more details on the functions of and benefits to muscles and joints used in twists, see Gudmestad (2003) and Cole (2005).

5. There is some debate over pressure on the head in Salamba Sirsasana I, with some insisting the pressure down through the crown of the head "will impinge on our intellectual development" along with "the possibility of damaging the subtle nadis in the brain." See Jois (2002, 126) and Maehle (2006, 122). Jois insists that the full weight of the body must be supported by the arms. This stands in stark contrast to Iyengar's emphasis on balanced grounding through the arms and the top of the head.

Chapter Four: Sequencing Asana Instructions

1. The ubiquitous sequence of Plank–Chaturanga–Up Dog–Down Dog should be demonstrated on a fairly regular basis. See Chapter Seven for the instructions.

2. A script of cues can be very helpful in the early experience of teaching yoga. However, every body is different and everyone experiences yoga in somewhat different ways. While some styles and systems of yoga propose universal movements, alignment principles, and energetic actions, it is best to consider any such notions of universality as a very rough starting place, instead giving greater emphasis to guiding students based on the actual reality of their individual condition and intention.

Chapter Five: Surya Namaskara—Sun Salutations

1. Prostrations to the sun are found in cultures around the globe and date back thousands of years. But Surya Namaskara as part of yoga asana practice came about as part of the larger renaissance of physical culture in India in the 1930s (Singleton 2010, 179–84).

Chapter Six: Introductory and Beginning-Level Classes

1. This movement is often referred to as "Cat and Cow." Most teachers agree on the term Cat (Bidalasana), in which the spine is arched into flexion, but not on the reversed position, in which the pelvis rotates forward, the sit bones reach toward the sky, and the heart center pulls through the window of the arms. The latter position has no resemblance to the cow-related asanas in yoga but very much anticipates Adho Mukha Svanasana (Downward-Facing Dog Pose), including the anterior rotation of the pelvis. Thus we use "Dog Tilt" to refer to this position. If you need any further validation of this terminology, ask any five-year-old to watch you in these movements and describe what animal you look like in Cat Tilt. Most will say a cat. Then reverse position and ask, "If the first position was a cat, what's this?" None will say a cow. Thus, Cat and Dog Tilts, as defined by Erich Schiffmann (1996, 89–94).

Chapter Eight: Advanced-Level Classes

1. This perspective came to me when walking through the woods with Joel Kramer and Diana Alstad a few years ago and discussing Joel's reemergence as a public teacher after a thirty-year sabbatical. One of the great American yoga pioneers, he was humored to discover many of his former students referring to themselves as yoga masters. He asked, "How can there be a yoga master when there's nothing to master?" This question came from a man who, a generation earlier, was among the most adept practitioners of physical yoga in the world, whose seminal 1970s *Yoga Journal* article, "Yoga as Self-transformation," gave us many of the central concepts at the heart of yoga as an unending process of change.

Chapter Nine: Yoga Sequencing for Kids

1. Research data also show higher rates of obesity are strongly correlated with economic poverty. For further information, see Ogden et al. (2010).

2. This trend is associated with increased rates of suicide among youth, especially when correlated with high rates of obesity. For more, see Substance Abuse and Mental Health Services Administration (2010).

3. While the ratio is only five percent, this represents approximately 3.75 million kids. For further information, see U.S. Department of Health and Human Services (1999).

4. Tanner stage 5 is approximately age fifteen. It should be noted that the Tanner stage model is controversial. Quoted in "Fitness and Exercise Guide" on the Keep Kids Healthy website (http://www.keepkidshealthy.com/welcome/treatmentguides/exercise.html), accessed August 26, 2011.

5. An excellent source on Indian mythology is *Ganesha Goes to Lunch* (Kapur 2007).

Chapter Ten: Sequencing for Special Conditions of Women

1. Gates goes on to discuss the powerful emergence of women in yoga that continues today as the leading source of creativity in yoga.

2. Menstrual egress can be blocked by endometriosis, primary dysmenorrhea (menstrual cramps), cervical stenosis (scarring around the cervical opening), congenital anomalies of the reproductive tract, or adenomyosis (the growth of glands in the uterine muscles that, when the tissue is sloughed, has nowhere to go). For further exploration, see Porth and Martin (2008, 1056–65) and Moore and Dalley (2006, 105–12 and 410–42).

3. Many yoga teachers make a further case against inverting during menstruation based on the movement of and effects of prana, specifically the idea that *apana-vayu*'s role in expelling unneeded materials from the body (urine, feces, menses) is disrupted. This is a curious proposition given that all prana-vayus manifest as part of subtle energetics that are generally posited as functioning beyond material forces such as gravity.

4. For fascinating stories of how fear can limit a woman's cervical dilation in labor, see Gaskin (2003, 133–42).

5. For specific exercises, see Calais-Germain (2003). This book should be required reading for all prenatal and postnatal yoga teachers; all women should be encouraged to read it as well.

6. For specific modifications of asanas in working with these two classes of students, there are excellent prenatal and postnatal books that closely correspond to the two groups: for more basic prenatal and postnatal classes, see

Balaskas (1994); for regular yoga classes and experienced students, see Freedman (2004).

7. The term *menopause* is often used interchangeably to describe the very different conditions and phases of perimenopause and postmenopause, the former marking the onset of hormonal shifts that will eventually lead to postmenopause, when there is no longer a menstrual cycle. The distinction is vitally important as there are different treatment symptoms and treatment protocols that, if confused, can create a variety of problems. For an excellent source on menopause in general, see Edelman (2009). For a more holistic perspective, see Boice (2007).

8. A wonderful resource on yoga and menopause written from the Iyengar perspective, see Francina (2003).

Chapter Eleven: Yoga Sequencing for Seniors

1. This characterization is given by the researchers in Duke University Medicine's Therapeutic Yoga for Seniors project. The sequencing suggestions given here draw significantly from their findings. See Krucoff and Peterson (2010, 899–905).

2. Responding to a reader's question about teaching aging students in Ashtanga Vinyasa and in doing Matsyasana (Fish Pose) in particular, *Yoga Journal* "mentor expert" Maty Ezraty (2011) wisely counsels, "not every pose is appropriate for every student." A devout Ashtangi, she then goes on to indicate that even Setu Bandhasana (Supported Bridge Pose), the final pose in the beginning Ashtanga sequence can be done safely as long as the neck has sufficient strength from doing poses such at Utthita Trikonasana (Extended Triangle Pose), despite the extreme hyperextension of the cervical spine. This is an example of an experienced teacher who is committed to a specific style of yoga finding ways to make it more appealing to all ages and levels of students, even when the advice runs counter to voluminous medical evidence contraindicating the recommended sequence or asana. In the case of Setu Bandhasana, a good case can be made for not doing or teaching this asana at all because of the severe risks involved in supporting half or more of one's body weight on the top of the head when the cervical spine is hyperextended.

3. See Cohen (2006) pages 4 and 95–114 for further exploration.

4. Basiphobia—the fear of falling—is entirely valid given seniors' greater difficulty with balance and the life-threatening consequences of a fall: women over age fifty have a twenty-five percent mortality rate in the first year following a hip fracture. See Kado et al. (2003). On the fear of falling, see Schmid et al. (2010).

5. Kramer's (1977) timeless article, "Yoga as Self-transformation," published in *Yoga Journal* in 1977, is the original source for this concept and method. Erich Schiffmann (1996) devotes a chapter of his book to this method; Stephens (2010) offers further guidance to teachers in using this method in their teaching.

6. While it is important to emphasize the life-affirming quality of yoga, the reality that we all eventually die is important to accept as a means of being freer in the present. For a variety of practices—asana, pranayama, mudra, kosha awareness, and meditation—see Taylor (2008).

Chapter Twelve: Cultivating Emotional and Mental Health

1. To explore this perspective, see Keedwell (2008).

Chapter Thirteen: Chakra Sequences

1. Finger (2005) gives specific physical locations and attributes for each chakra. As noted earlier, many others, including Johari (1987), dispute this specific association of chakras with physical elements.

2. For a fascinating discussion of pineal gland as explored in Cartesian philosophy, see Stanford Encyclopedia of Philosophy (2008).

Chapter Fifteen: Further Tips on Yoga Sequencing

1. Donna Farhi (2006) makes a clear case for having stronger standards of student attendance in public yoga classes.

2. The terms *passive* and *active* are often used in different ways depending on the context of the discussion. See Ganga White's (2007, 119–21) discussion of active and passive holding.

3. The value of dynamic practice for beginners is emphasized by Desikachar (1995, 29–31).

References

Aldous, Susi Hately. 2004. *Anatomy and Asana: Preventing Yoga Injuries.* Calgary: Functional Synergy.

Alter, Michael J. 1996. *Science of Flexibility* 2nd ed. Champaign, IL: Human Kinetics.

American Psychological Association. 2010. *Stress in America Findings.* Washington, DC: APA. http://www.stressinamerica.org.

Avalon, Arthur. 1974. *The Serpent Power: Being the Sat-Cakra-Nirupana and Paduka-Pancaka.* New York: Dover.

Avari, Burjor. 2007. *India: The Ancient Past.* Abingdon, UK: Routledge.

Ayyanga, T. R. S. 1952. *The Yoga Upanishads.* Adyar, India: Adyar Library.

Bailey, James. 2003. "Balancing Act." *Yoga Journal* 176 (September-October 2003), http://www.yogajournal.com/wisdom/927.

———. 2006. *Living Ayurveda Reader.* Santa Monica, CA: self-published.

Balaskas, Janet. 1994. *Preparing for Birth with Yoga.* Boston: Element.

Bandy, William D., and Jean M. Irion. 1994. "The Effect of Time on Static Stretch on the Flexibility of the Hamstring Muscles." *Physical Therapy* 74(9): 845–50.

Baptiste, Baron. 2003. *Journey into Power: How to Sculpt Your Ideal Body, Free Your True Self, and Transform Your Life with Yoga.* New York: Fireside.

Benagh, Barbara. 2003. "Inversions and Menstruation." *Yoga Journal.* http://yogajournal.com/practice/546_1.cfm.

Bhajan, Yogi. "Kundalini Research Institute." http://www.kundaliniresearchinstitute.org/teachertraining.htm.

Birch, Beryl Bender. 1995. *Power Yoga: The Total Strength and Flexibility Workout.* New York: Fireside.

———. 2000. *Beyond Power Yoga: 8 Levels of Practice for Body and Soul.* New York: Fireside.

Boice, Judith. 2007. *Menopause with Science and Soul: A Guidebook for Navigating the Journey.* Berkeley, CA: Celestial Arts.

Bouanchaud, Bernard. 1999. *The Essence of Yoga: Reflections on the Yoga Sutras of Patanjali*. New York: Sterling.

Briggs, Tony. 2001. "The Gift of Assisting." *Yoga Journal*. http://www.yogajournal.com/for_teachers/1024.

Broad, William J. 2012. *The Science of Yoga: The Risks and the Rewards*. New York: Simon and Schuster.

Calais-Germain, Blandine. 1991. *Anatomy of Movement*. Seattle: Eastland.

———. 2003. *The Female Pelvis: Anatomy and Exercises*. Seattle: Eastland.

———. 2005. *Anatomy of Breathing*. Seattle: Eastland.

California Department of Education. 2009. *Physical Education Framework for California Public Schools: Kindergarten through Grade Twelve*. Sacramento, CA: California Department of Education.

Campbell, Joseph. 1949. *The Hero with a Thousand Faces*. New York: Pantheon.

Chinmayananda, Swami. 1987. *Glory of Ganesha*. Bombay: Central Chinmaya Mission Trust.

Choudhury, Bikram. 2000. *Bikram's Beginning Yoga Class*. New York: Penguin Putnam.

Clennell, Bobby. 2007. *The Woman's Yoga Book: Asana and Pranayama for All Phases of the Menstrual Cycle*. Berkeley, CA: Rodmell.

Cohen, Gene D. 2006. *The Mature Mind: The Positive Power of the Aging Brain*. Cambridge, MA: Perseus Books.

Cole, Roger. 2005. "With a Twist." *Yoga Journal* (November 2005). http://www.yogajournal.com/practice/1923.

———. "Protect the Knees in Lotus and Related Postures." *Yoga Journal*. http://www.yogajournal.com/for_teachers/978.

Cope, Stephen. 1999. *Yoga and the Quest for the True Self*. New York: Bantam.

———. 2006. *The Wisdom of Yoga: A Seeker's Guide to Extraordinary Living*. New York: Bantam-Bell.

Courtright, Paul B. 1985. *Ganesa: Lord of Obstacles, Lord of Beginnings*. New York: Oxford University Press.

Daumal, René. 2004. *Mount Analogue: A Novel of Symbolically Authentic Non-Euclidean Adventures in Mountain Climbing*. Woodstock, NY: Overlook Press. First published 1960 by Pantheon.

Davidson, Ronald M. 2003. *Indian Esoteric Buddhism: A Social History of the Tantric Movement*. New York: Columbia University Press.

———. 2005. *Tibetan Renaissance: Tantric Buddhism in the Rebirth of Tibetan Culture.* New York: Columbia University Press.

DeNoon, Daniel J. 2011. "The 10 Most Prescribed Drugs." *WebMD.* http://www.webmd.com/news/20110420/the-10-most-prescribed-drugs.

Desikachar, T. K. V. 1995. *The Heart of Yoga: Developing a Personal Practice.* Rochester, VT: Inner Traditions.

———. 1998. *Health, Healing, and Beyond: Yoga and the Living Tradition of Krishnamacharya.* New York: Aperture.

Devereux, Godfrey. 1998. *Dynamic Yoga: The Ultimate Workout That Chills Your Mind as It Charges Your Body.* New York: Thorsons.

Dharma, Krishna. 1999. *Mahabharata: The Greatest Spiritual Epic of All Time.* Badger, CA: Torchlight.

Easwaran, Eknath, trans. 1987. *The Upanishads.* Tomales, CA: Nilgiri.

Edelman, Carole Lium, and Carol Lynn Mandle. 2010. *Health Promotion throughout the Life Span.* St. Louis: Mosby.

Eliade, Mircea. 1958. *Yoga: Immortality and Freedom.* New York: Pantheon.

Espinoza, Fernando. 2005. "An Analysis of the Historical Development of Ideas about Motion and Its Implications for Teaching." *Physical Education* 40(2).

Ezraty, Maty. 2006. *Yoga Journal.* http://www.yogajournal.com/for_teachers/1880.

———. 2011. "Teaching an Aging Population." *Yoga Journal.* http://www.yogajournal.com/for_teachers/2343.

Farhi, Donna. 1996. *The Breathing Book: Good Health and Vitality through Essential Breath Work.* New York: Henry Holt.

———. 2006. *Teaching Yoga: Exploring the Teacher-Student Relationship.* Berkeley, CA: Rodmell.

Finger, Alan. 2005. *Chakra Yoga: Balancing Energy for Physical, Spiritual, and Mental Well-being.* Boston: Shambhala.

Fishman, Loren, and Ellen Saltonstall. 2008. *Yoga for Arthritis.* New York: W. W. Norton.

———. 2010. *Yoga for Osteoporosis.* New York: W. W. Norton.

Folan, Lilias. 1976. *Lilias Yoga and You.* New York: Bantam.

Forbes, Bo. 2011. *Yoga for Emotional Balance: Simple Practices to Help Relieve Anxiety and Depression.* Boston: Shambhala.

Francina, Suza. 2003. *Yoga and the Wisdom of Menopause: A Guide to Physical, Emotional, and Spiritual Health at Midlife and Beyond.* Deerfield Beach, FL: Health Communications.

Frawley, David. 1999. *Yoga and Ayurveda: Self-healing and Self-realization.* Twin Lakes, WI: Lotus.

Freedman, Françoise Barbira. 2004. *Yoga for Pregnancy, Birth and Beyond.* New York: Dorling Kindersley.

French, Roger Kenneth. 2003. *Medicine Before Science: The Rational and Learned Doctor from the Middle Ages to the Enlightenment.* Cambridge, UK: Cambridge University Press.

Friend, John. 2006. *Anusara yoga teacher training manual* 9th ed. The Woodlands, TX: Anusara.

Gambhirananda, Swami. 1989. *Taittiriya Upanishad.* Calcutta: Advaita Ashram.

Gannon, Sharon, and David Life. 2002. *Jivamukti yoga: Practices for Liberating Body and Soul.* New York: Ballantine.

Gardner, Howard. 1993. *Frames of Mind: The Theory of Multiple Intelligences.* New York: Basic.

Gaskin, Ina May. 2003. *Ina May's Guide to Childbirth.* New York: Bantam.

Gates, Janice. 2006. *Yogini: The Power of Women in Yoga.* San Rafael, CA: Mandala Publications.

Getty, Alice. 1936. *Ganesa: A Monograph on the Elephant-faced God.* Repr., Oxford: Clarendon, 1992.

Ghosh, Aurobindo Akroyd. 1914. *The Synthesis of Yoga.* Pondicherry, India: SABDA.

Grilley, Paul. 2002. *Yin Yoga: Outline of a Quiet Practice.* Ashland, OR: White Cloud.

Gudmestad, Julie. 2003. "Let's Twist Again." *Yoga Journal* (January-February 2003).

Hanh, Thich Nhat. 1975. *The Miracle of Mindfulness: A Manual on Meditation.* Boston: Beacon.

Hardy, L., R. Lye, and A. Heathcote. 1983. "Active Versus Passive Warm-up Regimes and Flexibility." *Research Papers in Physical Education* 1(5): 23–30.

Hirschi, Gertrud. 2000. *Mudras: Yoga in Your Hands.* Boston: Weiser.

Hittleman, Richard. 1982. *Richard Hittleman's Yoga: 28-day Exercise Plan.* New York: Bantam.

Hoff, Benjamin. 1982. *The Tao of Pooh.* New York: Dutton.

Holleman, Dona, and Orit Sen-Gupta. 1999. *Dancing the Body Light: The Future of Yoga.* Amsterdam: Pandion.

Huxley, Aldous. 1962. *Island*. New York: Harper and Row.

Iyengar, B. K. S. 1966. *Light on Yoga*. New York: Schockten.

———. 1985. *Light on Pranayama: The Yogic Art of Breathing*. New York: Crossroad.

———. 1988. *The Tree of Yoga*. Boston: Shambhala.

———. 2001. *Yoga: The Path to Holistic Health*. London: Dorling Kindersley.

———. 2009. *Yoga Wisdom and Practice*. London: Dorling Kindersley.

Iyengar, Geeta S. 1995. *Yoga: A Gem for Women*. Spokane, WA: Timeless.

Johari, Harish. 1987. *Chakras: Energy Centers of Transformation*. Rochester, VT: Destiny.

Jois, Sri K. Pattabhi. 2002. *Yoga Mala*. New York: North Point.

Jung, Carl. 1953. "Yoga and the West." *The Collected Works of Carl Jung* vol. 1, ed. Sir Herbert Read, Michael Fordham, and Gerard Adler. New York and Princeton, NJ: Bollingen.

Kado, Deborah M., T. Duong, K. L. Stone, K. E. Ensrud, M. C. Nevitt, G. A. Greendale, and S. R. Cummings. 2003. "Incident Vertebral Fractures and Mortality in Older Women: A Prospective Study." *Osteoporosis International* 14(7): 589–94.

Kaminoff, Leslie, and Amy Matthews. 2011. *Yoga Anatomy* 2nd ed. Champaign, IL: Human Kinetics.

Kapur, Kamla K. 2007. *Ganesha Goes to Lunch: Classics from Mystic India*. San Rafael, CA: Mandala.

Keedwell, Paul. 2008. *How Sadness Survived: The Evolutionary Basis of Depression*. Oxford, UK: Radcliffe.

Kempton, Sally. 2010. *Meditation for the Love of It*. Boulder, CO: Sounds True.

Kramer, Joel. 1977. "A New Look at Yoga: Playing the Edge of Mind and Body." *Yoga Journal* (January 1977).

———. 1980. "Yoga as Self-Transformation." *Yoga Journal* (May–June 1980).

Kramer, Joel, and Diana Alstad. 2009. *The Passionate Mind Revisited: Expanding Personal and Social Awareness*. Berkeley, CA: North Atlantic.

———. 1993. *The Guru Papers: Masks of Authoritarian Power*. Berkeley, CA: North Atlantic.

Krishnamacharya, Tiramulai. 1934. *Yoga Makaranda*. Madurai, India: Madurai CMV Press.

Kriyananda, Swami (J. Donald Walters). 1967. *Ananda Yoga for Higher Awareness*. Nevada City, NV: Crystal Clarity.

Krucoff, Carol, and Matthew Peterson. 2010. "Teaching Yoga to Seniors: Essential Considerations to Enhance Safety and Reduce Risk in a Uniquely Vulnerable Age Group." *The Journal of Alternative and Complementary Medicine* 16(8): 899–905.

Lad, Vasant. 1984. *Ayurveda: The Science of Self-healing.* Twin Lakes, WI: Lotus.

Lasater, Judith. 1995. *Relax and Renew: Restful Yoga for Stressful Times.* Berkeley, CA: Rodmell.

Levine, Stephen. 1979. *A Gradual Awakening.* Garden City, NJ: Anchor.

Little, Tias. 2001. "From the Ground Up." *Yoga Journal* (November 2001).

Maehle, Gregor. 2006. *Ashtanga Yoga: Practice and Philosophy.* Novato, CA: New World Library.

Mallinson, James, trans. 2004. *The Gheranda Samhita.* Woodstock, NY: YogaVidya.com.

Manchester, Frederick. 2002. *The Upanishads: Breath of the Eternal.* New York: Signet Classics.

McCall, Timothy. 2007. *Yoga as Medicine: The Yogic Prescription for Health and Healing.* New York: Bantam Dell.

Miller, Elise Browning. 2003. *Yoga for Scoliosis.* Menlo Park, CA: self-published.

Mittelmark, Raul Artal, Robert A. Wiswell, and Barbara L. Drinkwater, eds. 1991. *Exercise in Pregnancy,* 2nd ed. Baltimore: Williams and Wilkins.

Mohan, A. G. 1993. *Yoga for Body, Breath, and Mind: A Guide to Personal Reintegration.* Portland, OR: Rudra.

Mohan, A. G., and Indra Mohan. 2004. *Yoga Therapy: A Guide to the Therapeutic Use of Yoga and Ayurveda for Health and Fitness.* Boston: Shambhala.

Moore, Keith L., and Arthur F. Dalley. 2006. *Clinically Oriented Anatomy,* 5th ed. Baltimore: Lippincott Williams and Wilkins.

Morrison, Judith. 1995. *The Book of Ayurveda.* London: Gaia.

Muktananda, Swami. 1997. *Nothing Exists That Is Not Siva: Commentaries on the Siva Sutra, Vijnanabhairava, Gurugita, and Other Sacred Texts.* South Fallsburg, NY: Siddha Yoga Publications.

Muktibodhananda, Swami, trans. 1993. *Hatha Yoga Pradipika: Light on Yoga.* Munger, India: Bihar School of Yoga.

Narayanananda, Swami. 1979. *The Primal Power in Man, or the Kundalini Shakti,* 6th rev. ed. Gylling, Denmark: Narayanananda Universal Yoga Trust.

Netter, Frank H. 1997. *Atlas of Human Anatomy,* 2nd ed. East Hanover, NJ: Novartis.

Newton, Isaac. 1999. *The Principia: Mathematical Principles of Natural Philosophy.* Trans. I. Bernard Cohen and Anne Whitman. Berkeley, CA: University of California Press.

Ogden, Cynthia L., Margaret D. Carroll, Lester R. Curtin, Molly M. Lamb, and Katherine M. Flegal. 2010. "Prevalence of High Body Mass Index in U.S. Children and Adolescents, 2007–2008." *Journal of the American Medical Association* 303(3): 242–49.

Porth, Carol Mattson, and Genn Martin. 2008. *Pathophysiology : Concepts of Altered Health States.* Philadelphia: Wolters Kluwer Health/Lippincott Williams & Wilkins.

Powers, Sarah. 2008. *Insight Yoga.* Boston: Shambhala.

Prabhavananda, Swami, and Christopher Isherwood, trans. 1944. *Bhagavad-Gita.* Los Angeles: The Vedanta Society.

Ramaswami, Srivatsa. 2000. *Yoga for the Three Stages of Life: Developing Your Practice as an Art Form, a Physical Therapy, and a Guiding Philosophy.* Rochester, VT: Inner Traditions.

———. 2005. *The Complete Book of Vinyasa Yoga.* New York: Marlowe.

Rea, Shiva. 1997. *Hatha Yoga as a Practice of Embodiment.* Master's thesis, Univ. of California, Los Angeles, World Arts and Cultures (Dance) Department.

Rosen, Richard. 2002. *The Yoga of Breath: A Step-by-Step Guide to Pranayama.* Boston: Shambhala.

———. 2006. *Pranayama Beyond the Fundamentals: An In-depth Guide to Yogic Breathing.* Boston: Shambhala.

Satchidananda, Swami. 1970. *Integral Hatha Yoga.* Austin, TX: Holt, Rinehart and Winston.

———, trans. 1978. *The Yoga Sutras of Patanjali.* Buckingham, VA: Integral Yoga.

Scaravelli, Vanda. 1991. *Awakening the Spine: The Stress-free New Yoga That Works with the Body to Restore Health, Vitality and Energy.* New York: HarperCollins.

Schatz, Mary Pullig. 2002. "A Woman's Balance: Inversions and Menstruation." http://www.yoga.com/ydc/enlighten/enlighten_document. asp?ID=74&section=9&cat=93.

Schiffmann, Erich. 1996. *Yoga: The Spirit and Practice of Moving into Stillness.* New York: Pocket.

Schmid, A., M. Van Puymbroeck, and D. Koceja. 2010. "Effect of a 12-week Yoga Intervention on the Fear of Falling and Balance in Older Adults—a Pilot Study."

Archives of Physical Medicine and Rehabilitation 91: 576–83.

Shamdasani, Sonu, ed. 1996. *The Psychology of Kundalini Yoga: Notes of the Seminar Given in 1932 by C. G. Jung.* Princeton: Princeton University Press.

Shrier, Ian, and Kav Gossal. 2000. "The Myths and Truths of Stretching: Individualized Recommendations for Healthy Muscles." *Physician and Sportsmedicine* 28(8).

Singer, Charles A. 1957. *A Short History of Anatomy and Physiology from the Greeks to Harvey.* New York: Dover.

Singleton, Mark. 2010. *Yoga Body: The Origins of Modern Postural Practice.* New York: Oxford University Press.

Sivananda Yoga Center. 1983. *The Sivananada Companion to Yoga.* Repr., New York: Fireside, 2000.

Sjoman, N. E. 1996. *The Yoga Tradition of the Mysore Palace.* New Delhi: Abhinav.

Stanford Encyclopedia of Philosophy. 2008. "Descartes and the Pineal Gland." http://plato.stanford.edu/entries/pineal-gland.

Stenhouse, Janita. 2001. *Sun Yoga: The Book of Surya Namaskar.* St.-Christophe, France: Innerspace.

Stephens, Anastasia. 2005. "Health: The Bikram Backlash." London: *The Independent,* January 25.

Stephens, James, Joshua Davidson, Joseph DeRosa, Michael Kriz, and Nicole Saltzman. 2006. "Lengthening the Hamstring Muscles without Stretching Using 'Awareness through Movement.'" *Physical Therapy* 86(12): 1641–50.

Stephens, Mark. 2010. *Teaching Yoga: Essential Foundations and Techniques.* Berkeley, CA: North Atlantic.

———. 2011. "Art of Asana: Effort and Ease in Handstand." *Yoga International* 113 (Spring 2011).

———. 2011. "Art of Asana: Divine Expression—the Path to Natarajasana." *Yoga International* 114 (Spring 2011).

———. 2012. "How Yoga Will Not Wreck Your Body." *Elephant Journal.* http://www.elephantjournal.com/2012/01/how-yoga-will-not-wreck-your-body—mark-stephens/.

Stryker, Rod. 2011. *The Four Desires: Creating a Life of Purpose, Happiness, Prosperity, and Freedom.* New York: Delacorte.

Substance Abuse and Mental Health Services Administration, Office of Applied Studies. 2010. *The NSDUH Report: Major Depressive Episode among Youths*

Aged 12 to 17 in the United States: 2004 to 2006. Rockville, MD: SAMHSA.

Svoboda, Robert. 1988. *Prakriti: Your Ayurvedic Constitution*. Bellingham, WA: Sadhana.

Svoboda, Robert, and Arnie Lade. 1995. *Tao and Dharma: Chinese Medicine and Ayurveda*. Twin Lakes, WI: Lotus.

Swatmarama, Swami. 2004. *Hatha Yoga Pradipika*. Woodstock, NY: YogaVidya.com.

Swenson, David. 1999. *Ashtanga Yoga: The Practice Manual*. Austin, TX: Ashtanga Yoga Productions.

Taylor, Jennifer. 2008. "End-of-life Yoga Therapy: Exploring Life and Death." *International Journal of Yoga Therapy* 18: 97–103.

Thompson, Marcia, and David Harsha. 1984. "Our Rhythms Still Follow the African Sun." *Psychology Today* 12 (January 1984): 50–54.

Tigunait, Pandit Rajmani. 1999. *Tantra Unveiled: Seducing the Forces of Matter and Spirit*. Honesdale, PA: Himalayan Institute Press.

Tirtha, Swami Sada Shiva. 2006. *The Ayurvedic Encyclopedia*. Coconut Creek, FL: Educa.

Todd, Mabel. 1937. *The Thinking Body*. Repr., New York: Dance Horizons, 1972.

Tolle, Eckhart. *The Power of Now: A Guide to Spiritual Enlightenment*. Novato, CA: New World Library, 1999.

Troels, B. 1973. "Achilles Heel Rupture." *Acta Orthopaedica Scandinavica*. 152(suppl.): 1–126.

U.S. Department of Health and Human Services. 1999. *Mental Health: A Report of the Surgeon General*. Rockville, MD: HHS.

Vasu, Rai B. Chandra, trans. 2004. *The Siva Samhita*. New Delhi: Munshiram Manoharial.

Vaughan, Kathleen. 1951. *Exercises Before Childbirth*. London: Faber.

Watts, Alan. 1980. *Om: Creative Meditations*. Berkeley, CA: Crystal Arts.

Weintraub, Amy. 2004. *Yoga for Depression: A Compassionate Guide to Relieve Suffering through Yoga*. New York: Broadway.

White, David Gordon. 1996. *The Alchemical Body: Siddha Traditions in Medieval India*. Chicago: University of Chicago Press.

———, ed. 2000. *Tantra in Practice*. Princeton, NJ: Princeton University Press.

———. 2003. *Kiss of the Yogini: "Tantric Sex" in Its South Asian Contexts*. Chicago: University of Chicago Press.

———. 2009. *Sinister Yogis*. Chicago: University of Chicago Press.

White, Ganga. 2007. *Yoga Beyond Belief: Insights to Awaken and Deepen Your Practice*. Berkeley, CA: North Atlantic.

Woolery, Alison, Hector Myers, Beth Sternlieb, and Lonnie Zeltzer. 2004. "A Yoga Intervention for Young Adults with Elevated Symptoms of Depression." *Alternative Therapies in Health and Medicine* 10(2): 60–63.

Yesudian, Selvarajan, and Elisabeth Haich. 1958. *Sport and Yoga*. Paris: Albin Michel.

Yogananda, Paramhansa. 1946. *Autobiography of a Yogi*. Los Angeles: Self-Realization Fellowship.

Zimmer, Heinrich. 1972. *Myths and Symbols in Indian Art and Civilization*. New York: Bollingen Foundation.

Index

A

action in the body, as class theme, 37

actions, integrating the effects of, 25–26

Active Reversal Pose. *See* Viparita Karani

active warming *vs.* passive warming, 39

Adho Mukha Svanasana (Downward-Facing Dog Pose)

  breech birth presentation and, 261

  constituent elements of, 360

  deeper refining cues, 108 (t)

  evolutionary approach to, 20–21

  as foundational arm support asana, 115–16

  as hip opener, 83

  in Surya Namaskara, 134, 136–37

  as warming asana, 41

Adho Mukha Vrksasana (Handstand), 132, 361

advanced classes

  arm balances, 68–69

  arm support sequence, 217–22

  back bends, 74, 203–8

  forward bends, 222–25

  hip opening sequence, 208–11

  inversions, focus on, 225–27

  mastery, Joel Kramer on, 474n1

  mildly stimulating class, 292–94

  pacing an advanced class, 331–32

  relax deeply class, 290

  sequences for, creating and teaching, 200–202

  Soulful Vinyasa yoga class sequences, 339–46

  standing balance, focus on, 214–16

  teaching advanced students, 197–200

  twisting, focus on, 211–14

aging. *See* seniors

Agnistambhasana (Two-Footed King Pigeon Pose or Fire Log Pose), 362

ajna chakra and class sequence, 311–13

Akarna Dhanurasana (Shooting Bow Pose), 362–63

alignment principles

  guiding students into alignment, 104

  of the peak asana, 46–47

anahata chakra and class sequence, 306–8

Anahatasana (Extended Puppy or Heart Chakra Pose), 363–64

anandamaya kosha, 14

Angelou, Maya, 197

anjali mudra, 28, 34, 65

Anjaneyasana (Low Lunge Pose), 72, 364–65

ankles, inside-outside balancing cue for, 106 (t)

annamaya kosha (sheath of the physical self), 13

Anusara sequence template, 461 (t)

anxiety, reducing, 80, 288–89

apana-vayu (downward-moving prana), 475n3

aparigraha (noncovetousness), 26

Arambha Avastha (Beginning Stage), 11, 12

archetypes and mythology, as class theme, 37–38

arc structure of yoga classes
  basic template applied to different-level flow classes, 89–91 (t)
  basic template for, 32 (t)
  description of, 29–32
  integrating the practice, 50–53
  the peak, exploring, 49–50
  the peak, pathway to, 43–48
  theme-oriented classes, creating, 36–38
  warming and awakening the body, 39–43
  yogic process, initiating, 32–36

Ardha Baddha Padmottanasana (Half Bound Lotus Intense Stretch Pose), 365–66

Ardha Chandrasana (Half Moon Pose), 109 (t), 266–67

Ardha Matsyendrasana (Half Lord of the Fishes Pose), 367–68

Ardha Uttanasana (Half Standing Forward Bend Pose), 134–36, 368

arm balances. *See* arm support asanas

arm support asanas
  for advanced classes, 217–22
  basic arc template for different-level flow classes, 90 (t)
  beginning level, 160–62
  foundational asanas, 115–16
  inside-outside balancing cue, 106 (t)
  intermediate-level classes, 187–91

for peak or theme classes, shoulder openers and, 60
roots and extension cues, 108 (t)
sequencing, 63–65, 67–69
sequencing cues for, 113–14

arthritis, sequences for, 278–79

asana
  duration and pacing of, 330–34
  foundation and essential elements of, 98
  history of, 471n4
  Patanjali on, 10
  See also specific asanas

asana families
  as class theme, 38
  distinguishing elements of, 56 (t), 57
  sequencing cues within, 112–22

asana instruction, sequencing
  absorbing and integrating the effects of, 111–12
  asana families, sequencing cues within, 112–22
  asanas, demonstrating, 95–96
  cueing oppositional actions, 105–6 (t)
  refining asanas, 102–4
  refining cues, deeper, 108–9 (t)
  roots and extension, 107–8 (t)
  teaching what you know, 94–95
  transitioning into asanas, 97–102
  transitioning out of asanas, 109–11
  See also sequencing

Ashta Chandrasana (High Lunge Pose or Crescent Pose), 137, 368–69

Ashtanga Pranam, 40–41

Ashtanga Vinyasa
  advanced series, 198
  integrated level 1–2 class, 335–38
  integrated level 2–3 class, 339–43
  integrated level 3+ class, 343–46

intermediate-level poses in, 168
older yoga practitioners and, 276,
    476n2
pace and flow of, 331
sequence (Primary Series) template,
    462–63 (t)
set order of poses, 8–9
Astavakrasana (Eight-Angle Pose),
    369–70
aum, chanting, 35, 472n3
avidya (ignorance), injury and, 26
awakening the body, 39–43
awakening the chakras, 296
ayurvedic yoga sequencing
    doshas, balancing, 317–19
    kapha dosha, 323–25
    pitta dosha, 321–23
    vata dosha, 319–21

B

back bend asanas
    advanced classes, 203–8
    basic arc template for different-
        level flow classes, 91 (t)
    beginning level, 153–55
    focus classes, using standing
        asanas, 60
    intermediate-level classes, 173–78
    sequencing, 69–75
    sequencing cues for, 117–18
back-front oppositional balances,
    cueing, 105 (t)
Baddha Konasana (Bound Angle Pose),
    370–71
Bakasana (Crane Pose), 371
Balanced Standing Pose. *See* Samastihi
    balance problems, sequences for,
        282–83, 476n4
Balasana (Child's Pose)
    in beginning classes, 145
    constituent elements of, 372

nurturing aspect of, 78
transitioning to, 74
basiphobia (fear of falling), 476n4
beautiful sequencing, 19
"beginner's mind," 144–45
beginning classes
    arm balances, 67
    arm support, focus on, 160–62
    back bends, focus on, 153–55
    Basic Introduction to Yoga class,
        149–50
    benefits of, 168
    Bikram sequence template, 463 (t)
    duration of poses, 334
    forward bends, focus on, 163–64
    hip opening, focus on, 156
    Introduction to Yoga workshop
        for more physically fit students,
        151–52
    inversion, focus on, 165–66
    mildly stimulating class, 291–92
    new students, teaching, 143–45
    pacing a beginning class, 331
    sequences for, creating and
        teaching, 147–48
    simple relaxation class, 289
    Soulful Vinyasa yoga class
        sequence, 335–38
    standing asanas, sequencing, 59
    standing balance, focus on,
        159–60
    twisting, focus on, 157–58
Benagh, Barbara, 246
Bharadvajrasana A, B (Sage
        Bharadvaj's Pose A, B), 372–74
Bhekasana (Frog Pose), 374
Bhujangasana (Cobra Pose), 375
Bhujapidasana (Shoulder-Squeezing
        Pose), 375–76
Bidalasana (Cat Pose), 376–77
Big Toe Pose. *See* Padangusthasana

Bikram Yoga
    passive warming, 39
    sequence for beginning class,
        463 (t)
    set order of poses, 8–9
birth. *See* labor, yoga poses to ease
bliss, Patanjali's Yoga Sutras and,
    10
Boat Pose. *See* Navasana
bodymind, 471n5
bone health, yoga for, 270–71
Both Big Toes Pose. *See* Ubhaya
    Padangusthanasana
Bound Angle Pose. *See* Baddha
    Konasana
Bow Pose. *See* Dhanurasana
brain balance of seniors, 276
breathing
    at the beginning of class, 34
    cueing, for transitioning into
        asanas, 98–99
    See also pranayama
breech birth presentation, 261
Bridge Pose. *See* Setu Bandha
    Sarvangasana
Bridge Rolls, for exploring supine back
    bends, 72

C

Camel Pose. *See* Ustrasana
carpal tunnel syndrome. *See* Healthy
    Wrist Sequence
"Cat and Cow," 474n1
Cat and Dog Tilts, 40
Cat Pose. *See* Bidalasana
Cat Tilts, 40, 474n1
causal body *(karana sharira),* 14
Chair Pose. *See* Utkatasana
chakras
    ajna chakra and class sequence,
        311–13

anahata chakra and class sequence,
    306–8
as class theme, 38
manipura chakra and class
    sequence, 303–6
muladhara chakra and class
    sequence, 297–99
sahasrara chakra and class
    sequence, 313–15
standing asanas and, 61
svadhisthana chakra and class
    sequence, 299–303
understanding, 295–97
vishuddha chakra and class
    sequence, 309–11
change, the constancy of
    (parinamavada), 15–16, 17
chanting Aum, 35, 472n3
Chaturanga Dandasana (Four-Limbed
    Staff Pose)
    in Ashtanga Vinyasa, 331
    constituent elements of, 377
    in Surya Namaskara, 131–32, 138
children
    elementary school–age children,
        sequencing for, 234–36
    high school–age youth, sequencing
        for, 239–41
    mental and emotional health of,
        475n2–3
    middle school–age children,
        sequencing for, 237–38
    yoga and physical fitness, 231–33
Child's Pose. *See* Balasana
cleansing, internal (shatkarma), 473n6
Clennell, Bobby, 244–45
Cobra Pose. *See* Bhujangasana
Cohen, Gene D., 276
Complete Arc Class, basic template for,
    32 (t)
contraction back bends, 70

core activation
    abdominals, basic arc template for
        different-level flow classes, 90 (t)
    sequencing for, 61–63
    to warm up the body, 43
corona capitis (top of the head),
        balancing cues for, 106 (t)
Corpse Pose. *See* Savasana
Cow Face Pose. *See* Gomukhasana
Crane Pose. *See* Bakasana
creativity, random, 8
Crescent Pose. *See* Ashta Chandrasana
cross-legged positions, moving into, 84
cueing
    Classical Surya Namaskara, breath
        and movement cues, 129 (t)
    oppositional actions, 105–6 (t)
    refining asanas, 102–4, 108–9 (t)
    roots and extension cues, 107–8 (t)
    scripts for, 474n2
    sequencing cues within asana
        families, 112–22
    transitioning into asanas, 97–102
    transitioning out of asanas, 109–11

D

Dancing Warrior series, 140–41
Dandasana (Staff Pose), 79, 80, 378
Dangling Earring Pose. *See* Lolasana
Daumal, René, 29
dedicating a class, 35
demonstrating asanas, 95–97, 111
depression, yoga and, 232, 288–89, 475n2
Desikachar, 109, 334, 477n3
Dhanurasana (Bow Pose), 378–79
discomfort in asanas, 334
disk injuries, forward bends and, 78
Divine Monkey Pose. *See*
        Hanumanasana
Dog Tilts, 40, 474n1
Dolphin Pose. *See* Shishulasana

doshas, balancing, 317–19
    See also specific doshas
Downward-Facing Dog pose. *See* Adho
        Mukha Svanasana
Downward-Facing Tree Pose. *See* Adho
        Mukha Vrksasana
duration and pace of yoga classes,
        330–34
Dvicakravahanasana (Yogic Bicycles),
        456
Dwi Pada Koundinyasana (Two-Leg
        Sage Koundinya's Pose), 379–80
Dwi Pada Sirsasana (Two Legs behind
        Head Pose), 380–81
dynamic to static exploration,
        movement sequences of, 21–22

E

Eagle Pose. *See* Garudasana
Ear-Squeezing Pose. *See*
        Karnapidasana
East Intense Stretch Pose. *See*
        Pursvottanasana
Easy Cobra. *See* Salabhasana
Eight-Angle Pose. *See* Astavakrasana
eightfold path, 471n3
Eka Pada Koundinyasana A, B
        (One-Leg Sage Koundinya's Pose
        A, B), 381–82
Eka Pada Raj Kapotasana (One-Leg
        King Pigeon Pose)
    constituent elements of, 383
    as hip opener, 83
    preparation for, 73
Eka Pada Sirsasana (One Leg behind
        Head Pose), 384
Eka Pada Urdhva Dhanurasana, 70
eka pada (one-leg) variations of back
        bends, 72
elementary school–age children,
        sequencing for, 234–36

Embryo in the Womb Pose. *See* Garbha
      Pindasana
Embryo Pose. *See* Pindasana
emotional health, sequencing for,
      287–89
energetic actions
of the peak asana, 47
transitioning into asanas and, 99–100
energetic balance, cultivating, 22–24,
      53, 288–89
evolutionary stages of yoga,
      traditional, 10–12
Extended Hand to Foot Pose. *See*
      Utthita Hasta Padangusthasana
      I, II
Extended Leg Pose. *See* Uttana
      Padasana
Extended Puppy Pose. *See*
      Anahatasana
Extended Side Angle Pose. *See* Utthita
      Parsvakonasana
Extended Triangle Pose. *See* Utthita
      Trikonasana
extension and roots cues, 107–8 (t)
externally rotated standing asanas, 57,
      58–59, 71
external rotators, 82
Ezraty, Maty, 476n2

F

falling, fear of, 476n4
Farhi, Donna, 477n1
Feathered Peacock Pose. *See* Pincha
      Mayurasana
feet
   front-back balancing cue, 105 (t)
   inside-outside balancing cue,
      106 (t)
   positioning, in Adho Mukha
      Svanasana, 116

roots and extension cues, 107 (t)
upper-lower balancing cue for,
      105 (t)
fingers, upper-lower balancing cue
      for, 105 (t)
Firefly Pose. *See* Tittibhasana
Fire Log Pose. *See* Agnistambhasana
first trimester of pregnancy, guidelines
      and sequences for, 251–55
Fish Pose. *See* Matsyasana
flow-style classes
   arm balances in, 68
   templates for, different-level,
      89–91 (t)
   transitional asanas in, 99
Flying Crow Pose. *See* Galavasana
Flying Fish Pose. *See* Uttana Padasana
Flying Lizard Pose. *See* Uttana
      Prasithasana
forward bending asanas
   advanced classes, 222–25
   basic arc template for different-
      level flow classes, 91 (t)
   beginning level, 163–64
   intermediate-level sequences,
      192–94
   sequencing, 77–81
   sequencing cues for, 119–20
Four-Limbed Staff Pose. *See*
      Chaturanga Dandasana
Frawley, David, 24
Frog Pose. *See* Bhekasana
front-back oppositional balances,
      cueing, 105 (t)

G

Galavasana (Flying Crow Pose), 385
Garbha PIndasana (Embryo in the
      Womb Pose), 385–86
Garland Pose. *See* Malasana

Garudasana (Eagle Pose), 59, 386–87
Gate Pose. *See* Parighasana
Gates, Janice, 244
gather-around demonstrations, 95–97
gender differences and yoga practice,
    243–44
general active warming, 39
Ghata Avastha (Vessel Stage), 11, 13
Gomukhasana (Cow Face Pose), 66,
    75, 83, 387–88
greeting your class, 33
gunas (qualities of mind and emotion),
    22–24

H

Halasana (Plow Pose), 86–87, 388
Half Bound Lotus Intense Stretch
    Pose. *See* Ardha Baddha
    Padmottanasana
Half Lord of the Fishes Pose. *See*
    Ardha Matsyendrasana
Half Moon Pose. *See* Ardha
    Chandrasana
Half Standing Forward Bend Pose. *See*
    Ardha Uttanasana
Hamilton, Alexander, 248
hamstrings, warming and releasing, 79
hands
    Hand dance, 65
    position of, in Adho Mukha
        Svanasana, 115
    roots and extension cues, 107 (t)
Handstand. *See* Adho Mukha
    Vrksasana
Hand to Foot Pose. *See* Pada
    Hastasana
Hanumanasana (Divine Monkey Pose),
    73, 389
Harrison, George, 125

Hatha yoga, 10–12, 471n1
Hatha Yoga Pradipika, 199, 472n4
head
    front-back balancing cue, 105 (t)
    roots and extension cues, 108 (t)
Headstand. *See* Sirsasana I, II
    (Headstand I, II)
Headstand, Supported. *See* Salamba
    Sirsasana (Supported Headstand)
Head to Knee Pose. *See* Janu Sirsasana
health challenges for seniors, 277
Healthy Shoulder Sequence, 65–66
Healthy Wrist Sequence, 64–65
Heart Chakra Pose. *See* Anahatasana
heart disease, sequences for, 283–84
Heron Pose. *See* Krounchasana
Hero Pose. *See* Virasana
Hesse, Herman, 287
High Lunge Pose. *See* Ashta
    Chandrasana
high school–age youth, sequencing for,
    239–41
hip muscles, 81–82
hip opening sequences
    advanced classes, 208–11
    basic arc template for
        different-level flow classes, 91 (t)
    beginning level, 156
    during first trimester of pregnancy,
        251
    intermediate-level classes, 179–81
    during second trimester of
        pregnancy, 256
    sequencing, 81–84
    during third trimester of
        pregnancy, 262
hips, upper-lower balancing cue for,
    105 (t)
hot flashes, yoga for symptoms of, 269

I

imbalances, energetic, 288–89

informed sequencing, 17–18

inhalation, cueing, for transitioning into asanas, 98

initiating the yogic process, 32–36

injuries, 26–28, 333

inside-outside oppositional balances, cueing, 106 (t)

integrated sequencing
  integrated level 2–3 class, 339–43
  integrated level 3+ class, 343–46
  level 1–2 class, 335–38
  understanding, 19

integrating the practice
  four stages of, 50–51
  ideas for deepening, 52–53
  Savasana, 88–89
  ways to, 111–12
  See also pratikriyasana (integrating actions)

Intense Extended Side Stretch Pose. *See* Parsvottanasana

intentions for classes, 35

intermediate-level classes
  arm balances, 67–68
  arm support sequences, 187–91
  in Ashtanga Vinyasa, 168
  back bends, 74, 173–78
  challenges of teaching, 167–68
  criteria for students, 169
  forward bending sequences, 192–94
  hip opening sequences, 179–81
  inversions, focus on, 194–95
  mildly stimulating classes, 291–94
  the plateau, 169–70
  relaxation classes for, 289–90
  sequences for, creating and teaching, 170–73

Soulful Vinyasa yoga class sequences, 335–38, 339–43

standing asanas, sequencing, 59

standing balance sequences, 184–86

twisting sequences, 181–83

internal cleansing (shatkarma), 473n6

internally rotated femurs, 57, 71

internal rotators, 82

in-the-flow demonstrations, 95

introductory-level classes. *See* beginning classes

inversion asanas
  advanced classes, 225–27
  basic arc template for different-level flow classes, 91 (t)
  beginning level, 165–66
  intermediate-level classes, 194–95
  sequencing, 84–88
  sequencing cues for, 120–22

Inverted Staff Pose. *See* Viparita Dandasana

Iyengar, Geeta, 244

Iyengar yoga, 99, 464 (t)

J

Janu Sirsasana (Head to Knee Pose), 390

Jathara Parivartanasana (Revolving Twist Pose), 390–91

Joan of Arc, 243

Johari, Harish, 296

Jung, Carl, 296

K

kapalabhati pranayama, 40, 472n4

kapha dosha, balancing, 318, 323–25

Kapotasana (Pigeon Pose), 391–92

Karnapidasana (Ear-Squeezing Pose), 392–93

Keller, Helen, 329
kids, sequencing for. *See* children
King Dancer Pose. *See* Natarajasana
King Pigeon Pose. *See* Raj Kapotasana
knees, balancing cues for, 105 (t),
    106 (t)
koshas, 12–14, 472n6
Kramer, Joel, 474n1, 477n5
Kripalu sequence, Sun flow, 464 (t)
Krishnamurti, J., 55
Krounchasana (Heron Pose), 393
Kukkutasana (Rooster Pose), 394
Kurmasana (Tortoise Pose), 394–95

L

labor, yoga poses to ease, 265, 475n4
Laghu Vajrasana (Little Thunderbolt
    Pose), 395–96
Lao Tzu, 167
legs
    in Adho Mukha Svanasana, 116
    front-back balancing cues, 105 (t)
    inside-outside balancing cue,
        106 (t)
    roots and extension cues, 107 (t)
leverage back bends, 70
Levine, Stephen, 33
Little Thunderbolt Pose. *See* Laghu
    Vajrasana
Locust Pose. *See* Salabhasana
Lolasana (Dangling Earring Pose),
    396–97
Lotus Pose. *See* Padmasana
lower-upper oppositional balances,
    cueing, 105–6 (t)
Low Lunge Pose. *See* Anjaneyasana

M

Malasana (Garland Pose), 397
manipura chakra and class sequence,
    303–6

manomaya kosha, 13
Marichyasana A, C (Sage Marichi's
    Pose A, C), 398–99
mat, moving off of, 53
Matsyasana (Fish Pose), 400
meditation
    basic arc template for different-
        level flow classes, 89 (t)
    creating space for, 53
    at the end of class, 51
menopause
    bone health, yoga for, 270–71
    hot flashes, yoga for symptoms of,
        269
    mood swings, yoga for reducing,
        272–73
    processes and symptoms of,
        267–68
    resources for, 476n7–8
menstruation, yoga practice during,
    244–47, 475n2–3
mental health, sequencing for, 287–89
middle school–age children,
    sequencing for, 237–38
mind and body, 471n5
mindfulness, 472n2
mirroring students, 95
mood swings, yoga for reducing,
    272–73
Mountain Pose. *See* Tadasana
mudras. *See* specific mudras
mula bandha, 105 (t), 106 (t), 250
muladhara chakra and class,
    297–99
mythology, Indian, 475n5

N

Natarajasana (King Dancer Pose)
    constituent elements of, 400–401
    Prana Flow Sequence for, 466 (t)
    preparation for, 73

nature and the cosmos, as class theme, 37

Navasana (Boat Pose), 401–2

neck

front-back balancing cue, 105 (t)

position, in Adho Mukha Svanasana, 116

risk of injury, in inversion poses, 120, 476n2

tension, releasing, 86

Nin, Anaïs, 143

Niralamba Sirsasana (headstand without support), 86

Nispattia Avastha (Consummation Stage), 11–12, 14

numbness during pregnancy, 256, 257, 261

O

O'Keeffe, Georgia, 295

One Leg behind Head Pose. *See* Eka Pada Sirsasana

One-Leg King Pigeon Pose. *See* Eka Pada Raj Kapotasana

One-Leg Sage Koundinya's Pose A. *See* Eka Pada Koundinyasana A, B

opening toward peak of a practice, 45–46

oppositional actions, cueing, 105–6 (t)

osteoporosis, 270–71, 280–81

outside-inside oppositional balances, cueing, 106 (t)

P

pace and duration of yoga classes, 330–34

pada bandha, balancing cues for, 105 (t), 106 (t), 473n1

Pada Hastasana (Hand to Foot Pose), 402–3

Padangusthasana (Big Toe Pose), 403

Padmasana (Lotus Pose), 404

palate, balancing cues for, 105 (t)

Parichaya Avastha (Increase Stage), 11, 13

Parighasana (Gate Pose), 404–5

parinamavada (inherent nature of change), 15–16, 17

Parivrtta Ardha Chandrasana (Revolved Half Moon Pose), 405–6

Parivrtta Hasta Padangusthasana (Revolved Hand to Big Toe Pose), 406–7

Parivrtta Janu Sisasana (Revolved Head to Knee Pose), 407–8

Parivrtta Parsvakonasana (Revolved Extended Side Angle Pose), 408

Parivrtta Trikonasana (Revolved Triangle Pose), 409

Parivrtta Utkatasana (Revolved Chair Pose), 410

Parsva Bakasana (Side Crane Pose), 411

Parsvottanasana (Intense Extended Side Stretch Pose), 110, 412

Paschimottanasana (West Stretching Pose or Seated Forward Bend Pose), 75, 77–78, 80, 413

passive warming *vs.* active warming, 39, 477n2

Patanjali's Yoga Sutras, eight-stage process of, 10

peak of a practice

constituent elements of, 45–48

exploring, 49–50

the pathway to, 43–48

peak pratikriyasana, 50–51

pelvis

front-back balancing cue for, 106 (t)

inside-outside balancing cue, 106 (t)

pregnancy and yoga practice, 250, 251

upper-lower balancing cue for, 105 (t)

Phalakasana (Plank Pose), 131, 414

physical fitness of children, 231–33

Pigeon Pose. *See* Kapotasana

Pincha Mayurasana (Feathered Peacock Pose), 414–15

Pindasana (Embryo Pose), 415–16

pineal gland, 477n2

pitta dosha, balancing, 318, 321–23

Plank–Chaturanga–Up Dog–Down Dog, 41–42

Plank Pose. *See* Phalakasana

plateau, 169–70

playing the edge, 278, 477n5

Plow Pose. *See* Halasana

postpartum yoga, 265–67

postural forms of the peak asana, 46–47

Power Yoga Sequence, 465 (t)

prakriti (nature/matter), 22

Prana Flow Sequence for Natarajasana, 466 (t)

pranamaya kosha (energy sheath), 13, 472n6

prana-vayus, 475n3

pranayama
  in advanced classes, 199
  in Ashtanga Vinyasa practice, 331, 332
  to balance the ajna chakra, 311–12
  at the beginning of class, 36
  at the end of class, 51
  during the first trimester of pregnancy, 251
  kapalabhati and bhastrika, 472n4

for kapha imbalance, 323
  for pitta imbalance, 321
  postpartum, 265
  for vata imbalance, 319
  to warm up the body, 39–40
  when and whom to teach, 146–47 (t)
  See also breathing; specific types of pranayama

Prasarita Padottanasana (Spread-Leg Forward Fold Pose)
  variation A, 68, 416–17
  variation B, 417
  variation C, 66, 72, 418
  variation D, 418–19

pratikriyasana (integrating actions), 25–26, 50–51, 74

pregnancy and yoga practice
  categories of students, 250, 475n6
  first trimester, guidelines and sequences for, 251–55
  history of, 248–49
  during labor, 265
  mula bandha and the pelvis, 250
  postpartum reintegration, 265–67
  second trimester, guidelines and sequences for, 255–61
  third trimester, guidelines and sequences for, 261–64

prescription drugs, stress and, 288

principles of sequencing
  action, integrating the effects of, 25–26
  energetic balance, cultivating, 22–24
  moving from dynamic to static exploration, 21–22
  moving from simple to complex, 19–21

principles of sequencing *(continued)*
  self-transformation, cultivating,
    26–28
  See also sequencing
properties of asanas, general, 56 (t), 57
Pursvottanasana (Upward-Facing
    Plank Pose or East Intense Stretch
    Pose), 419–20
purusha (consciousness), 22

R

rajas, 23, 289
raja yoga, 471n1
Raj Kapotasana (King Pigeon Pose),
    420–21
Reclined Big Toe Pose. *See* Supta
    Padangusthasana
Reclined Bound Angle Pose. *See* Supta
    Baddha Konasana
Reclined Hero Pose. *See* Supta
    Virasana
refining asanas, 102–9
relaxation poses
  for beginning-intermediate
    students, 289
  for intermediate-advanced
    students, 290
  during second trimester of
    pregnancy, 257
repetitive sequences, and the potential
    for strain, 9
resources for teachers, 469–70
resting, creating space for, 52
Revolved Chair Pose. *See* Parivrtta
    Utkatasana
Revolved Extended Side Angle Pose.
    See Parivrtta Parsvakonasana
Revolved Half Moon Pose. *See*
    Parivrtta Ardha Chandrasana
Revolved Hand to Big Toe Pose. *See*
    Parivrtta Hasta Padangusthasana
Revolved Head to Knee Pose. *See*
    Parivrtta Janu Sisasana
Revolved Triangle Pose. *See* Parivrtta
    Trikonasana
Revolving Twist Pose. *See* Jathara
    Parivartanasana
risk of transitional movements,
    understanding, 110
Roosevelt, Eleanor, 275
Rooster Pose. *See* Kukkutasana
roots and extension cues, 107–8 (t)
Rousseau, Jean-Jacques, 231

S

safe space, the need to create, 33
Sage Bharadvaj's Pose A, B. *See*
    Bharadvajrasana A, B
Sage Marichi's Pose A. *See*
    Marichyasana A, C (Sage
    Marichi's Pose A, C)
sahasrara chakra and class, 313–15
Salabhasana (Locust Pose or "Easy
    Cobra")
  version B, in Surya Namaskara,
    132–33
  versions A, B, and C (constituent
    elements of), 421
Salamba Sarvangasana (Supported
    Shoulder Stand), 121–22, 422
Salamba Sirsasana (Supported
    Headstand)
  at beginning of class, 42
  demonstrating, 97
  preparing the base of, 86
  pressure on the head, 473n5
  sequencing cues for, 120–21
  sequencing inversions and, 85–87
  versions I and II, constituent
    elements of, 422–24
Samastihi (Balanced Standing Pose),
    424–25

sattva, 23
Savasana (Corpse Pose)
    at conclusion of class, 51, 53
    constituent elements of, 425
    for integration, 88–89
    in the third trimester of pregnancy,
        262
Scales Pose. *See* Tolasana
scapula, stabilizing, 67
Scaravelli, Vanda, 334
Schiffmann, Erich, 472n8, 477n5
Scorpion Pose. *See* Vrschikasana
Seated Forward Bend Pose. *See*
    Paschimottanasana
second trimester of pregnancy,
        guidelines and sequences for,
        255–61
self-acceptance, importance of, 15–16
self-assessment, creating space for, 52
self-discovery and self-transformation,
    2
self-limitation, releasing, 198
self-transformation, cultivating,
        26–28
seniors
    arthritis, sequences for, 278–79
    balance problems, sequences for,
        282–83
    fear of falling, 476n4
    heart disease, sequences for,
        283–84
    Maty Ezraty on specific poses,
        476n2
    osteoporosis, sequences for,
        280–81
    yoga sequencing for, 275–78
sequencing
    actions, integrating the effects of,
        25–26
    advanced-level, 200–202
    Anusara sequence template, 461 (t)

Ashtanga Vinyasa sequence
    (Primary Series) template,
    462–63 (t)
Avurvedic, 317–19
beginning-level, 147–48
Bikram sequence, beginning class,
    463 (t)
cues for, in Classical Surya
    Namaskara, 129 (t)
cues for, within asana families,
    112–22
effective and efficient, 18
for elementary school–age children,
    234–36
energetic balance, cultivating,
    22–24
for the first trimester of pregnancy,
    251
for high school–age youth,
    239–41
intermediate-level, 170–73
Iyengar basic class template,
    464 (t)
Kripalu sequence, Sun flow, 464 (t)
for mental and emotional health,
    287–89
for middle school–age children,
    237–38
moving from dynamic to static
    exploration, 21–22
moving from simple to complex,
    19–21
Parinamavada and Vinyasa
    Krama, 15–19
philosophy and principles of, 7–9
Power Yoga Sequence, 465 (t)
Prana Flow Sequence for
    Natarajasana, 466 (t)
for the second trimester of
    pregnancy, 255–57
for seniors, 277–78

sequencing *(continued)*
    set sequences, positive and negative aspects of, 8–9
    Sivananda Sequence, 467 (t)
    sustainable self-transformation, cultivating, 26–28
    for the third trimester of pregnancy, 261–62
    tips on, 329–35, 477n1
    traditional approaches to, 10–14
    White Lotus Sequence, 467–68 (t)
    worksheet for, 458–60
    See also specific sequences
Setu Bandhasana (Supported Bridge Pose), 425–26, 476n2
Setu Bandha Sarvangasana (Bridge Pose), 98–99, 426–27
shatkarma practices (internal cleansing), 12, 473n6
Shishulasana (Dolphin Pose), 427–28
Shiva Rea, 12, 140, 472n7
Shooting Bow Pose. *See* Akarna Dhanurasana
shoulders
    in Adho Mukha Svanasana, 115
    front-back balancing cue for, 105 (t)
    healthy shoulder sequence, 65–66
    inside-outside balancing cue, 106 (t)
    opening, in preparation for inverted poses, 85
    shoulder extension and shoulder flexion back bends, 70
    upper-lower balancing cue for, 105 (t)
Shoulder-Squeezing Pose. *See* Bhujapidasana
Side Crane Pose. *See* Parsva Bakasana
Side Plank Pose. *See* Vasisthasana
    simplicity to complexity,

movement sequences, 19–21
Sirsasana I, II (Headstand I, II)
    deeper refining cues, 109 (t)
    transitioning out of, cueing, 111
    version II, in advanced classes, 68–69
    sitting bones, roots and extension cues, 107 (t)
sitting practice, 33–34, 35–36
    See also meditation
Sivananda Sequence, 467 (t)
soulful Vinyasa yoga
    integrated level 1–2 class, 335–38
    integrated level 2–3 class, 339–43
    integrated level 3+ class, 343–46
spine
    front-back balancing cue for, 105 (t)
    inside-outside balancing cue, 106 (t)
    upper-lower balancing cue for, 105 (t)
Spread-Leg Forward Fold Pose. *See* Prasarita Padottanasana
stability, elements of, 46
Staff Pose. *See* Dandasana
standing asanas
    basic arc template for different-level flow classes, 90 (t)
    beginning level, 159–60
    as hip openers, 83
    during second trimester of pregnancy, 256
    sequencing, 57–61
    sequencing cues for, 112–13
    to warm up the body, 42, 48
standing balance sequences
    advanced classes, 214–16
    intermediate-level classes, 184–86
Standing Forward Bend Pose. *See* Uttanasana

starting classes, the yogic process and, 32–36

sthira (steadiness), 32

stillness, moving into, 22

stimulating classes, mild, 291–94

strain, potential for in repetitive sequences, 9

Streep, Meryl, 317

strength building, and asana duration, 333

stress levels, yoga and, 287–88

Strom, Max, 143

subtleties of practice, 198–99

sukham (ease), 32

Sun Flow, Kripalu sequence template, 464 (t)

Sun Salutations. See Surya Namaskaras

Supported Bridge Pose. See Setu Bandhasana

Supported Headstand. See Salamba Sirsasana

Supta Baddha Konasana (Reclined Bound Angle Pose)
    constituent elements of, 428
    to open hips and thighs, 72
    in the third trimester of pregnancy, 262

Supta Padangusthasana (Reclined Big Toe Pose), 79, 80, 120, 429

Supta Virasana (Reclined Hero Pose), 429–30

Surya Namaskaras (Sun Salutations)
    asanas in, 126–27 (t)
    backward bending poses and, 71
    basic arc template for different-level flow classes, 89 (t)
    Classical Surya Namaskara, 128–30
    as dynamic movement, 22
    general properties of, 127–28
    as hip opener, 83
    history of, 474n1

neutralizing asanas after, 61

during the second trimester of pregnancy, 256

Surya Namaskara A, 131–36

Surya Namaskara B, 136–39

to warm up the body, 41, 48

svadhisthana chakra and class sequence, 299–303

Swenson, David, 168

T

Tadasana (Mountain Pose)
    constituent elements of, 430–31
    deeper refining cues, 108 (t)
    as foundation of standing asanas, 58
    to Urdhva Dhanurasana, preparation for, 73–74
    as wrist therapy, 64

tamas, 23, 289

Tanner levels of development, 233, 475n4

tantric model of the chakras, 295–96

targeted active warming, 39

teaching yoga
    advanced classes, 197–202
    as art and science, 2–3
    intermediate-level classes, 167–73
    new students, 143–45, 147–48
    pranayama, when and whom to teach, 146–47 (t)
    resources for, 469–70
    role of teachers, 17
    sequencing worksheet, 458–60
    teach what you know, 94–95, 199
    tips for, 329–35

temperature of class, warming up, 39

templates
    Anusara sequence, 461 (t)
    Ashtanga Vinyasa sequence (Primary Series), 462–63 (t)

templates *(continued)*

    basic template for arc structure of classes, 32 (t)

    Bikram sequence, beginning class, 463 (t)

    for different-level flow classes, 89–91 (t)

    Iyengar basic class template, 464 (t)

    Kripalu sequence, Sun flow, 464 (t)

    Power Yoga Sequence, 465 (t)

    Prana Flow Sequence for Natarajasana, 466 (t)

    Sivananda Sequence, 467 (t)

    White Lotus Sequence, 467–68 (t)

    tension

    neutralizing practice, 25

    peak asana and, 47

theme-oriented classes, 36–38, 332

thighs, front-back balancing cue for, 105 (t)

third trimester of pregnancy, guidelines and sequences for, 261–64

Thread the Needle, 83

Three Limbs Facing One Foot West Stretching Pose. *See* Tiriang Mukha Eka Pada Paschimottanasana

Tilts, Cat and Dog, 40, 474n1

time constraints, 332

Tiriang Mukha Eka Pada Paschimottanasana (Three Limbs Facing One Foot West Stretching Pose), 431–32

Tittibhasana (Firefly Pose), 432

Tolasana (Scales Pose), 433

Tortoise Pose. *See* Kurmasana

traction back bends, 70

traditional approaches to sequencing, 10–14

transitioning into asanas, 97–102

transitioning out of asanas, 109–11

Tree Pose. *See* Vrksasana

tridoshic constitution, 318

trimesters of pregnancy. *See* pregnancy and yoga practice

Twain, Mark, 93

twisting asanas

    advanced classes, 211–14

    basic arc template for different-level flow classes, 91 (t)

    beginning level, 157–58

    during first trimester of pregnancy, 251

    intermediate-level classes, 181–83

    sequencing, 75–77

    sequencing cues for, 118–19

    standing, sequencing with other standing asanas, 59–60

Two-Footed King Pigeon Pose. *See* Agnistambhasana

Two-Leg Sage Koundinya's Pose. *See* Dwi Pada Koundinyasana

Two Legs behind Head Pose. *See* Dwi Pada Sirsasana

U

Ubhaya Padangusthanasana (Both Big Toes Pose), 433–34

ujjayi pranayama

    basic arc template for different-level flow classes, 89 (t)

    as basic breathing technique, 16

    during first trimester of pregnancy, 251

    to warm the body, 39–40

Upavista Konasana (Wide-Angle Forward Fold Pose), 434–35

upper-lower oppositional balances, cueing, 105–6 (t)

Upward-Facing Bow Pose. *See* Urdhva Dhanurasana

Upward-Facing Dog Pose. *See* Urdhva
    Mukha Svanasana
Upward-Facing Plank Pose. *See*
    Pursvottanasana
Upward-Facing West
    Intense Stretch Pose. *See* Urdhva
    Mukha Paschimottanasana
Upward Hands Pose. *See* Urdhva
    Hastasana
Upward Lotus Pose. *See* Urdhva
    Padmasana
Upward Rooster Pose. *See* Urdhva
    Kukkutasana
Urdhva Dhanurasana (Upward-
    Facing Bow Pose, or Wheel
    Pose)
    constituent elements of, 435–36
    potential tensions in, 25
    transitioning to Tadasana,
        preparation for, 73–74
Urdhva Hastasana (Upward Hands
    Pose), 436–37
Urdhva Kukkutasana (Upward
    Rooster Pose), 437
Urdhva Mukha Paschimottanasana
    (Upward-Facing West Intense
    Stretch Pose), 438
Urdhva Mukha Svanasana (Upward-
    Facing Dog Pose)
    constituent elements of, 439
    deeper refining cues, 108 (t)
    in Surya Namaskara, 132–34
Urdhva Padmasana (Upward Lotus
    Pose), 440
Ustrasana (Camel Pose), 441
Utkatasana (Chair Pose), 136, 442
Uttana Padasana (Extended Leg
    Pose or Flying Fish Pose),
    442–43
Uttana Prasithasana (Flying Lizard
    Pose), 443–44

Uttanasana (Standing Forward Bend
    Pose)
    constituent elements of, 444
    deeper refining cues, 108 (t)
    in Surya Namaskara, 136
Uttanasana wrist pratikriyasana,
    64–65
Utthita Hasta Padangusthasana I, II
    (Extended Hand to Foot Pose),
    445
Utthita Parsvakonasana (Extended Side
    Angle Pose), 446
Utthita Trikonasana (Extended
    Triangle Pose)
    constituent elements of, 447
    refining cues, 103–4
    transitioning out of, cueing, 110

V
Vasisthasana (Side Plank Pose), 448
vata dosha, balancing, 318, 319–21
Vaughan, Kathleen, 248–49
vijnanamaya kosha, 13–14
vinyasa krama, 15, 16–17, 19–20, 27,
    30–32
Vinyasa Yoga. *See* Ashtanga Vinyasa
Viparita Dandasana (Inverted Staff
    Pose), 87–88, 449
Viparita Karani (Active Reversal Pose),
    85, 450
Virabhadrasana (Warrior Pose)
    constituent elements of versions I,
        II, and III, 451–53
    cues for transitioning into version
        II, 100–102
    deeper refining cues, 109 (t)
        to teach internal rotation of the
            back leg, 73
    transitioning in, 59
    version I, in Surya Namaskara,
        137, 138

Virasana (Hero Pose)
   constituent elements of, 453–54
   as preparation for forward bends,
      79
   to teach internal rotation of the
      femurs, 71
vishuddha chakra and class sequence,
   309–11
Vrksasana (Tree Pose), 454
Vrschikasana (Scorpion Pose), 455

W

warming the body, 39–43, 89 (t)
Warrior Pose. *See* Virabhadrasana
welcoming new students, 145
West Stretching Pose. *See*
   Paschimottanasana
Wheel Pose. *See* Urdhva Dhanurasana
White Lotus Sequence, 467–68 (t)
Wide-Angle Forward Fold Pose. *See*
   Upavista Konasana
winding down, integrative
   pratikriyasana and, 27
women, sequencing for special
   conditions of
   first trimester yoga sequences,
      251–55
   gender differences and yoga
      practice, 243–44

labor, yoga sequence during, 265
menopause, yoga sequences for,
   267–73
menstruation, yoga practice
   during, 243–44, 244–47,
   475n2–3
postpartum reintegration, 265–66
pregnancy, yoga practice during
   and after, 248–50
second trimester yoga sequences,
   255–61
third trimester yoga sequences,
   261–64
worksheet for sequencing, 458–60
wrists, 26–27, 64–65

Y

yoga
   Hatha yoga, origins of, 10–12
   and the koshas, 12–14
   mastery of, 474n1
   Patanjali's Yoga Sutras, 10, 471n2
   yoga chikitsa ("yoga therapy"),
      144, 473n7
   yogic process, initiating, 32–36
Yogic Bicycles, 456

About the Author

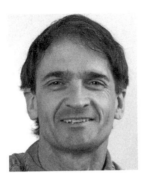

An esteemed yoga guide and author who has trained over a thousand yoga teachers, Mark Stephens conducts classes, workshops, retreats, and teacher trainings worldwide. Practicing yoga since 1991 and teaching since 1996, Stephens has sought out complementary approaches along his path as student and teacher, studying Ashtanga Vinyasa, Iyengar, Vinyasa Flow, tantra, yoga therapy, functional yoga anatomy and kinesiology, traditional yoga philosophy, and modern philosophies of being and consciousness.

The author of the best-selling *Teaching Yoga: Essential Foundations and Techniques* and *Yoga Adjustments: Philosophy, Principles, and Techniques* and recently the "Art of Asana" columnist for *Yoga International* magazine, Stephens has taught yoga at conferences, in traditional studios, and in alternative settings across the United States (in inner city schools, juvenile institutions, treatment centers, prisons, and mental hospitals). In 2000, he received *Yoga Journal*'s first annual Karma Yoga Award for his non-profit work with Yoga Inside Foundation. He lives and teaches in Santa Cruz, California, and is the founder and director of teacher training at Santa Cruz Yoga.

Stephens's website provides extensive resources for yoga students and teachers, including videos giving detailed guidance on how to practice and guide students in each of 108 asanas, guided audio classes, slideshows showing how to transition in and out and of over 100 asanas, articles, teaching tips, practice tips, poems, and a calendar of his workshops.

Visit www.markstephensyoga.com

About North Atlantic Books

North Atlantic Books (NAB) is an independent, nonprofit publisher committed to a bold exploration of the relationships between mind, body, spirit, and nature. Founded in 1974, NAB aims to nurture a holistic view of the arts, sciences, humanities, and healing. To make a donation or to learn more about our books, authors, events, and newsletter, please visit www.northatlanticbooks.com.

North Atlantic Books is the publishing arm of the Society for the Study of Native Arts and Sciences, a 501(c)(3) nonprofit educational organization that promotes cross-cultural perspectives linking scientific, social, and artistic fields. To learn how you can support us, please visit our website.